Hypertension

Physiological Basis and Treatment

Edited by

Helen H. Ong

Chemical Research Department
Hoechst–Roussel Pharmaceuticals Inc.
Somerville, New Jersey

John C. Lewis

Department of Drug Safety
Hoechst–Roussel Pharmaceuticals Inc.
Somerville, New Jersey

1984

ACADEMIC PRESS, INC.
(Harcourt Brace Jovanovich, Publishers)
Orlando   San Diego   San Francisco   New York   London
Toronto   Montreal   Sydney   Tokyo   São Paulo

Academic Press Rapid Manuscript Reproduction

ACADEMIC PRESS, INC.
Orlando, Florida 32887

United Kingdom Edition published by
ACADEMIC PRESS, INC. (LONDON) LTD.
24/28 Oval Road, London NW1 7DX

Library of Congress Cataloging in Publication Data
Main entry under title:

Hypertension : physiological basis and treatment.

Includes index.
1. Hypertension--Congresses. 2. Hypertension--
Chemotherapy--Congresses. 3. Hypotensive agents--Testing
--Congresses. I. Ong, Helen H. II. Lewis, John C.
[DNLM: 1. Hypertension--physiopathology--congresses.
2. Hypertension--drug therapy--congresses. WG 340 H9964
1983]
RC685 .H8H918 1984   616.1'32   84-9181
ISBN 0-12-526850-5 (alk. paper)

PRINTED IN THE UNITED STATES OF AMERICA

84 85 86 87   9 8 7 6 5 4 3 2 1

Contents

Contributors

Numbers in parentheses indicate the pages on which the authors' contributions begin.

Richard C. Allen (123), *Chemical Research Department, Hoechst–Roussel Pharmaceuticals Inc., Somerville, New Jersey 08876*

Michael J. Brody (1), *Department of Pharmacology and Cardiovascular Center, University of Iowa College of Medicine, Iowa City, Iowa 52242*

James E. Faber[1] (1), *Department of Pharmacology and Cardiovascular Center, University of Iowa College of Medicine, Iowa City, Iowa 52242*

Stephen F. Flaim (269), *Department of Biological Research, McNeil Pharmaceutical, Spring House, Pennsylvania 19477*

Catherine E. Johnson[2] (193), *Miles Institute for Preclinical Pharmacology, Miles Laboratories, Inc., New Haven, Connecticut 06509*

John H. Laragh (49), *Cardiovascular and Hypertension Center, The New York Hospital–Cornell Medical Center, New York, New York 10021*

Michael M. Mangiapane[3] (1), *Department of Pharmacology and Cardiovascular Center, University of Iowa College of Medicine, Iowa City, Iowa 52242*

James P. Porter (1), *Department of Pharmacology and Cardiovascular Center, University of Iowa College of Medicine, Iowa City, Iowa 52242*

Paul H. Ratz (269), *Division of Cardiology, M. S. Hershey Medical Center, The Pennsylvania State University, Hershey, Pennsylvania 17033*

Rudyard J. Ress (269), *Division of Cardiology, M. S. Hershey Medical Center, The Pennsylvania State University, Hershey, Pennsylvania 17033*

---

[1]*Present address: Department of Physiology, University of North Carolina, Chapel Hill, North Carolina 27514.*
[2]*Present address: E. I. duPont de Nemours and Co., Stine Laboratory, Newark, Delaware 19711.*
[3]*Present address: Department of Pharmacology, School of Medicine and Dentistry, University of Rochester, Rochester, New York 14642.*

Alexander Scriabine (193), *Miles Institute for Preclinical Pharmacology, Miles Laboratories, Inc., New Haven, Connecticut 06509*

Gregory M. Shutske (123), *Chemical Research Department, Hoechst–Roussel Pharmaceuticals Inc., Somerville, New Jersey 08876*

Louis Tobian (95), *Hypertension Section, Department of Medicine, University of Minnesota Hospital and School of Medicine, Minneapolis, Minnesota 55455*

David J. Triggle (233), *Department of Biochemical Pharmacology, School of Pharmacy, State University of New York at Buffalo, Buffalo, New York 14260*

Preface

The past 20 years have witnessed significant progress in our understanding of the physiological basis of hypertension as well as its treatment. These advances are reflected to some extent by the changing outlook of antihypertensive therapy which now includes the possible reversal of structural alterations in addition to pressure reduction and a heightened sensitivity to side effects.

To attain such goals undoubtedly requires a multidisciplinary approach and closer communication among the clinicians, pharmacologists, biochemists, molecular biologists, and medicinal chemists. The present volume, evolving from a recent symposium sponsored by Hoechst–Roussel Pharmaceuticals Inc., constitutes a medium that enables the contributors to summarize the most significant developments in their areas of expertise. Additionally, it also serves as a forum for the enunciation of general principles and the formulation of new concepts. The result is a book consisting of seven in-depth and timely reviews covering six major areas of hypertension research.

The inaugural chapter deals with the central neurohumoral regulations of arterial pressure. Dr. Brody and his colleagues review a large body of evidence supporting the interdependence of neural and humoral factors and evidence coupling neural mechanisms with the development and maintenance of hypertension in a variety of experimental models. Highlighted in the discussion are recent findings that the anteroventral third ventricle region (AV3V) plays a major role in interfacing the neurohumoral aspects of cardiovascular control with fluid–electrolyte homeostasis.

Dr. Laragh's authoritative treatise of the renin–angiotensin system begins with a historical account of the renal–adrenal axis. Experimental and clinical studies using β-blockers, renin antagonists, and converting enzyme inhibitors have collectively revealed the heterogeneity of hypertensive diseases, as related to the differences in renin profile and drug responsiveness. From this framework emerges the vasoconstriction–volume hypothesis which enables the analysis of virtually all human hypertensive phenomena. The chapter concludes with a detailed scheme offering systematic approaches to the diagnosis and treatment of hypertension, thus setting apart some potentially fertile areas for future research.

From a somewhat different perspective, Dr. Tobian examines numerous lines of evidence linking sodium chloride to human essential hypertension, the form of hypertension closely associated with a hereditary factor. With data drawn from clinical as well as experimental sources, the first link in the chain of causal events is established to be some initial accumulation of sodium, followed by increased arteriolar narrowing and a resetting of the regulatory system. Of special interest are findings that potassium exerts a protective effect against nephrosclerosis in the Dahl S rats during severe sodium chloride-induced hypertension; this could have some important implications in man in terms of both diet therapy and drug treatment.

A discussion of the mechanism underlying human essential hypertension is logically followed by a chapter on agents that directly alter salt and water balance. For more than 20 years diuretics have been the mainstay of therapy for hypertension of all levels of severity, despite controversy regarding their mechanisms and debate over long-term benefits. In this substantial chapter by Drs. Shutske and Allen, the therapeutic advantages of diuretics are reviewed, along with other considerations that collectively justify their continued dominance as the first-step drug of choice. The remainder of this chapter is devoted to current theories as to how changes in water and salt balance are related to the antihypertensive effect of diuretics: the complex interplay involving vascular autoregulation, neurogenic control, hormonal regulation of the kidney, and a circulating sodium-transport inhibitor. Consolidation of knowledge on these frontiers will undoubtedly lead to the development of diuretics with improved profiles.

It has been said that vasoconstriction is the ultimate mechanism operating in sustained hypertension. Agents that reverse this condition have thus assumed primary importance in antihypertensive therapy. Dr. Scriabine's contribution on this topic begins with an overview of the direct-acting vasodilators: their hemodynamic effects, therapeutic advantages versus disadvantages, and the proposed cellular sites of action. This is followed by a survey of major vasodilator drugs now in clinical use, including those with a sympatholytic component and selective renal dopamine agonists. The discussions close with an interesting projection that one of the focal points for future research will be the endothelial vasodilator factor and agents involved in its release.

The final two chapters are devoted to calcium antagonists, with emphasis on the slow channel blockers which dilate the smooth muscle vasculature by inhibiting transmembrane Ca^{2+} influx. This heterogeneous class of compounds, hailed as the drugs of the eighties, represents the most significant development in cardiovascular drug therapy since the β-blockers. In the chapter by Dr. Triggle, a brief introduction on the cellular regulation of calcium sets the stage for a comprehensive review in which the author examines the various biochemical and pharmacological aspects of leading calcium channel blockers, from the viewpoint of specificity, SAR, and mechanisms of action. The discussions by Dr. Flaim and coauthors, on the other hand, delve into the calcium handling mechanisms in vascular smooth muscle, the pathophysiology of angina, and the comparative effects of major calcium channel blockers (nifedipine, verapamil, and diltiazem) on cardiovascular hemodynamics. Together, the two reviews provide a sound scientific rationale for the clinical effectiveness of calcium antagonists in three major therapeutic areas: arrythmias, angina, and hypertension.

We hope the advances detailed in this book will be of value to investigators in hypertension research for many years to come. For future readers, this concise yet broadly based volume may provide some historical insights into the pioneering work which sets the basis for recognition of hypertension as a multifactorial disease.

HELEN H. ONG
JOHN C. LEWIS

Acknowledgments

Although not as apparent as those of the contributors and editors, the efforts of many people were required to take this book from conception to publication. Dr. Grover C. Helsley, Vice President of Research, Hoechst–Roussel Pharmaceuticals Inc., sponsored the seminar and provided the resources and personnel to see the book to completion. In addition, Dr. Helsley applied the initial impetus and continuous encouragement throughout the project.

Much of the success of the original seminar should be attributed to Dr. Jan M. Kitzen for his suggestions during the organization of the program. Rigorous and welcome technical assistance was provided by Drs. Lawrence L. Martin and John J. Tegeler, who helped proofread countless drafts and index chapters.

For the preparation of the photo-ready manuscripts, we were fortunate to have the skillful assistance of Mrs. Rose Marie Boysen, Miss Grace Naumovitz, Ms. Dolores Koziol, Mrs. Ursula Effland, and Mrs. Patricia Leicht. We would also like to acknowledge the assistance of the staff of the Hoechst–Roussel Pharmaceuticals Inc. Library for tracing references and performing literature surveys. Without the talents and abilities of these and other individuals, this work would not have been possible.

Central Neural and Humoral Regulation of Arterial Pressure in Hypertension

Michael J. Brody, James E. Faber,[1]
Michael M. Mangiapane,[2] and James P. Porter

Department of Pharmacology and Cardiovascular Center
University of Iowa College of Medicine
Iowa City, Iowa

The mechanisms underlying the pathogenesis and maintenance of hypertension are exceptionally complex. Numerous physiological regulatory mechanisms serve to maintain arterial pressure within normal limits. The appearance of high arterial pressure can often be attributed to a single cause such as elevated
blood levels of a vasoconstrictor such as angiotensin or a catecholamine. What has fascinated investigators interested in the
causes of hypertension is how such relatively simple etiologic
factors can disrupt the complex system of homeostatic mechanisms whose purpose is to defend against changes in the level of
arterial pressure.

From a historical standpoint early hypertension research
was focused on humoral vasoconstrictor mechanisms and abnormalities of vascular smooth muscle and its responsiveness. The
high degrees of efficacy of the first antihypertensive agents
such as ganglionic blockers began to draw attention to the possibility that the nervous system was intimately involved in the

[1]*Present address: Department of Physiology, University of North Carolina, Chapel Hill, North
Carolina 27514.*
[2]*Present address: Department of Pharmacology, School of Medicine and Dentistry, University of
Rochester, Rochester, New York 14642.*

hypertensive process. As knowledge about the peripheral and
central neural mechanisms of arterial pressure regulation increased, the number of experimental approaches to understanding the participation of the nervous system in hypertensive states
enlarged.

In recent years, an appreciation of the fact that neural and
humoral mechanisms are interdependent has developed. The
nervous system has been demonstrated to be intimately involved
in the release of a variety of humoral factors that have been
implicated in hypertension, and conversely, a number of humoral
factors thought to owe their hypertensive properties to direct
actions on vascular muscle have been demonstrated to exert
prominent effects on neural control of the circulation. The purpose of this chapter is to review the evidence for the interdependence of neural and humoral factors in the pathogenesis of hypertensive disease. The review is organized into consideration of the
most prominently studied experimental models of hypertension.

I. RENIN-DEPENDENT RENAL HYPERTENSION

It is well recognized that virtually all forms of hypertension
which involve disturbances in renal blood flow depend in large
part on increased release of renin from the stenosed kidney for
the initial elevation in peripheral resistance. What is less clearly
understood and a matter of much current debate is the mechanism
which accounts for the maintenance of renal hypertension (RH)
after circulating renin and angiotensin levels return to normal.
There is evidence that elevated sympathetic vascular tone (i.e.,
neurogenic tone) may be a key factor. It is now evident that
neurogenic tone may be altered as well during the initial, high
renin phase of RH. The following discussion will review evidence
regarding mechanisms by which the renin-angiotensin (RAS) and
sympathetic nervous systems are believed to interact and whether
such interactions participate in the elevation of blood pressure
during renin-dependent hypertension.

A. Early Renal Hypertension: Renin-Angiotensin Dependency

Many studies have documented that circulating renin and
angiotensin (AII) levels are elevated during the onset of experimental RH in association with peripheral vasoconstriction. Liard
et al., (1974) subjected conscious instrumented dogs to acute
stenosis of the renal artery to the sole remaining kidney and

observed an immediate (within minutes) sustained increase in
arterial pressure and plasma renin activity (PRA). Similar results following acute renal stenosis have been reported by others
in dogs with or without unilateral nephrectomy (Freeman et al.,
1977; Anderson et al., 1979; Gavras and Liang, 1980; Dzau et al.,
1981; Faber and Brody, 1983a), and in the conscious two-kidney
(2K) rat where regional vascular resistance was observed to increase along with arterial pressure (Faber and Brody, 1983a).
Blockade of AII receptors with [Sar^1-Ala^8]-AII (saralasin) prevents or largely reverses this acute stage of RH (Freeman, et al.,
1977; Faber and Brody, 1983a). In general, high blood pressure in
most experimental models of RH including Goldblatt (renal artery
stenosis), Page (perinephritis), Grollman (renal compression), and
aortic ligation/coarctation models remains largely dependent on
activation of the renin-angiotensin system for several days to
weeks after the initial surgical procedure (Miller et al., 1975;
Carretero and Romero, 1977; Barger, 1979). Subsequently, depending on such factors as the severity of the reduction in renal
blood flow, presence of an untouched contralateral kidney, and
fluid-electrolyte status of the animal, a direct contribution of
the RAS may become reduced or absent (Davis, 1977; Carretero
and Romero, 1977).

B. Peripheral Sympathetic-Angiotensin Interactions

During renin-dependent RH the mechanism by which angiotensin elevates vascular resistance and blood pressure may include,
in addition to a direct vasoconstrictor effect, indirect effects
directed at the central and peripheral sympathetic nervous system.
Several points of interaction with the peripheral sympathetic
nervous system have been described. Angiotensin has been shown
to act on the adrenal medulla to release catecholamines (Feldberg
and Lewis, 1964; Peach, 1977) by apparently producing a direct
depolarization of adrenal chromaffin cells (Douglas et al., 1976a).
However, there is little evidence favoring a significant role for
the mechanism in the pressor response to AII in vivo (Peach,
1977). Moreover, in renin-dependent or renin-independent RH
adrenal medullectomy does not alter the time course or severity
of the hypertension (Finch and Leach, 1970; deChamplian et al.,
1977; Antonaccio et al., 1980).
There is also evidence that AII can potentiate ganglionic
transmission by a non-nicotinic mechanism. Feldberg and Lewis
(1964) demonstrated that administration of AII into the arterial
supply to the superior cervical ganglion of the cat caused con-

traction of the nictitating membrane which was not prevented by ganglionic blockade or decentralization of the ganglion; the effect was interrupted when postganglionic fibers were cut (Lewis and Reit, 1965). This non-nicotinic ganglionic stimulating action of AII may be species-specific, as evidenced by a weak or absent effect in rabbits (Peach, 1977). Tachycardia can be elicited by a direct action of AII on the stellate ganglion in cats (Aiken and Reit, 1968) and costocervical ganglion in dogs (Farr and Grupp, 1971). It has not yet been shown that AII facilitates ganglionic transmission during high renin RH, or that this contributes to the rise in blood pressure.

An indirect action of AII on vascular adrenergic endings to faciliate impulse-mediated vasoconstriction has been intensely studied. Zimmerman (1962) demonstrated that the AII vasoconstrictor response in the canine hindlimb was reduced by acute lumbar sympathectomy, whereas responses to exogenous norepinephrine were unaffected. Stimulation of the peripheral end of the cut sympathetics reestablished the full response to AII. At the same time McCubbin and Page (1962) found that low doses of AII increase the pressor response to tyramine and the splanchnic vasoconstrictor response to carotid occlusion. In dogs with C_6 spinal transection or ganglionic blockade, and in pithed cats, AII failed to elicit the effect. Since these early studies, the hypothesis that has received the greatest support proposes that AII facilitates a greater release of norepinephrine with each nerve impulse; reuptake mechanisms and neurotransmitter synthesis may also be affected, however, and some controversy persists (Peach, 1977; Zimmerman, 1981). This presynaptic facilitatory action of AII is most pronounced at low frequencies of sympathetic nerve stimulation and at physiologic concentrations of the peptide. However, it has been difficult to prove that presynaptic facilitation participates in renin-dependent hypertension because the potent direct vasoconstrictor action of AII would act in concert with the indirect effect, and AII receptor antagonists do not distinguish between the pre- and postsynaptic sites of action.

C. Central Nervous System Actions of Angiotensin

Bickerton and Buckley (1961) found in cross-perfusion studies that a pressor response occurred in the recipient dog upon administration of AII into the blood supply of the vascularly isolated head of the recipient. Later it was shown by others that small doses of the peptide, which had no effect when given intravenously, elevated arterial pressure in the conscious rabbit when administered into the vertebral artery (Gildenberg et al., 1973). Since these early studies AII has been demonstrated to exert a number of actions on the brain of significance to cardiovascular control, including an increase in peripherally directed sympathetic drive, vasopressin and ACTH release, reduced renin secretion, and activation of thirst mechanisms (for detailed reviews see Severs and Daniels–Severs, 1973; Dickinson and Ferrario, 1974; Buckley, 1977; Brody and Johnson, 1980; and Ganong, 1981). These central actions of AII have been found in all species tested.

It now appears that the diverse central actions of AII depend on binding to receptors localized in or near specialized regions of the brain, the circumventricular organs. These structures, including the area postrema, neurohypophysis, median eminence, subfornical organ and organum vasculosum of the lamina terminalis (OVLT), have an imperfect blood-brain barrier (Phillips et al., 1977) to the central nervous system. In the dog, cat, and rabbit the area postrema in the lower medulla is the critical site mediating the central pressor response to AII; the pressor response occurs primarily as a result of increased efferent sympathetic nerve activity and peripheral resistance (Ferrario et al., 1972; Buckley, 1977). In contrast, in the rat AII exerts its central actions through more rostral circumventricular organs. The central pressor response to AII is elicited in the rat via carotid rather than vertebral artery administration, and lesions of the area postrema which abolish the response in other species have no effect in the rat (Haywood et al., 1980). The AII receptor fields for this response are located in periventricular tissue of the antero-ventral region of the third ventricle (AV3V region) which is adjacent to the OVLT (Brody et al., 1978; Brody and Johnson, 1980), and in the subfornical organ (SFO) (Mangiapane and Simpson, 1980). Stimulation of these receptors in the AV3V region, but not SFO, may also be achieved by cerebrospinal fluid (CSF)-borne AII. When an electrolytic lesion is placed in the region of the AV3V, the central pressor response to blood- or CSF-borne AII is abolished, whereas lesions placed outside of this region are ineffective. Pharmacological blockade of central AII receptors with administration of intracerebroventricular (ivt) saralasin also effectively reduces or eliminates elevation of blood pressure via ivt AII.

The central pressor response to blood- or CSF-borne AII is produced, in part, by an increase in neurogenic vascular tone. In conscious rats chronically instrumented for regional Doppler flowmetry, the centrally mediated pressor action of AII, estimated by the magnitude of the difference evoked when AII is infused via the carotid versus aortic routes, was accompanied by vasoconstriction in the renal, mesenteric, and hindquarters vasculatures (Lappe and Brody, 1981). The greater vasoconstrictor responses to intracarotid AII are significantly attenuated by ivt saralasin or peripheral ganglionic blockade. Direct measurement of peripheral sympathetic nerve activity supports a sympatho-excitatory action of blood-borne AII. Infusion of AII into the canine vertebral artery increased splanchnic nerve activity, although renal nerve activity was reduced (Ferrario et al., 1976).

Baroreflex alterations also occur with intravertebral AII infusion or reduced renal perfusion pressure. These alterations involve facilitation of reflex vasoconstriction and attenuation of reflex vasodilatation (Sweet and Brody, 1970; Goldstein et al., 1974). Recently Guo and Abboud (1982) demonstrated that step-wise increases in arterial pressure with vertebral artery infusion of AII in anesthetized rabbits produced smaller reductions in lumbar sympathetic nerve activity and heart rate than for similar pressure elevation with infusion of phenylephrine. There is evidence that the pressor response produced by ivt AII administration also depends on the release of vasopressin into the periphery (Severs and Daniels-Severs, 1973; Brody and Johnson, 1980). Whether this action extends to blood-borne AII at physiological concentrations is not clear.

D. Sympathetic–Renin–Angiotensin Interaction in Hypertension

From the preceding discussion it would appear that ample evidence exists to support the concept that high circulating levels of angiotensin could participate, through peripheral and particularly central interactions with the sympathetic nervous system, in the elevation of vascular resistance during high-renin hypertension. In accordance with this hypothesis attempts have been made to analyze points of interaction of the renin-angiotensin and sympathetic nervous systems during high-renin models of hypertension. While the most direct means for testing this hypothesis, i.e., recording of efferent sympathetic nerve activity along peripheral nerves innervating blood vessels, has not been possible due to inherent technical difficulties, various indirect approaches have been utilized.

1. INDIRECT INDICES OF SYMPATHETIC NERVE ACTIVITY. Evidence suggests that increased tissue norepinephrine (NE) turnover and plasma NE levels provide an index, albeit sometimes insensitive, of elevated peripheral adrenergic

nerve activity. Tanaka et al. (1977) failed to observe changes in the disposition of NE in peripheral tissues of 2K, 1-clip Goldblatt hypertension in any phase of the disease. In the same study, however, 1K, 1-clip hypertensive rats demonstrated increased NE turnover in heart and blood vessel tissue, although it was not clear whether this coincided with the early renin-dependent phase. However, plasma NE was increased in 1K, 1-clip hypertensive rats at 1, 7, 14 and 28 days after clipping (Dargie et al., 1977a), covering the typical early period of renin dependency in this model. During hypertension induced by acute renal artery stenosis in conscious dogs, circulating levels of both NE and epinephrine increased significantly (Gavras and Liang, 1980). Although these data are consistent with an increased level of sympathetic nerve activity, conclusions must be drawn cautiously since alterations in handling of NE at peripheral neuroeffector junctions, such as reduced NE reuptake or degradation, could alone provide for an increase in functional neurogenic tone without an increase in nerve traffic per se.

The drop in blood pressure following ganglionic blockade has been used to estimate peripheral sympathetic tone. Using this approach, Bellini and coworkers (1979) found an accentuated drop in blood pressure during infusion of pentolinium in rats at 5 and 12 days after interrenal aortic ligation, a hypertensive model characterized by very high circulating levels of renin (Sweet et al., 1976). That the hypertension was renin-dependent was evidenced by sensitivity to saralasin on both days. While these data clearly indicate an enhanced dependency of blood pressure on ganglionic nerve transmission, they do not identify whether interruption of neurogenic tone to resistance vessels underlies the effect, since ganglionic blockade reduces cardiac output as well as peripheral resistance. Also, an increased vascular responsiveness to NE which is known to occur as early as 3 to 4 days following clipping (Ichikawa et al., 1978; Greenberg, 1981), rather than increased nerve traffic per se, could alone lead to an accentuated response to ganglionic blockade.

Recently we have observed in conscious rats chronically instrumented with miniature Doppler flow probes that peripheral neurogenic vascular tone is inappropriately high during acute renal hypertension coincident with high circulating renin and sensitivity to saralasin (Faber and Brody, 1983a). After several hours of hypertension produced by acute unilateral renal artery stenosis with an implanted vascular occluder, neurogenic tone was assessed by measuring the decrease in regional resistance following hexamethonium administration. Surprisingly, ganglionic blockade produced large reductions in regional resistance and arterial pressure indicating that, relative to normotensive animals, neurogenic vascular tone was maintained in the renal and mesenteric beds and significantly increased in the hindquarters during acute renal hypertension. In contrast, during acute hypertension produced by infusion of the "purely" peripherally acting adrenergic agonist phenylephrine, complete -- presumably baroreflex-mediated -- withdrawal of neurogenic tone occurred, as evidenced by an absence of the effect of ganglionic blockade on blood pressure. These data indicate that, during acute RH, vascular resistance is elevated not only by the direct action of AII, but also by an inappropriately high level of sympathetic vascular tone. That this occurs at the onset of RH, well before alterations in other factors such as vascular reactivity and structural geometry and fluid-electrolyte balance, suggests actual nerve traffic may be maintained at a relatively high level.

2. CENTRAL CATECHOLAMINE DEPLETION AND PERIPHERAL SYMPATHECTOMY. Another technique that has been used to evaluate the importance of the sympathetic nervous system or central neural mechanisms involves the use of neurotoxins such as 6-hydroxydopamine (6-OHDA) and guanethidine to destroy catecholaminergic nerve endings in the central or peripheral nervous system. In dogs with 2K, 1-clip renal hypertension of 16 days duration with only a minimal dependency on AII-mediated vasoconstriction, peripheral administration of guanethidine had a small (-14 mmHg) effect on blood pressure (Zimmerman et al., 1980). Although the degree of functional denervation was not assessed, vascular tissue catecholamine content was reduced by 75%. However, significant functional sympathetic tone may still have been present in these animals as adrenal medullectomy, which was not performed, is necessary for more complete peripheral sympathectomy. In the rat, 2K, 1-clip renal hypertension is often characterized by plasma levels of AII that remain high for some time. In such rats peripherally sympathectomized with intravenous 6-OHDA treatment and adrenal medullectomy, hypertension failed to develop when measured at 6 and 12 weeks after clipping, although plasma renin levels were increased to the same extent as the sham-sympathectomized hypertensive animals (Antonaccio et al., 1980).

In a recent study we examined the response to acute renal artery stenosis in conscious rats that were peripherally sympathectomized by adrenal medullectomy and intravenous 6-OHDA treatment (Faber and Brody, 1983a). Since our other studies revealed a sympathetic component during acute renal hypertension, it was expected that sympathectomy would attenuate the acute hypertension provided that compensation by another system did not occur. Despite good evidence for functional sympathectomy, this procedure had little effect on hemodynamic responses during acute renal hypertension. However, circulating renin levels increased 3-fold more in the sympathectomized animals during acute stenosis, suggesting compensation by the RAS may have occurred. These results point out a major problem in interpreting data on chronic destruction of the peripheral sympathetic nervous system, i.e., failure of sympathectomy to alter arterial pressure does not imply that neurogenic mechanisms do not contribute when the nervous system is intact. It must be demonstrated that a deficit created by removal of a neurogenic component is not replaced by another system before lack of importance of neurogenic mechanism can be concluded.

Depletion of brain or spinal cord catecholamines has also been utilized to examine central mechanisms in 2K, 1-clip renal hypertensive rats. Intraventricular 6-OHDA prevented hypertension from developing in one study (Kubo et al., 1978) but was without effect in another (Dargie et al., 1977a). Selective interruption of spinal catecholamine pathways with intraspinal 6-OHDA failed to block the development of 2K renal hypertension (Kubo et al., 1978), although the onset was delayed one week (Bosland et al., 1981). Conclusions drawn from these studies must be viewed cautiously, however, since spinal catecholaminergic transmission may not be essential to activate preganglionic sympathetic nerves (Bosland et al., 1981), and brain as well as other spinal neuronal pathways could compensate for the loss of catecholaminergic pathways.

Evidence from local section of peripheral autonomic nerves suggests neurogenic vascular tone is elevated during high renin hypertension produced by suprarenal aortic coarctation (Overbeck, 1980). Blood pressure below the coarctation is normal. Denervation of the hindlimb causes a greater drop in resistance relative to control animals, and this enhanced neurogenic component is not evident in animals with guanethidine-induced peripheral sympathectomy (Overbeck, 1980).

In summary, although inconsistencies exist, the weight of the indirect evidence suggests that efferent sympathetic nerve activity to resistance vessels is maintained at a high level during renal hypertension at a time when a contribution of the RAS is also clearly evident. The following sections will address evi-

Denervation of the remaining kidney in this model will also reverse the hypertension, and is accompanied by a decrease in
circulating norepinephrine and hypothalamic norepinephrine
content (Katholi et al., 1982; Winternitz et al., 1982). Finally,
work in our laboratory has shown that in the rat the integrity of
the anteroventral third ventricle (AV3V) is required for the development and maintenance of this form of hypertension.

B. Effect of AV3V Lesions on 1-Kidney Hypertension

As mentioned previously, the AV3V region plays an important role in the maintenance of fluid and electrolyte homeostasis. Lesions in this region prevented the development of 1-
kidney Grollman hypertension (Buggy et al., 1977). Sham lesion
animals developed a sustained hypertension and significantly
increased water intake. The animals with AV3V lesions failed to
increase water intake. However, the increase in water intake
was not necessary for the development of hypertension since
another group of rats with intact neural tissue still increased
blood pressure after the renal wrap, even though they were restricted to 35 ml of water per day (the approximate amount
drunk by AV3V lesion rats).

In subsequent studies, the effect of the AV3V lesions on the
maintenance phase of 1-kidney Grollman hypertension was investigated (Buggy et al., 1978). Lesions were placed in the AV3V
at 1 and 6 weeks after the renal wrapping. At 1 week, AV3V
lesions prevented any further increase in blood pressure; at 6
weeks, most of the lesion animals died due to post-lesion adipsia.
However, another group of rats which were trained to drink 35 ml
of water daily survived the post-lesion hydrational crisis and, in
these animals, the AV3V lesions returned blood pressure to control levels.

C. Mechanism of Antihypertensive Action of AV3V Lesion

The mechanism by which AV3V lesions prevent renal hypertension is currently under investigation. Recent evidence suggests that the lesions may interrupt a reflex arc that originates
with renal afferent activation. The lesions may also interfere
with central osmoreception. Finally, the lesions may prevent
synthesis, storage, or release of a natriuretic hormone.

1. RENAL AFFERENT NERVE INVOLVEMENT. The increased sympathetic activity present in 1-kidney hypertension

may be a reflex response resulting from activation of renal me-mechano- or chemoreceptors. The mechanoreceptors are present on the surface of the kidney and in the parenchyma associated with blood vessels (Niijima, 1975). Increases in renal perfusion pressure or direct manual compresson produced an increase in renal afferent firing. The location of the chemoreceptors is not known, but renal ischemia or local release of substances due to ischemia have been hypothesized to activate these receptors (Recordati et al., 1980).

While renal afferent nerve activity has not been monitored during the development of 1-kidney hypertension, it is possible that constriction of the renal artery or wrapping of the kidney results in activation of one or both kinds of these receptors. This suggestion is supported by the finding that electrical stimu-laton of renal afferents produced vasoconstriction in the me-senteric and renal vascular beds (Webb et al., 1981). In addi-tion, complete renal denervation accomplished by kidney auto-transplantation delayed for ten weeks the development of 1-kidney Grollman hypertension (Haywood et al., 1983). Surgical renal denervation also reversed chronic 1-kidney hypertension (Katholi et al., 1981). As mentioned above, this was accom-panied by a decrease in circulating norepinephrine and hypo-thalamic norepinephrine content. In these studies removal of renal afferent influences probably accounted for the antihyper-tensive effect, because in this model of hypertension renal sym-pathetic nerves (efferents) have been shown to be depleted of norepinephrine and the vasoconstrictor response to electrical stimulation of the renal nerves is reduced (Barajas et al., 1976; Fink and Brody, 1980).

Recently, the involvement of the renal afferent nerves in this model of hypertension has come under question. Freeman et al. (1983) reported that moderate and severe hypertension pro-duced by renal artery clips of different diameters was not af-fected by renal denervation. The completeness of denervation was assessed by measuring kidney norepinephrine content which was shown to be greatly decreased. However, as mentioned above, renal norepinephrine content decreases in renal hyper-tension even with intact renal nerves, so the degree of denerva-tion in this study may be subject to question. Moreover, selective renal afferent denervaton accomplished by dorsal rhizotomy also had no affect on the hypertension in this model (Pan et al., 1983; Lappe and Brody, unpublished observation). It may be that in this model both renal afferents and renal efferents must interact to produce the hypertension.

An increase in renal afferent activity may also account for part of the hypertension produced by unilateral renal artery constriction. Under normal conditions, blockade of the renin-angiotensin system prevents the elevation in blood pressure. However, Faber and Brody (1983b) investigated the possibility that renal nerve-dependent cardiovascular effects produced by the constriction were masked by baroreflex function. In conscious rats with sino-aortic baroreceptor denervation, renal artery constriction produced an elevation in blood pressure even after pretreatment with a converting enzyme inhibitor. Denervation of the kidney, carried out before constriction of its artery, significantly attenuated the increase in blood pressure. These data suggest that the renal nerves participate in the acute hypertension produced by renal artery constriction.

The cardiovascular response produced by renal afferent stimulation is qualitatively similar to the response obtained during electrical stimulation of the AV3V region (Fink et al., 1978; Webb et al., 1982). This similarity led to the hypothesis that renal afferent activity relays through the AV3V region. Mahoney et al. (1981) tested this hypothesis functionally by stimulating the renal afferent nerves before and after acute lesions of the AV3V region. The blood pressure and vascular resistance changes were essentially abolished by the lesions. In addition, electrophysiologic data have provided direct evidence for a neural connection between the renal afferent nerves and the AV3V region. Spontaneously active neural units in the preoptic region of cats and rats have been identified which change their firing rate in response to electrical stimulation of the renal afferent nerves (Ciriello and Calaresu, 1980; Knuepfer et al., 1980).

a. Afferent Pathways. Recent work in our laboratory has identified the putative central neural pathways which are activated by renal afferent nerve stimulation. Spinal section at T-6 abolishd the cardiovascular response to renal afferent nerve stimulation, and lesions in the nucleus tractus solitarius (NTS) significantly attenuated all responses except mesenteric vasoconstriction. However, NTS lesions did not prevent the typical response to AV3V stimulation (Webb et al., 1981). These data suggest that the ascending information passes through the spinal cord to NTS, but efferent information descending from AV3V does not pass through NTS. Acute or chronic bilateral lesions in the lateral parabrachial nucleus also blocked the response produced by renal afferent stimulation (Webb et al., 1982, 1983).

This suggests that rostral to NTS the pathway activated by renal afferent stimulation ascends to the parabrachical nucleus. Anatomical techniques have been used to identify a dense neural projection from NTS to parabrachial nucleus (Norgren, 1980). Projections from the parabrachial nucleus to the median preoptic nucleus, or nucleus medianus (Saper and Loewy, 1980), a specific site within the AV3V region, probably complete the afferent side of the reflex arc.

b. Efferent Pathways. As described earlier, two separate vasoconstrictor pathways which descend from the AV3V region have been identified (Hartle and Brody, 1982a). One pathway follows a midline route and mediates responses produced by activation of the AV3V area with AII and participates in renin-dependent forms of renal hypertension. A second constrictor pathway travels laterally through the medial forebrain bundle (MFB). This lateral pathway appears to be important for non-renin-dependent renal hypertension since a knife cut which transected the MFB bilaterally in the anterior hypothalamus prevented 1-kidney Grollman hypertension (Hartle and Brody, 1982a). From this lateral area, the descending projections of this pathway converge toward the midline and pass through the ventromedial basal hypothalamus. Electrolytic lesions in this region blocked the cardiovascular response to electrical stimulation of the AV3V and also prevented 1-kidney Grollman hypertension (Johnson et al., 1981). From here, the vasoconstrictor pathway from the AV3V descends through the periaqueductal gray (Kneupfer et al., 1983); however, chronic lesions in this region proved to be fatal, so the importance of the periaqueductal gray pathway in 1-kidney hypertension could not be determined (unpublished observations).

2. INTERRUPTION OF CENTRAL OSMORECEPTION.
Early studies showed that AV3V lesions blocked the increase in blood pressure produced by central infusions of hypertonic saline (Johnson et al., 1978). This blockade presumably occurred because important osmosensitive receptors or pathways were destroyed by the lesion. Since alterations in fluid and electrolytes may occur in 1-kidney hypertension, the possibility that central changes in osmolality contributed to the elevated pressure was investigated (Brody et al., 1978). During the first three days after 1-kidney Grollman wrapping, CSF osmolality and sodium concentration were elevated without a concomitant increase in blood pressure. However, by seven days, both CSF osmolality

pressinergic pathways must also be postulated to account for the hypertension of DOC-salt animals.

C. Plasma Sodium

In rats with DOC-salt hypertension, plasma sodium is elevated (Villamil et al., 1982). This electrolyte derangement may increase arterial pressure through an interacton with the CNS. Injection of hypertonic saline into the cerebral ventricles produces a pressor response, and this may be due to stimulation of osmoreceptors in or near the AV3V region. These responses are attenuated by ablation of the AV3V (Johnson et al., 1978). These same lesions also attenuated antidiuretic responses to intraventricular hypertonic saline, indicating that vasopressin responses to the hypertonic injections may also have been impaired. Intravenous administration of hypertonic saline also increases arterial pressure. This increase is at least partly dependent on vasopressin (Hatzinikalaou et al., 1981), because vasopressin blockade reduces the pressor response significantly. Lesions of the AV3V block both this increased arterial pressure and the vasopressin response (Haywood et al., 1982).

D. Suppression of the Sodium–Potassium Pump

The contractility of arterial smooth muscle may depend, in part, on the activity of the cellular electrogenic sodium pump. Decreases in the activity of the pump have been reported in DOC-salt hypertension (Pamnani et al., 1978). Further, there is evidence that the decrease in pump activity is mediated by a circulating substance (Gruber et al., 1980) that may be of central origin (Haupert and Sancho, 1979). Ablation of the AV3V region blocks the development of DOC-salt hypertension (Berecek et al., 1982a), and rats with these lesions also fail to show suppression of Na-K pump activity (Songu-Mize et al., 1982), indicating that there may be a lack of the putative circulating inhibitor of the pump in these animals. Protection of the AV3V-ablated rat from hypertension may therefore be partly due to the lack of a natriuretic factor which has been proposed as the putative circulating inhibitor of the sodium–potassium pump.

E. Central Catecholamines

Depletion of central catecholamines by intraventricular injection of 6-hydroxydopamine prevents the development or maintenance of DOC-salt hypertension. The fact that AV3V lesions also have this effect is only one example of the many similarities between the AV3V lesion syndrome and the syndrome following central 6-OHDA treatment. The AV3V region is innervated by catecholamine terminals (Olson and Fuxe, 1972; Kobayashi et al., 1974), and subregions of the AV3V have a relatively high catecholamine content (Palkovits et al., 1974; Saavedra et al., 1976). It may be the case, then, that destruction of catecholamine nerves in the AV3V region is the critical factor in both the AV3V lesion and in central catecholamine depletion studies. The critical area within the AV3V which must be depleted of catecholamines may be the nucleus medianus (median preoptic nucleus; personal communication, Bellini and Johnson). Nonetheless, the AV3V region may not be the only important region involved in DOC-salt hypertension. A recent study by Richardson (1983) has implicated the septum in catecholamine mediation of DOC-salt hypertension. Electrolytic lesions of septum blocked the development of this model of hypertension in rats, and central 6-OHDA treatment produced the largest catecholamine depletions in the septum. Subsequently, it was shown that local injectons of a small dose of 6-OHDA into the septum also blocked DOC-salt hypertension. Thus, both the septum and the AV3V region have been implicated in CNS mediation of DOC-salt hypertension.

IV. DAHL SALT-SENSITIVE MODEL

Dahl selectively bred two strains of rat, one sensitive (S) and one resistant (R) to the hypertensive effects of dietary salt (Dahl et al., 1962). The response to dietary salt is inherited as a polygenic trait (Knudsen et al., 1970). This is another model of hypertension in which renin is not elevated (Rapp et al., 1978). Several mechanisms are involved in the generaton of hypertension in this model, including unidentified plasma factors, the kidney, the adrenal, and the central nervous system.

Takeshita and Mark (1978) showed that S rats have a greater neurogenic component of hindlimb vascular resistance than do R rats. Sympathetic nerve stimulation increased perfusion pressure more in S rats than in R rats, and sympathetic denervation decreased perfusion pressure in S rats on high salt. Gordon et al. (1981) found that S rats showed abnormal baroflex control of the heart. These investigators found that for any change in arterial pressure, R rats changed heart rates more than did S rats.

Takeshita, Mark, and Brody (1979) found that administration of intraventricular 6-hydroxydopamine attenuated the severity of DOC-salt hypertension in Dahl rats. Thus, these studies suggest central nervous participation in the hypertension of S rats.

The anterior hypothalamus has been the focus of several lesion studies attempting to prevent hypertension in S rats. Lesions of the AV3V region prevented S rats from developing the severe hypertension seen in sham-ablated rats. The AV3V-ablated S rats had pressures which were intermediate between the very high pressures of sham-ablated S rats and the normal pressures of R rats (Brody and Johnson, 1980; Goto et al., 1982). These studies provide additional evidence of AV3V involvement in salt-induced hypertension.

Other studies have shown that lesions of the paraventricular nuclei (Goto et al., 1981) or of the region from the suprachiasmatic nuclei to the paraventricular nuclei (Azar et al., 1981) have effects on Dahl strain hypertension similar to that of the AV3V lesion. However, the Azar et al. (1981) lesion clearly overlaps the tissue destroyed in the AV3V lesion, and paraventricular lesions may be interrupting a medial pathway from the AV3V to the brainstem. It is clear, however, that the anterior hypothalamus is necessary for the complete expression of the hypertensive potential in the Dahl rat strain.

V. NEUROGENIC HYPERTENSION

A full appreciation of the role of the sympathetic nervous system in hypertensive states is best determined by examining models that depend, at least on theoretical grounds, solely on increased sympathetic nervous sytem activity for the increase in arterial pressure. The increase in pressure in these models is referred to as neurogenic hypertension and is ordinarily produced by interrupting the inhibitory influence of the high pressure baroreceptors. If in any model hypertension is produced by the vasoconstrictor action of the sympathetic nerves, it should be possible to produce sustained hypertension by allowing sympathetic activity to remain elevated chronically. Several models of neurogenic hypertension have been developed and have been examined in a number of species. There is common agreement that interventions which block the baroreceptor input to the central nervous sytem raise arterial pressure acutely and produce large spontaneous variations in pressure referred to as lability. There is much less agreement about the question of whether arterial pressure is sustained at hypertensive levels in animals deprived of normal baroreceptor reflexes.

The major techniques for producing neurogenic hypertension are denervation of the sino-aortic baroreceptor nerves (reviewed by Ito and Scher, 1981) or bilateral lesion of the nucleus tractus solitarius (NTS), the major termination site for primary baroreceptor afferent nerves (Doba and Reis, 1973). Both of these procedures produce acute elevations of arterial pressure; however, there are significant differences between the effects produced by the two procedures. Despite the similarities and the magnitude of pressure increment (e.g., in the rat they are virtually identical), hypertension produced by NTS lesions is usually lethal, whereas animals routinely survive the increase in arterial pressure produced by deafferentation of the sino-aortic nerves (SAD). Rats with NTS lesions develop pulmonary edema and severe respiratory embarrassment, whereas no evidence of these pulmonary malfunctions occurs in rats with SAD. Finally, the increase in arterial pressure produced by SAD is seen under anesthesia, whereas reinstatement of the conscious state is required before arterial pressure increases after NTS lesion. These differences suggest that NTS lesion may not be selective for baroreceptor afferent systems and may produce a complex syndrome that involves interruption of a number of other visceral afferent projections which terminate in the NTS.

Several studies have indicated that long term survival after NTS lesions is possible if animals are treated vigorously with antihypertensive interventions (Zandberg et al., 1978) or are maintained under anesthesia for long periods of time (Buchholz and Nathan, 1983). These rats with chronic hypertension produced by NTS lesions are an important model for future study on the mechanisms of neurogenic hypertension. Survival after NTS lesions is found in other species such as cat (Nathan and Reis, 1977) and dog (Carey et al., 1979; Laubie and Schmitt, 1979). In these latter species, the pulmonary distress seen in rats with NTS lesions is not observed. Arterial pressure is increased modestly in the cat and to a greater extent in the dog.

A key characteristic of all animals with baroreceptor deafferentation, whether produced by NTS lesion or by SAD, is a high level of arterial pressure lability. Variations in arterial pressure occur spontaneously in resting awake animals and are also observed during sleep. These variations are exaggerated during normal behavior such as eating, drinking and grooming (Nathan and Reis, 1977). The central site(s) of origin of arterial pressure lability in neurogenic hypertensive animals is not known. In recent studies from our laboratories, we examined the possibility that forebrain structures might contribute. Rats with lesions of the AV3V region have attenuation or partial reversal of NTS or SAD hypertension (Brody and Johnson, 1980). Arterial pressure lability appears to be unchanged. This finding was confirmed in another recent study using midcollicular decerebration (Trapani et al., 1983). This procedure produced an attenuation of hypertenion elicited by SAD; however, arterial pressure lability was unchanged. These data suggest that the central origin of lability is in sites residing in brainstem. Since lability persists even in sleep, it probably originates in pacemakers for sympathetic discharge that exhibit wide variations in tonic activity. It is important for our understanding of arterial pressure regulation in hypertensive states to determine the central sites of origin of these large pressure variations.

The mechanism of neurogenic hypertension is an increase in total peripheral resistance that appears to be entirely neurogenic in origin. For example, the hypertension can be prevented by pretreatment with the peripheral sympathetic nerve toxin 6-hydroxydopamine or can be reversed completely with ganglionic blockade. We have noted in the rat an increase in circulating blood levels of vasopressin and angiotensin (Trapani, Barron, and Brody, unpublished observations). Since the release of vasopressin and renin are both under strong inhibitory control of the baroreceptors, the finding of increased circulating levels of these vasoconstrictor substances is not surprising. The increments are not sufficient, however, to contribute to the elevation in arterial pressure since treatment of rats with SAD hypertension with competitive antagonists of angiotensin and vasopressin fails to lower arterial pressure in the first days after cutting the baroreceptor nerves (Trapani, Barron, and Brody, unpublished observations).

An important consideraton in understanding the contribution of the central nervous system to the development and maintenance of neurogenic hypertension concerns the failure of hypertension to be sustained despite persistent loss of baroreceptor control. As reviewed by Ito and Scher (1981) and by Ferrario and Takeshita (1983), there are numerous reports of normalizaton or virtual normalization of arterial pressure in animals with either NTS lesions or SAD. Ferrario and Takeshita argue that several issues must be resolved before the answer to the mechanism is uncovered. These problems concern the adequacy of denervation, the need for 24 hour monitoring of arterial pressure, and the tests used to determine the adequacy of denervation. If it is assumed that denervation of the baroreceptors may in fact be complete and that arterial pressure returns towards normal, then it must be determined whether the loss of elevated vascular resistance and the fall in arterial pressure results from failure of vasoconstrictor tone to be maintained at a high level or rather is produced by a return of central sympathetic discharge towards normal levels.

We addressed this question in several ways. In cats, sympathetic nerve discharge was recorded from both pre- and postganglionic nerves continuously before and for several hours following SAD (Strait and Brody, 1983). The increase in sympathetic discharge produced by bilateral carotid artery occlusion was abolished by SAD which, in turn, produced approximately a doubling of integrated sympathetic nerve activity. This increase in central discharge was associated with elevations of arterial pressure to over 200 mmHg. In these cats, arterial pressure returned to control levels within 60 minutes following SAD; however, central sympathetic discharge remained elevated at its peak levels for the several additional hours in which it was recorded. The failure of arterial pressure to be maintained was not due to the presence of anesthetic since identical effects on arterial pressure were obtained in conscious cats. SAD was produced by previous aortic depressor nerve section and by injection of local anesthetic into the region of the carotid sinus at the time of experiment. In these unanesthetized animals arterial pressure rose to equivalent levels seen in the anesthetized cats and returned to normal within 60 minutes. In companion studies reactivity to norepinephrine and vasoconstrictor responses to peripheral sympathetic nerve stimulation were not significantly altered. These data indicate that local vascular adaptations to high sympathetic discharge prevent vasoconstrictor tone from being maintained at high levels. This phenomenon may be identical to "autoregulatory escape", described earlier by Folkow and colleagues (1964). No recordings of sympathetic discharge are available on animals with chronic SAD; however, if the results on acute SAD are applicable to the chronic state, they suggest that sympathetic discharge may be maintained at elevated levels for some time after baroreceptor deafferentation and that the failure to sustain high arterial pressure may be the result of local vascular adaptive mechanisms.

We have also examined the contribution of neurogenic vasoconstrictor tone to the maintenance of neurogenic hypertension in conscious rats at various stages after SAD (Trapani et al.,

1982). Using animals instrumented with miniaturized pulsed Doppler flow probes, we found that shortly after SAD the increase in vascular resistance is produced entirely by neurogenic mechanisms since resistance is normalized by interruption of sympathetic transmission with a ganglionic blocking agent. In our hands, rats with SAD return to near control arterial pressure levels within approximately 7 days after the procedure. Again, using ganglionic blockade as a test for the contribution of neurogenic mechanisms to the maintenance of vascular resistance, we found that despite the normalization of arterial pressure, neurogenic vasoconstrictor tone remained high compared to that of control animals for 1–4 weeks after SAD. In other words, although vascular resistance was at approximately the same level in control animals versus SAD rats, the magnitude of neurogenic vasoconstrictor tone was persistently higher in the deafferented animals and was maintained high in the absence of any changes in vascular reactivity to norepinephrine. These data suggest that in the rat central sympathetic discharge may be maintained at a high level for weeks following SAD; however, local adaptive mechanisms may shift the balance of neurogenic to non-neurogenic vasoconstrictor tone such that the total vascular resistance is normalized in the face of high sympathetic discharge.

The implication of these studies for understanding of hypertensive mechanisms is considerable. Since numerous forms of hypertension are associated with increased sympathetic activity, it is necessary to determine whether abnormalities in the autoregulatory or adaptive processes that tend to minimize the vasoconstrictor effects of high sympathetic discharge allow for an increase in functional neurogenic vasoconstrictor tone. Models of neurogenic hypertension allow for relatively uncompromised examination of the selective contribution of the sympathetic nervous system, whereas other models involve altered humoral or endocrine systems or salt ingestion. These additional factors may well interact with neurogenic control of the peripheral circulation and allow sympathetic vasoconstrictor tone to be maintained in hypertensive states.

Another model of neurogenic hypertension is worthy of mention. Partial baroreceptor denervation, produced by selective aortic depressor nerve deafferentation, results in a mild elevation of arterial pressure in dog (Ito and Scher, 1981) and rat (Fink et al., 1980). As is the case with total SAD, the increase in arterial pressure is entirely neurogenic in origin in its early stages (Touw et al., 1979) and remains largely neurogenic in its later stages. A recent report indicates that the development of hypertension produced by aortic baroreceptor deafferentation can be attenuated by renal sympathetic denervation (Kline et al., 1983). The protective effect of renal denervation was suggested to involve renal afferent systems postulated to participate in the pathogenesis of the hypertension.

VI. SPONTANEOUS HYPERTENSION

Several experimental forms of hypertension have been developed by selective inbreeding, especially in rats. These models are ordinarily created by breeding for the trait of high arterial pressure although several strains have been developed where high arterial pressure is the consequence of a genetically inbred susceptibility to other factors. High salt ingestion provokes hypertension in the case of the Dahl salt-sensitive strain, whereas rats of the Sabra strain are bred for susceptibility to DOC-salt (Ben-Ishay et al., 1972). The characteristics and pathophysiology of the various strains of spontaneously hypertensive rats have been reviewed recently (Yamori, 1983).

The most commonly used rat model of spontaneous hypertension is the spontaneously hypertensive rat (SHR) developed by Okamoto and Aoki (1963). There is now ample evidence for the participation of central neurogenic mechanisms in the development and maintenance of this important experimental model. In addition to findings on altered catecholamine metabolism, changes in plasma levels of catecholamines and other indirect estimates of the participation of the sympathetic nervous system, the most important evidence for neurogenic participation in SHR are the effects of destruction of the nervous system and the direct recordings of sympathetic nerve activity. Hypertension in SHR can be prevented by interventions that destroy sympathetic nerves such as anti-nerve growth factor or the selective sympathetic nerve terminal toxin 6-hydroxydopamine (Provoost and DeJong, 1978). There is not complete agreement about the effectiveness of these neurotoxic interventions since susceptibility to the agents is age- and dose-dependent. The prevention of hypertension in SHR was not achieved with guanethidine, an agent which produces a more permanent and complete sympathectomy than does anti-nerve growth factor or 6-hydroxydopamine (Johnson and Vacia, 1979). When anti-nerve growth factor was administered in conjunction with guanethidine, a complete sympathectomy which prevented the development of hypertension was achieved. It needs to be emphasized that the failure of peripheral sympathectomy to alter the development of hypertension does not necessarily rule out the participation of neurogenic mechanisms since local vascular factors or humoral mechanism could assume greater pressor significance in the absence of a functional sympathetic nervous system. Direct evidence for the participation of the central nervous system in the pathogenesis of spontaneous hypertension has been achieved with the use of central administration of 6-hydroxydopamine (Haeusler, 1976). Since the effects of the neurotoxin are restricted to the brain, central catecholaminergic systems can be implicated in the propagation of the hypertension. The difficulty with this interpretation, however, is that the neurotoxin is potentially nonspecific for catecholaminergic systems. Furthermore, catecholamines have diverse effects upon blood pressure regulation with both pressor and depressor mechanisms present in forebrain and brainstem, respectively.

Direct recordings of sympathetic activity have provided some conflicting results about the participation of central mechanisms in the development and maintenance of hypertension in SHR. A significant increase in discharge compared to normotensive control animals has been found in splanchnic and renal nerves (Judy et al., 1976; Ricksten and Thoren, 1979). No difference in discharge was observed in the lumbar sympathetic innervation (Lais et al., 1974). While the data demonstrating increased neural activity in SHR are compelling, they must be viewed with several reservations. First, with the exception of studies carried out in Thoren's laboratory, measurements of central sympathetic discharge in SHR have been made in the anesthetized state. Even in the case of the Thoren studies, the nerve recordings, while made in the conscious state, are carried out within only 24 hours following surgical implantation of the recording electrode. We must await the development of more sophisticated technology for evaluating the question of whether SHR in their basal state have a sympathetic discharge rate higher than that of normotensive rats.

Another significant factor to be considered is whether high sympathetic discharge, even if it exists, results in increased vascular resistance which is of neurogenic origin. Our laboratory has investigated this problem using SHR instrumented chronically with miniaturized pulsed Doppler flow probes. As described above in the section on neurogenic hypertension, if vascular resistance and arterial pressure are maintained at elevated levels

by neurogenic mechanisms, the neurogenic contribution can be uncovered with the use of ganglionic blockade. Thus in SAD rats, elevated arterial pressure and regional vascular resistance can be significantly reduced to levels not different from those seen in normotensive animals by the use of ganglionic blockade. When such studies were carried out in conscious SHR, only a modest reduction in vascular resistances was observed with ganglionic blockade, indicating that the elevated vascular resistance was maintained by a relatively small neurogenic component (Touw et al., 1980). Although our laboratory had routinely found increased vascular reactivity to several vasoconstrictor agents in perfused vascular beds of SHR (Lais and Brody, 1978), in the conscious animals no significant changes in vascular reactivity to norepinephrine or angiotensin were observed. These data suggest that in the conscious resting state any increase in sympathetic nerve discharge that may exist is not converted into the functional consequence of elevated vascular resistance of primarily neurogenic origin. There are numerous potential explanation for such findings, but work should focus on the possibility that the release of norepinephrine from sympathetic nerve terminals of intact SHR is impaired. Recent findings on this problem suggest that in SHR vessels studied in vitro (Galloway and Westfall, 1982) or in perfused vessels (Vanhoute, 1981), enhanced release of norepinephrine occurs.

The most important difference between SHR and normotensive animals that may help explain the role of neurogenic mechanisms is the observation that SHR exhibit exaggerated cardiovascular responsiveness to environmental stress (Hallback and Folkow, 1974). It is conceivable that SHR at rest might have normal sympathetic discharge and that arterial pressure is maintained by non-neurogenic vascular factors such as intrinsic contractile activity, structual alterations, and increased responsiveness to vasoconstrictor agents. If responses of the autonomic nervous system to changes in the environment were abnormal in SHR, sympathetic nerve discharge might be intermittently elevated. The recent studies of Lundin and Thoren (1982) provide direct evidence for the participation of exaggerated sympathetic discharge as a consequence of environmental stress. In these studies basal sympathetic discharge was slightly higher in SHR than in normotensive rats; however, the major difference observed was the increase in discharge seen in response to a blast of air on the face. In these studies, SHR not only increased renal sympathetic nerve discharge to a significantly greater extent, but they also retained more sodium .

   Central sites responsible for altered cardiovascular control
in SHR have been examined. Lesions of the AV3V region which
protect against the development of renal, mineralocorticoid, and
neurogenic models of hypertension were found to have no effect
on either the development or maintenance of hypertension in
SHR (Gordon et al., 1982). On the other hand, arterial pressure
has been lowered by lesions in pressor areas of the posterior
hypothalamus (Yamori and Okomoto, 1969; Bunag and Eferakeya,
1976), and the development of hypertension in SHR was attenuated by posterior hypothalamic lesions (Riley et al., 1979). Although the posterior hypothalamus is a major pressor region, it
receives substantial afferent input from other forebrain and
brainstem areas, so it is unclear whether this important hypothalamic area is of primary importance in the propagation of
hypertension in SHR. It should be noted that the widely quoted
study of Folkow and Rubenstein (1966) demonstrating the induction of hypertension by chronic stimulation of the hypothalamic
defense area was not confirmed (Bunag and Riley, 1979).
   The limbic system was examined by our laboratory for its
possible participation in the pathogenesis of spontaneous hypertension. Integration between sensory input from the environment
and the autonomic nervous system is believed to involve the
amygdala. We found that the lesions of the central nucleus of
the amygdala placed in weanling SHR attenuated the development
of hypertension (Galeno et al., 1982). This protective effect was
recently confirmed (Folkow et al., 1982). Since the amygdala
sends primary projections to major brainstem regions involved in
cardiovascular regulation, we further explored its role in the
control of regional vascular resistance and arterial pressure in
SHR. In studies on electrical activation of the amygdala, we
found that in conscious, but not in anesthetized rats, the classic
pattern of the "defense reaction" could be evoked. Stimulation
of the central nucleus produced hypertension, tachycardia, increased vascular resistance in the kidney and gut, and vasodilatation in the hindquarters, a vascular bed composed primarily of
skeletal muscle (Galeno and Brody, 1983). When consicous SHR
were exposed to an aversive noise stress, they exhibited exaggerated increases in arterial pressure compared to their normotensive
counterparts (Galeno et al., 1984). The regional hemodynamic
basis of this increased pressor effect was of some interest. The
vascular bed exhibiting the greatest increase in resistance was
the kidney, a finding that provides functional evidence for the
results of Lundin and Thoren (1982) that renal sympathetic nerve

discharge is exaggerated in SHR response to an acute environmental stress.

The participation of amygdaloid structures in exaggerated responsiveness of the cardiovascular system of SHR was explored (Galeno et al., 1984). In rats with chronic lesions of the central nucleus of the amygdala, the increases in arterial pressure and regional vascular resistances produced by the acute noise stress were reduced to levels seen in normotensive rats receiving the same lesion. Thus, the capacity of the nervous sytem to generate abnormally large increases in sympathetic discharge, vascular resistance, and arterial pressure appear to be dependent upon the amygdala, a critical limbic system structure. These results do not provide specific evidence that a primary abnormality in SHR resides in the amygdala; however, the data do provide a focus for future studies on the central neural mechanisms that participate in the pathogenesis of spontaneous hypertension.

ACKNOWLEDGEMENT

Portions of the work reported here were supported by HHS grants HLB-14388, 2F32 HL-06597, 2F32 HL-06101, HLB-07121 and a gift from the Searle Family Trust.

REFERENCES

Aiken, J. W., and Reit, E. (1968). Stimulation of the cat stellate ganglion by angiotensin. J. Pharmacol. Exp. Ther. 159, 107-114.

Anderson, W. P., Korner, P. I., and Johnston, C. I. (1979). Acute angiotensin II-mediated restoration of distal renal artery pressure in renal artery stenosis and its relationship to the development of sustained one-kidney hypertension in conscious dogs. Hypertension 1, 292-298.

Antonaccio, M. J., Ferron, R. A., Waugh, M., Harris, D., and Rubin, B. (1980). Sympathoadrenal and renin-angiotensin system in the development of two-kidney, one clip renal hypertension in rats. Hypertension 2, 723-731.

Ayitey-Smith, E., and Varma, D. R. (1970). An assessment of the role of the sympathetic nervous system in experimental hypertension using normal and immunosympathectomized rats. Brit. J. Pharmacol. 40, 175-185.

Azar, S., Ernsberger, P., Livingston, S., Azar, P., and Iwai, J.

(1981). Paraventricular-suprachiasmatic lesions prevent salt-induced hypertension in Dahl rats. Clin. Sci. **61**, 495.

Barajas, L., Wang, P., Bennett, C. M., and Wilburn, R. L. (1976). The renal sympathetic system and juxtaglomerular cells, in experimental renovascular hypertension. Lab. Invest. **35**, 574-587.

Barger, A. C. (1979). Experimental renovascular hypertension. Hypertension, 447-445.

Bealer, S. L. Haywood, J. R., Gruber, K. A., Buckalew, V. M., Jr., Fink, G. D., Brody, M. J., and Johnson, A. K. (1983). Preoptic-hypothalamic periventricular lesions reduce natriuresis to volume expansion. Am. J. Physiol. **244**, R51-R57.

Bellini, G., Fiorentini, R., Fernandez, M., Onestic, G., Hesson, H., Gould, A. B., Bianchi, M., Kim, K. H., and Swartz, C. (1979). Neurogenic activity-angiotensin II interaction during the development and maintenance of renal hypertension in the rat. Clin. Sci. **57**, 25-29.

Ben-Ishay, D., Saliternick, R., and Welnes, A. (1972). Separation of two strains of rats with inbred dissimilar sensitivity to DOCA-salt hypertension. Experientia **28**, 1321-1322.

Berecek, K. H., Barron, K. W., Webb, R. L., and Brody, M. J. (1982a). Vasopressin-central nervous system interactions in the development of DOCA hypertension. Hypertension **4** (Suppl. II), II-131-II-137.

Berecek, K. H., Murray, R. D., Gross, F., and Brody, M. J. (1982b). Vasopressin and vascular reactivity in the development of DOCA hypertension in rats with hereditary diabetes insipidus. Hypertension **4**, 3-12.

Berecek, K. H., Webb, R. L., and Brody, M. J. (1983). Evidence for a central role for vasopressin in cardiovascular regulation. Am. J. Physiol. **244**, H852-H859.

Bickerton, R. K., and Buckley, J. P. (1961). Evidence for a central mechanism in angiotensin induced hypertension. Proc. Soc. Exp. Biol. Med. **106**, 834-836.

Bosland, M. C., Versteeg, D. H. G., van Put, J., and deJong, W. (1981). Effect of depletion of spinal noradrenaline by 6-hydroxydopamine on the development of renal hypertension in rats. Clin. Exp. Pharmacol. Physiol. **8**, 67-77.

Brody, M. J., and Johnson, A. K. (1980). Role of the anteroventral third ventricle region in fluid and electrolyte balance, arterial pressure regulation, and hypertension. In "Frontiers in Neuroendocrinology", Vol. 6 (L. Martini and W. F. Ganong, eds.), pp. 249-292. Raven Press, New York.

Brody, M. J., Barron, K. W., Berecek, K. H., Faber, J. E., and Lappe, R. W. (1983). Neurogenic mechanisms of experimental hypertension. In "Hypertension" (J. Genest, O. Kuchel, P. Hamet and M. Cantin, eds.), pp. 117-140. McGraw-Hill, New York.

Brody, M. J., Fink, G. D., Buggy, J., Haywood, J. R., Gordon, F. J., and Johnson, A. K. (1978). The role of the anteroventral third ventricle (AV3V) region in experimental hypertension. Circ. Res. 43 (Suppl. I), I-2-I-13.

Buchholz, R. A., and Nathan, M. A. (1983). Short vs. long term blood pressure recording in rats with NTS lesions. Fed. Proc. 42, 1120.

Buckley, J. P. (1977). Central vasopressor actions of angiotensin. Biochem. Pharmacol. 26, 1-3.

Buckley, J. P., and Jandhyala, B. S. (1977). Central cardiovascular effects of angiotensin. Life Sci. 20, 1485-1494.

Buggy, J., Fink, G. D., Johnson, A. K., and Brody, M. J. (1977). Prevention of the development of renal hypertension by anterovental third ventricle tissue lesions. Circ. Res. 40 (Suppl. I), I-110-I-117.

Buggy, J., Fink, G. D., Haywood, J. R., Johnson, A. K., and Brody, M. J. (1978). Interruption of the maintenance phase of established hypertension by ablation of the anteroventral third ventricle (AV3V) in rats. Clin. Exp. Hypertension I, 337-353.

Bumpus, F. M., Sen, S., Smeby, R. R., Sweet, C., Ferrario, C. M. and Khosla, M. C. (1973). Use of angiotensin II antagonist in experimental hypertension. Circ. Res. (Suppl I), I-150-I-158.

Bunag, R. D., and Eferakeya, A. E. (1976) Immediate hypotensive after effects of posterior hypothalamic lesions in awake rats with spontaneous, renal, or DOCA hypertension. Cardiovasc. Res. 10, 663-671.

Bunag, R. D., and Riley, E. (1979). Chronic hypothalamic stimulation in awake rats fails to induce hypertension. Hypertension, 498-507.

Carey, R. M., Dacey, R. G., Jane, J. A., Winn, H. R., Ayers, C. R., and Tyson, G. W. (1979). Production of sustained hypertension by lesions in the nucleus tractus solitarii of the American foxhound. Hypertension, 246-254.

Carretero, O. A., and Romero, J. C. (1977). Production and characteristics of experimental hypertension in animals. In: "Hypertension" (J. Genest, E. Koiw and O. Kuchel, eds.), pp. 485-507. McGraw-Hill, New York.

Ciriello, J., and Calaresu, F. R. (1980). Hypothalamic projections of renal afferent nerves in the cat. Can. J. Physiol. Pharmacol. **58**, 574–576.

Cowley, A. W., Monos, E., and Guyton, A. C. (1974). Interaction of vasopressin and the baroreflex system in the regulation of arterial blood pressure in the dog. Circ. Res. **34**, 505–514.

Crofton, J. T., Share, L., Shade, R. E., Lee-Kwon, W. J., Manning, M., and Sawyer, W. H. (1979). The importance of vasopressin in the development and maintenance of DOC-salt hypertension in the rat. Hypertension **1**, 31–38.

Dahl, L. K., Heine, M., and Tassinar, L. (1962). Effects of chronic excess salt ingestion. Evidence that genetic factors play an important role in susceptibility to experimental hypertension. J. Exp. Med. **115**, 1173–1190.

Dargie, H. J., Franklin, S. S., and Reid, J. L. (1977a). Central and peripheral noradrenalin in the two-kidney model of renovascular hypertension in the rat. Brit. J. Pharmacol. **61**, 213–215.

Dargie, H. J., Franklin, S. S., and Reid, J. L. (1977b). Plasma noradrenaline concentration in experimental renovascular hypertension in the rat. Clin. Sci. Mol. Med. **52**, 477–483.

Davis, J. O. (1977). The pathogenesis of chronic renovascular hypertension. Circ. Res. **40**, 439–444.

deChamplain, J., and van Ameringen, M. R. (1972). Regulation of blood pressure by sympathetic nerve fibers and adrenal medulla in normotensive and hypertensive rats. Circ. Res. **31**, 617–628.

deChamplain, J., Cousineau, D., van Amerigan, M. R., and Marc-Aurele, J. (1977). The role of the sympathetic system in experimental and human hypertension. Postgrad. Med. J. **53** (Suppl. 3), 15–30.

Dickinson, C. J., and Ferrario, C. M. (1974). Central neurogenic effects of angiotensin. In "Angiotensin" (I. H. Page and F. M. Bumpus, eds.), pp. 408–416. Springer Verlag, New York.

Doba, N., and Reis, D. J. (1973). Acute fulminating neurogenic hypertension produced by brainstem lesions in the rat. Circ. Res. **32**, 584–593.

Douglas, J., Saltman, S., and Fredlund, P. (1976a). Receptor binding of angiotensin II and antagonist: correlation with aldosterone production by isolated canine adrenal glomerulosa cells. Circ. Res. **38** (Suppl. II), II-108–II-112.

Douglas, J. R. Jr., Johnson, E. M., Jr., Heist, J. F., Marshall, G. R., and Needleman, P. (1976b). Is the peripheral sympathoadrenal nervous system necessary for renal hypertension? J.

Pharmacol. Exp. Ther. **196**, 35–43.

Dzau, V. J., Sivek, L. G., Rosen, S., Fahri, E. R., Mizoguchi, H., and Berger, A. C. (1981). Sequential renal hemodynamics in experimental benign and malignant hypertension. Hypertension **3** (Suppl. I), I-63–I-68.

Faber, J. E., and Brody, M. J. (1982). Enhanced neurogenic vasoconstrictor tone during initiation of 2-kidney 1-clip Goldblatt hypertension in conscious rats. Fed. Proc. **41**, 1094.

Faber, J. E., and Brody, M. J. (1983a). Neural contribution to renal hypertension following acute renal artery stenosis in conscious rats. Hypertension **5** (Suppl. I), I-55 – II-164.

Faber, J. E., and Brody, M. J. (1983b). Renal nerve-dependent hypertension (HT) following acute renal artery stenosis (RS) in the conscious sinoarotic deafferented (SAD) rat. Fed. Proc. **42**, 873.

Farr, W. C., and Grupp, G. (1971). Ganglionic stimulation: mechanism of the positive inotropic and chronotropic effects of angiotensin. J. Pharmacol. Exp. Ther. **177**, 48–55.

Feldberg, W., and Lewis, G. P. (1964). The action of peptides on the adrenal medulla. Release of adrenalin by bradykinin and angiotensin. J. Physiol. **171**, 98.

Ferrario, C. M., and Takishita, S. (1983). Baroreceptor reflexes and hypertension. In "Hypertension", Second Edition (J. Genest, O. Kuchel, P. Hamet and M. Cantin, eds.), pp. 161–170. McGraw-Hill, New York.

Ferrario, C. M., Gildenberg, P. L., and McCubbin, J. W. (1972). Cardiovascular effects of angiotensin mediated by the central nervous system. Cir. Res. **30**, 257–262.

Ferrario, C. M., McCubbin, J. W., and Berti, G. (1976). Centrally mediated hemodynamic effects of angiotensin. In "Regulation of Blood Pressure by the Central Nervous System" (G. Onesti, M. Fernandes, and K. E. Kim, eds.), pp. 175–182. Grune and Stratton, New York.

Finch, L., and Leach, F. G. H. (1970). Does the adrenal medulla contribute to the maintenance of experimental hypertension? Eur. J. Pharmacol. **11**, 388–391.

Finch, L., Haeusler, G., and Thoenen, H. (1972). Failure to induce experimental hypertension in rats after intraventricular injection of 6-hydroxydopamine. Brit. J. Pharmacol. **44**, 356.

Fink, G. D., and Brody, M. J. (1980). Impaired neurogenic control of renal vasculature in renal hypertensive rats. Am. J. Physiol. **238**, H770–H775.

Fink, G. D., Buggy, J., Haywood, J. R., Johnson, A. K., and
    Brody, M. J. (1978). Hemodynamic effects of electrical
    stimulation of forebrain angiotensin and osmosensitive sites.
    Am. J. Physiol. **235**, H445-H451.
Fink, G. D., Kennedy, F., Bryan, W. J., and Werber, A. (1980).
    Pathogenesis of hypertension in rats with chronic aortic
    baroreceptor deafferentation. Hypertension **2**, 319.
Folkow, B., and Rubenstein, E. H. (1966). Cardiovascular effects
    of acute and chronic stimulation of the hypothalamic
    defense area in the rat. Acta Physiol. Scand. **68**, 48-57.
Folkow, B., Lewis, D. H., Lundgren, O., Mellander, S., and
    Wallentin (1964). The effect of graded vasoconstrictor fibre
    stimulation on the intestinal resistance of capacitance
    vessels. Acta Physiol. Scand. **61**, 445-451.
Folkow, B., Nordlander-Hallback, M., Martner, J., and Nordborg,
    C. (1982). Influence of amygdala lesions on cardiovascular
    responses to alerting stimuli, on behaviour and on blood
    pressure development in spontaneously hypertensive rats.
    Acta Physiol. Scand. **116**, 133-139.
Freeman, R. H., Davis, J. O., Watkins, B. E., and Lohmeier, T. E.
    (1977). Mechanism involved in two-kidney renal
    hypertension induced by constriction of one renal artery.
    Circ. Res. **40** (Suppl. I), I-29-I-35.
Freeman, R. H., Davis, J. O. Watkins, B. E., Stephens, G. A., and
    DeForrest, J. M. (1979). Effects of continous converting
    enzyme blockade on renovascular hypertension in the rat.
    Am. J. Physiol. **236**, F21-F24.
Freeman, R. H., Villarreal, D., Davis, J. O., and Garoutee, G.
    (1983). Effect of renal denervation in rats with 1-clip, 1-
    kidney Goldblatt hypertension. Fed. Proc. **42**, 766.
Friedman, S. M., Friedman, C. L., and Nakashima, M. (1960).
    Accelerated appearance of DOCA hypertension in rats
    treated with pitressin. Endocrinology **67**, 752-759.
Galeno, T. M., and Brody, M. J. (1983). Hemodynamic responses
    to amygdaloid stimulation in the spontaneously hypertensive
    rat. Am. J. Physiol., in press.
Galeno, T. M., Van Hoeson, G. W., Maixner, W., Johnson, A. K.,
    and Brody, M. J. (1982). Contribution of the amygdala to
    the development of sponaneous hypertension. Brain Res.
    246, 1-6.
Galeno, T. M., Van Hoesen, G. W., and Brody, M. J. (1984).
    Central amygdaloid nucleus lesion attenuates exaggerated
    hemodynamic responses to noise stress in the spontaneously

hypertensive rat. Brain Res., **91**, 249-259.

Galloway, M. P., and Westfall, T. C. (1982). The release of endogenous norepinephrine from the coccygeal artery of spontaneously hypertensive and Wistar-Kyoto rats. Circ. Res. **51**, 225-232.

Ganong, W. F. (1981). The brain and the renin-angiotensin system. In "Central Nervous System Mechanisms in Hypertension" (J. P. Buckley and C. M. Ferrario, eds.), pp. 283-292. Raven Press, New York.

Gavras, H., and Liang, C.-S. (1980). Acute renovascular hypertension in conscious dogs. Circ. Res. **47**, 356-365.

Gavras, H., Brunner, H. R., Laragh, J. J., Vaughan, E. D., Koss, M., Cote, L. J., and Gavras, I. (1975). Malignant hypertension resulting from deoxycorticosterone acetate and salt excess. Circ. Res. **36**, 300-309.

Gildenberg, P. L., Ferrario, C. M., and McCubbin, J. W. (1973). Two sites of cardiovascular action of angiotensin II in the brain of the dogs. Clin. Sci. **44**, 417-420.

Goldstein, B. M., Heitz, D. C., Shaffer, R. A., and Brody, M. J. (1974). Modulation of baroreceptor reflex by central administration of angiotensin. Eur. J. Pharmacol. **26**, 212.

Gordon, F. J., Matsuguchi, H., and Mark, A. L. (1981). Abnormal baroreflex control of heart rate in prehypertensive and hypertensive Dahl genetically salt-sensitive rats. Hypertension 3 (Suppl. I), I-135-I-141.

Gordon, F. J., Haywood, J. R., Brody, M. J., and Johnson, A. K. (1982). Effect of lesions of the anteroventral third ventricle (AV3V) on the development of hypertension in spontaneously hypertensive rats. Hypertension 4, 387-393.

Goto, A., Ikeda, T., Tobian, L., Iwai, J., and Johnson, M. A. (1981). Brain lesions in the paraventricular nuclei and catecholaminergic nuclei neurons minimize salt hypertension in Dahl salt-sensitive rats. Clin. Sci. **61**, 535.

Goto, A., Ganguli, M., Tobian, L., Johnson, M. A., and Iwai, J. (1982). Effect of an anteroventral third ventricle lesion on NaCl hypertension in Dahl salt-sensitive rats. Am. J. Physiol. **243**, H614-H618.

Greenberg, S. (1981). Vascular responses of the perfused intestine to vasoactive agents during the development of two-kidney, one-clip Goldblatt hypertension in dogs. Circ. Res. **48**, 895-906.

Grewal, R. S., and Kaul, C. L. (1971). Importance of the sympathetic nervous system in the development of renal hypertension in the rat. Br. J. Pharmacol. 42, 497–504.

Gruber, K. A., Whitaker, J. M., and Buckalew, V. M., Jr. (1980). Endogenous digitalis-like substance in plasma of volume-expanded dogs. Nature 287, 743–745.

Guo, G. B., and Abboud, F. M. (1982). Inhibition by angiotensin II of baroreflex control of lumbar sympathetic nerve activity in rabbits. Circulation 66 (Suppl. II), II-33.

Haddy, F. J. (1982). Natriuretic hormone-the missing link in low renin hypertension? Biochem. Pharmacol. 31, 3159–3161.

Haeusler, G. (1976). Central adrenergic neurons in experimental hypertension. In "Regulation of blood pressure by the central nervous system" (Onesti, G., Fernandex, M., Kim, K. E. eds.), pp. 53–64. Grune and Stratton, New York.

Hallback, M., and Folkow, B. (1974). Cardiovascular responses to acute mental "stress" in spontaneously hypertensive rats. Acta Physiol. Scand. 90, 684–698.

Hartle, D. K. (1981). Studies on the role of the anterior hypothalamic angiotensin II pressor system in experimental renal hypertension. Ph.D. Thesis, University of Iowa, Iowa City, Iowa.

Hartle, D. K., and Brody, M. J. (1982a). Hypothalamic vasomotor pathways mediating the development of hypertension in the rat. Hypertension 4 (Suppl. III), III-68–III-71.

Hartle, D. K., and Brody, M. J. (1982b). Dissociation of central angiotensin II and sodium pressor systems from mechaniams of development of 1K-renal and steroid/salt hypertension in the rat. Neuro. Abs. 8, 431.

Hartle, D. K., Lind, R. W., Johnson, A. K., and Brody, M. J. (1982). Localization of the anterior hypothalamic angiotensin II pressor system. Hypertension 4 (Suppl. II), II-159–II-165.

Hatzinikalaou, P., Gavras, H., Brunner, H. R., and Gavras, I. (1981). Role of vasopressin catecholamines and plasma volume in hypertonic saline-induced hypertension. Am. J. Physiol. 240, H827–H831.

Haupert, G. T., Jr., and Sancho, J. M. (1979). Sodium transport inhibitor from bovine hypothalamus. Proc. Nat. Acad. Sci. USA 76, 4658–4660.

Haywood, J. R., Fink, G. D., Buggy, J., Phillips, M. I., and Brody, M. J. (1980). The area postrema plays no role in the pressor action of angiotensin in the rat. Am. J. Physiol. 239, H108–H113.

Haywood, J. R., Ball, N. W., Lifschitz, D., and Brennan, T. (1982). Contribution of the anteroventral third ventricle (AV3V) region in hypertonic sodium chloride induced hypertension. Neuro. Abs. 8, 431.

Haywood, J. R., Fink, G. D., Buggy, J., Boutelle, S., Johnson, A. K., and Brody, M. J. (1983). Prevention of two-kidney one-clip renal hypertension in the rat by ablation of antero-ventral third ventricle (AV3V) tissue. Am. J. Physiol., 245, H683-H689.

Huang, C. T., Cardona, R., and Michelakis, A. M. (1978). Existence of a new vasoactive factor in experimental hypertension. Am. J. Physiol. 234, E25-E31.

Huot, S. J., Pamnani, M. B., Glough, D. L., Buggy, J., Bryant, H. J., Harder, D. R., and Haddy, F. J. (1983). Sodium-potassium pump activity in reduced renal-mass hypertension. Hypertension 5 (Suppl. I), I-94-I-100.

Ichikawa, S., Johnson, J. A., Fowler, W. C., Payne, C. G., Kurz, K., and Keitzer, W. F. (1978). Pressor responses to nor-epinephrine in rabbits with 3-day and 30-day renal artery stenosis. Circ. Res. 43, 437-446.

Ito, C. S., and Scher, A. M. (1981). Hypertension following arterial baroreceptor denervation in the unanesthetized dog. Circ. Res. 48, 576-591.

Johnson, A. K., Hoffman, W. E., and Buggy, J. (1978). Attenu-ated pressor responses to intracranially injected stimuli and altered antidiuretic activity following preoptic hypo-thalamic periventricular ablation. Brain Res. 157, 161-166.

Johnson, A. K., Buggy, J., Fink G. D., and Brody, M. J. (1981). Prevention of renal hypertension and of the central pressor effect of angiotensin by ventromedial hypothalamic ablation. Brain Res., 205, 255-264.

Johnson, E. M., Jr., and Vacia, R. A. (1979). Unique resistance to guanethidine-induced chemical sympathectomy of spontaneously hypertensive rats. Circ. Res. 45, 243-249.

Judy, W. V., Watanabe, A. M., Henry, D. P., Besch, H. R., Jr., Murphy, W. R., and Hockel, G. M. (1976). Sympathetic nerve activity. Role in regulation of blood pressure in spontaneously hypertensive rat. Circ. Res. 38 (Suppl. II), II-21-II-29.

Katholi, R. E., Winternitz, S. R., and Oparil, S. (1981). Role of the renal nerves in the pathogenesis of one-kidney renal hypertension in the rat. Hypertension 3, 404-409.

Katholi, R. E., Winternitz, S. R., and Oparil, S. (1982). Decrease in peripheral sympathetic nervous system activity following renal denervation or unclippling in the one-kidney one-clip Goldblatt hypertensive rat. J. Clin. Invest. 69, 55-62.

Kline, R. L., Patel, K. P., Ciriello, J., and Mercer, P. F. (1983). Effect of renal denervation on arterial pressure in rats with aortic nerve transection. Hypertension 5, 468-475.

Knudsen, K. D., Dahl, L. K., Thompson, K., Iwai, J., Heine, M., and Leitl, G. (1970). Effects of chronic excess salt ingestion. Inheritance of hypertension in the rat. J. Exp. Med. 132, 976-1000.

Knuepfer, M. M., Mohrland, J. S., Shaffer, R. A., Gebhart, G. F., Johnson, A. K., and Brody, M. J. (1980). Effects of afferent renal nerve (ARN) stimulation and baroreceptor activation on unit activity (UA) in the anteroventral third ventricle (AV3V) region. Fed. Proc. 39, 837.

Knuepfer, M. M., Johnson, A. K., and Brody, M. J., (1983). Identification of brain stem projections mediating hemo-dynamic responses to stimulation of the anteroventral third ventricle (AV3V) region. Brain Research, in press.

Kobayashi, R. M., Palkovits, M., Kopia, I. J., and Jacobowitz, D. M. (1974). Biochemical mapping of noradrenergic nerves arising from the rat locus coeruleus. Brain Res. 77, 269-279.

Kubo, T., Hashimoto, M., and Ohashi, T. (1978). Effects of intraventricular and intraspinal 6-hydroxydopamine on blood pressure of renal hypertensive rats. Arch. Internat. Pharmacol. Therap. 234, 270-278.

Lais, L. T., and Brody, M. J. (1978). Vasoconstrictor hyper-responsiveness: an early pathogenic mechanism in the spontaneously hypertensive rat. Eur. J. Pharmacol. 47, 177.

Lais, L. T., Shaffer, R. A., and Brody, M. J. (1974). Neurogenic and humoral factors controlling vascular resistance in the spontaneously hypertensive rat. Circ. Res. 35, 764.

Lappe, R. W., and Brody, M. J. (1981). Regional vascular re-sistance changes to intracarotid vs. systemic angiotensin II (AII) in conscious rats. Federation Proc. 40, 528.

Laubie, M., and Schmitt, J. (1979). Destruction of the nucleus tractus solitarii in the dog: comparison with sinoaortic denervation. Am. J. Physiol. 236, H736.

Lewis, G. P., and Reit, E. (1965). The action of angiotensin and bradykinin on the superior cervical ganglion of the cat. J. Physiol. (London) 197, 538-553.

Liard, J. F., Cowley, A. W., McCaa, R. E., McCaa, C. S., and Guyton, A. C. (1974). Renin aldosterone body fluid volumes and the baroreceptor reflex in the development or reversal of Goldblatt hypertension in conscious dogs. Circ. Res. 34, 549-560.

Lundin, S., and Thoren, P. (1982). Renal function and sympathetic activity during mental stress in normotensive and spontaneously hypertensive rats. Acta Physiol. Scand. 115, 115-124.

Mahoney, L. T., Haywood, J. R., Corry, R., Patel, P. N., Johnson, A. K., and Brody, M. J. (1981). The role of the renal afferent nerves in the pathogenesis of experimental renal and mineralocorticoid hypertension. In "Hypertension" (H. Villarreal, ed.), pp. 195-198. John Wiley and Sons, New York.

Mangiapane, M. L., and Simpson, J. B. (1980). Subfornical organ: forebrain site of pressor and dipsogenic action of angiotensin II. Am. J. Physiol. 239, R382-R389.

Mann, J. F. E., Phillis, M. L, Dietz, R., Haebara, H., and Ganten, D. (1978). Effects of central and peripheral angiotensin blockade in hypertensive rats. Am. J. Physiol. 234, H629-H637.

Matsuguchi, H., and Schmid, P. G. (1982a). Acute interaction of vasopressin and neurogenic mechanisms in DOC-salt hypertension. Am. J. Physiol. 242, H37-H43.

Matsuguchi, H., and Schmid, P. G. (1982b). Pressor response to vasopressin and impaired baroreflex function in DOC-salt hypertension. Am J. Physiol. 22, H44-H49.

McCubbin, J. W., and Page, I. H. (1962). Neurogenic component of chronic renal hypertension. Science 139, 210-211.

Miller, E. D. Jr., Samuels, A. J., Haber, E., and Barger, A. C. (1975). Inhibition of angiotensin conversion and prevention of renal hypertension. Am. J. Physiol. 228, 448-453.

Mohring, J., Mohring, B., Petri, M., and Haack, D. (1977). Vasopressor role of ADH in the pathogenesis of malignant DOC hypertension. Am. J. Physiol. 232, F260-F269.

Mohring, J., Glanzer, K., Maciel, J. A., Jr., Dusing, R., Kramer, H. J., Arbogast, R., and Koch-Weser, J. (1980). Greatly enhanced pressor response to antidiuretic hormone in patients with impaired cardiovascular reflexes due to idiopathic orthostatic hypotension. J. Cardiovasc. Pharmacal. 2, 367-376.

Montani, J. P., Liard, J. F., Schoun, J., and Mohring, J. (1980). Hemodynamic effects of exogenous and endogenous vasopressin at low plasma concentrations in conscious dogs. Circ. Res. 47, 346-355.

Nathan, M. A. and Reis, D. J. (1977). Chronic labile hypertension produced by lesions of the nucleus solitarii in the cat. Cir. Res. 40, 72-81.

Niijima, A. (1975). Observation on the localization of mech-
    anoreceptors in the kidney and efferent nerve fibers in
    the renal nerves in the rabbit. J. Physiol. **78**, 339-369.
Norgen, R. (1980). The central organization of the gustatory and
    visceral afferent systems in the nucleus of the solitary
    tract. In "Brain Mechanisms of Sensation" (Y. Katsuki, R.
    Norgren and M. Sato, eds.), pp. 143-160. John Wiley and
    Sons, New York.
Okamoto, K., and Aoki, K. (1963). Development of a strain of
    spontaneously hypertensive rats. Jpn. Circ. J. **27**, 282-293.
Olson, L., and Fuxe, K. (1972). Further mapping out of central
    noradrenaline neuron systems: projections of the "sub-
    coeruleus" area. Brain Res. **43**, 289-295.
Overbeck, H. W. (1980). Pressure-independent increases in
    vascular resistance in hypertension: role of sympatho-
    adrenergic influences. Hypertension **2**, 780-786.
Overbeck, H. W., Pamnani, M. B., Akera, T., Brody, T. M., and
    Haddy, F. J. (1976). Depressed function of a ouabain-
    sensitive sodium-potassium pump in blood vessels from renal
    hypertensive dogs. Circ. Res. **38** (Suppl. II), II-48-II-52.
Palkovits, M., Brownstein, M., Saavedra, M. J., and Axelrod, J.
    (1974). Norephinephrine and dopamine content of the
    hypothalamic nuclei of the rat. Brain Res. **77**, 137-149.
Pamnani, M. B., Clough, D. C., and Haddy, F. J. (1978). Altered
    activity of the Na^+-K^+ pump in arteries with steroid
    hypertension. Clin. Res. **261**, 511A.
Pamnani, M. B., Clough, D., and Haddy, F. (1979). Na^+-K^+ pump
    activity in tail arteries of spontaneously hypertensive rats.
    Jpn. Heart J. **20** (Suppl. I), 228-230.
Pamnani, M. B., Huot, S., Buggy, J., Clough, D., and Haddy, F.
    (1981). Demonstration of a humoral inhibitor of the Na^+-K^+
    pump in some models of experimental hypertension.
    Hypertension **3** (Suppl. II), II-96-II-101.
Pamnani, M. B., Huot, S., Steffen, R., and Haddy, F. (1980).
    Evidence for a humoral Na^+ transport inhibiting factor in
    one-kidney, one wrapped hypertensive dogs. Physiologist **23**,
    91.
Pan, J. Y., Bishop, V. S., Ball, N., and Haywood, J. R. (1983).
    The inability of dorsal spinal rhizotomy to prevent or
    reverse one-kidney, one-wrap renal hypertension. Fed.
    Proc. **42**, 897.
Peach, M. J. (1977). Renin-angiotensin system: biochemistry
    and mechanisms of action. Physiol. Rev. **57**, 313-370.

Phillips, M. I., Felix, I. D., Hoffman, W. E., and Ganten, D. (1977). Angiotensin-sensitive sites in the brain ventricular system. In "Neurosciences Symposia", (W. Cowan and J. A. Ferendelli, eds.), pp. 308-399. Society for Neurosciences, Bethesda, Maryland.

Provoost, A. P., and DeJong, W. (1978). Differential development of renal, DOCA-salt, and spontaneous hypertension in the rat after neonatal sympathectomy. Clin. Exp. Hypertens. 1, 177-189.

Rabito, S. F., Carretero, O. A., and Scicli, A. G. (1981). Evidence against a role of vasopressin in the maintenance of high blood pressure in mineralocorticoid and renovascular hypertension. Hypertension 3, 34-38.

Rapp, J. P., Tan, S. Y., and Marolius, H. S. (1978). Plasma mineralocorticoids, plasma renin, and urinary kallikrein in salt-sensitive and salt-resistant rats. Endocr. Res. Comm. 5, 35-41.

Rascher, W., Lang, R. E. Taubitz, M., Meffle, H., Unger, T. H., Ganten, D., Gross, F. (1981). Vasopressin-induced increase is total peripheral resistance in deoxycorticosterone acetate hypertensive rats is buffered by the baroreceptor reflex. Clin. Sci. 61, 153S-156S.

Recordati, G. M., Moss, N. G., Genovesi, S., and Rogenes, P. R. (1980). Renal receptors in the rat sensitive to chemical alteration of their environment. Circ. Res. 46, 395-405.

Richardson, J. S. (1983). On the role of the septal area in the development of DOCA-salt hypertension in the rat. Clin. Exp. Hypertension A5, 469-478.

Ricksten, S. E., and Thoren, P. (1979). Characteristics of the sympathetic nervous activity in awake normotensive and hypertensive rats. Acta Physiol. Scand. 105, 31A-32A.

Riley, E., Takeda, K., and Bunag, R. (1979). Medial posterior hypothalamic lesions inhibit hypertension in spontaneously hypertensive rats. Neuro. Abs. 5, 49.

Saavedra, J. M., Brownstein, M. J., Kizer, J. S., and Palkovits, M. (1976). Biogenic amines and related enzymes in the circumventricular organs of the rat. Brain Res. 107, 412-417.

Saito, Y., Yajima, Y., and Watanabe, T. (1981). Involvement of AVP in the development and maintenance of hypertension in rats. In "Antidiuretic Hormone" (S Yoshida, L. Share, and K. Yagi, eds.), pp. 215-225. University Park Press, Baltimore, Maryland.

Saper, C. B., and Loewy, A. D. (1980). Efferent connections of
  the parabrachial nucleus in the rat. Brain Res. **197**, 291–
  317.
Scroop, G. C., Katic, F. P., Brown, M. J., Cain, M. D., and
  Zeegers, P. J. (1975). Evidence for a significant contribution from central effects of angiotensin in the development of acute renal hypertension in greyhound. Clin.
  Sci. Mol. Med. **48**, 115–119.
Severs, W. B., and Daniels-Severs, A. E. (1973). Effects of
  angiotensin on the central nervous system. Pharmacol.
  Rev. **25**, 415–449.
Songu-Mize, E., Bealer, S. C., and Caldwell, R. W. (1982). Effect
  of AV3V lesions on development of DOCA-salt hypertension
  and vascular Na^+-pump activity. Hypertension **4**, 575–580.
Strait, M. R., and Brody, M. J. (1983). Effects of sinoaortic
  deafferentation on sympathetic discharge and vascular
  resistance. Submittted to Am. J. Physiol.
Sweet, C. S., and Brody, M. J. (1970). Central inhibition of
  reflex vasodilation by angiotensin and reduced renal pressure. Am. J. Physiol. **219**, 1751–1758.
Sweet, C. S., Columbo, J. M., and Gaul, S. L. (1976). Central
  antihypertensive effects of inhibitors of the renin-angiotensin system in rats. Am. J. Physiol. **231**, 1794–1799.
Takeda, K., and Bunag, R. D. (1980). Augmented sympathetic
  nerve activity and pressor responsiveness in DOCA hypertensive rats. Hypertension **2**, 97–101.
Takeshita, A., and Mark, A. L. (1978). Neurogenic contribution
  to hindquarters vasoconstriction during high sodium intake
  in Dahl strain of genetically hypertensive rat. Circ. Res. **43**
  (Suppl. I), I-86.
Takeshita, A., Mark, A. L., and Brody, M. J. (1979). Prevention
  of salt-induced hypertension in the Dahl strain by 6-hydroxy-
  dopamine. Am. J. Physiol. **236**, H48–H52.
Tanaka, T., Seki, A., Fujii, J., Kurihara, H., and Ikeda, M. (1977).
  Norepinephrine turnover in two types of experimental
  renovascular hypertension of the rabbit. Jpn. Circ. J. **41**,
  881–881.
Touw, K., Fink, G., Haywood, J. R., Shaffer, R. A., and Brody,
  M. J. (1979). Elevated neurogenic vasoconstrictor tone is
  the mechanism of hypertension in rats with aortic baroreceptor deafferentation (ABD). Fed. Proc. **38**, 1232.
Touw, K. B., Haywood, J. R., Shaffer, R. A., and Brody, M. J.
  (1980). Contribution of the sympathetic nervous system to

vascular resistance in conscious young and adult spontaneously hypertensive rats. Hypertension 2, 408–418.

Trapani, A. J. Barron, K. W., and Brody, M. J. (1982). Regional
neurogenic basis of hypertension produced by sinoarotic
baroreceptor denervation (SAD). Fed. Proc. 41, 1094.

Trapani, A. J., Barron, K. W., and Brody, M. J. (1983). Analysis
of hemodynamic lability in hypertension produced by
sinoarotic baroreceptor denervation (SAD). Fed. Proc. 42,
2772.

Unger, T., Rockhold, R. W., Kaufmann-Buhler, Hubner, D.,
Schull, B., Speck, G., and Ganten, D. (1981). Effects of
angiotensin converting enzyme inhibitors on the brain. In
"Angiotensin Converting Enzyme Inhibitors" (Z. P. Horovitz,
ed.), pp. 55–79. Urban and Schwarzenberg, Baltimore.

Vanhoutte, P. M. (1981). Relase and disposition of noradrenaline
in the blood vessel wall of the spontaneously hypertensive
rat. In "New Trends in Arterial Hypertension, INSERM
Symposium #17", (M. Worcel, ed.), pp. 3–10. Elsevier, North
Holland.

Villamil, M. F., Amorena C., Ponce-Hornos, J., Muller, A., and
Taquini, A. C. (1982). Role of extracellular volume expansion in the development of DOC-salt hypertension in
the rat. Hypertension 4, 620–624.

Volicer, L., Scheer, E., Hilse, H., and Visweswaram, D. (1968).
The turnover of norephinephrine in the heart during
experimental hypertension in cats. Life Sci. 7, 525–532.

Webb, R. L., Knueper, M. M., and Brody, M. J. (1981). Central
projections of afferent renal nerves. Fed. Proc. 40, 545.

Webb, R. L., Johnson, A. K., and Brody, M. J. (1982). Role of
parabrachial nucleus in the hemodynamic effects of renal
afferent nerve stimulation (RANS). Fed. Proc. 41, 1258.

Webb, R. L. Boutelle, S., and Brody, M. J. (1983). Central relay
sites for cardiovascular reflexes elicited by renal afferent
nerve stimulation (RANS). Fed. Proc. 42, 583.

Winternitz, S. R., Katholi, R. E., and Oparil, S. (1982). Decrease
in hypothalamic norepinephrine content following renal
denervation in the one-kidney one-clip Goldblatt, hypertensive rat. Hypertension 4, 369–373.

Yamori, Y. (1983). Physiopathology of the various strains of
spontaneously hypertensive rats. In "Hypertension", Second
Edition (J. Genest, O. Kuchel, P. Hamet, and M. Cantin,
eds.). McGraw-Hill, New York.

Yamori, Y., and Okamoto, K. (1969). Hypothalamic tonic regulation of blood pressure in spontaneously hypertensive rats. Jpn. Circ. J. **33**, 509-519.

Zandberg, P., Palkovits, M., and DeJong, W. (1978). Effect of various lesions in the nucleus tractus solitari of the rat on blood pressure, heart rate and cardiovascular reflex responses. Clin. Exp. Hypertension **1**, 355.

Zimmerman, B. G. (1962). Effect of acute sympathectomy on responses to angiotensin and norepinephrine. Circ. Res. **11**, 780-787.

Zimmerman, B. G. (1981). Adrenergic fascilitation by angiotensin: does it serve a physiological function? Clin. Sci. **60**, 343-348.

Zimmerman, B. G., Mommsen, C., and Kraft, E. (1980). Sympathetic and renin-angiotensin system influence on blood pressure and renal blood flow of two-kidney, one clip Goldblatt hypertensive dog. Hypertension **2**, 53-62.

Biochemical and Physiological Aspects of the Renin–Angiotensin System: A Journey through Darkest Hypertension

John H. Laragh

Cardiovascular and Hypertension Center
The New York Hospital–Cornell Medical Center
New York, New York

As the topics assigned for discussion at this meeting signify, a not-so-distant thunder rumbles over the field of hypertension research. Its welcome portent is that the frustrating orthodoxy of useful but blind, trial-and-error treatment of the blood pressure level may have lingered beyond its time and that the basis already exists for discriminating among hypertensive patients not only on grounds of separate risk but of differentiable etiology, susceptible to more specific -- and increasingly available treatments.

I have been responsible for a certain share of that rumbling, all of which entitles me to speak particularly on the biochemical and physiological aspects of the renin-angiotensin system, a biologic control system for regulation of blood pressure and sodium balance, which to my mind is the keystone of a rational new approach to the understanding and treatment of hypertension now and in the future. The development of this point of view represents something of an odyssey which might best be presented historically.

HYPERTENSION: PHYSIOLOGICAL
BASIS AND TREATMENT

49

ALDOSTERONE SECRETION IN HYPERTENSIVE DISEASE

Our research had its beginnings some 25 years ago in a program examining hormonal mechanisms in salt metabolism (Laragh and Stoerk, 1957) and their involvement in hypertensive or in fluid-retaining states such as congestive heart failure (Laragh, 1962). We were particularly interested in the then newly discovered adrenocortical hormone, aldosterone, which acts at the distal renal tubule to retain sodium in an electrochemical exchange for potassium which is thereby excreted into the urine (Sonnenblick et al., 1961). We developed an accurate double isotope dilution assay for aldosterone (Ulick et al., 1958), and this made it possible for us to measure the hormone's secretion rate in the whole gamut of clinically encountered forms of hypertension.

We, like many others, were interested in the possible role of the sodium-retaining hormone in hypertension (Laragh et al., 1960). We expected to find, as we did, excessive aldosterone secretion with resultant sodium retention, hypertension and potassium depletion in primary aldosteronism, a rare form of hypertension that is cured by surgical removal of the culprit adrenocortical tumor. Nor did it stir us to find that, in contrast, patients with common essential hypertension had normal to near normal aldosterone secretion rates.

However, to our great surprise and excitement, we discovered that patients with malignant hypertension consistently exhibited massive oversecretion of aldosterone — far beyond that seen in any other form of clinical hypertension (Laragh et al., 1960). We were excited because this was the first finding of a biochemical abnormality of possible pathogenic relevance in this disease.

The puzzling thing was that, except for the high blood pressure, malignant hypertension in no way resembled primary aldosteronism. Surely it did not respond to the same treatment: in fact we found that total adrenalectomy failed to reverse it. But we learned something crucial from our surgical attempts. Although surgical exploration of all twelve patients showed no tumor, it did reveal that both adrenal glands were enlarged and hyperplastic (Laragh et al., 1960). Thus, this massive oversecretion of aldosterone was probably not arising in the adrenals themselves but was very likely a response of them to a chemical signal coming from another place in the body. It is perhaps not surprising that our first suspect candidate for that source was

the kidney because it is the most damaged organ in malignant hypertension.

DISCOVERING THE RENAL-ADRENAL AXIS
IN MALIGNANT HYPERTENSION

Postulation of a kidney secretion as the culprit in malignant hypertension revived a discarded concept. In 1898 Tigerstedt and Bergman (1898) produced hypertension in rabbits by injecting saline extracts of minced rabbit kidneys. They called the active substance renin. This work was not confirmed by more established investigators. In 1934 Goldblatt raised blood pressure in the dog by clamping a renal artery (Goldblatt et al., 1934). This reawakened interest in renin because of the numerous ensuing failures to find a relationship between plasma renin levels and blood pressure in either experimental or human forms of Goldblatt hypertension, renin did not quite make it as a scientifically respectable etiologic factor in high blood pressure and interest waned in it.

By the time we got to it, a few things were known about renin even though it had not yet been purified and it was not available for experiment or direct measurement. With no primary physiologic effects of its own, renin acted as an enzyme in the bloodstream to cleave the decapeptide angiotensin I from a plasma globulin substrate of hepatic origin. This product, too, was inactive but was converted rapidly by a pulmonary converting enzyme into the octapeptide angiotensin II, a most powerful vasoconstrictor. Both of these angiotensins had been isolated and synthesized and were available for experiment; moreover, their definition had furnished the basis for indirect assays of renin activity. Accordingly, it seemed reasonable for us to investigate angiotensin II's possible relationship to the massive aldosteronism that we had discovered in malignant hypertension.

In 1958 we began to infuse angiotensin II into normal volunteers. To our great excitement we observed an immediate and large rise in aldosterone secretion (Laragh et al., 1960). The aldosterone response was specific for angiotensin and was not just related to the state of vasoconstriction and blood pressure level since no other pressor substance tested had the capacity to stimulate aldosterone. We systematically studied epinephrine, norepinephrine, vasopressin, and serotonin, and their synthetic analogues.

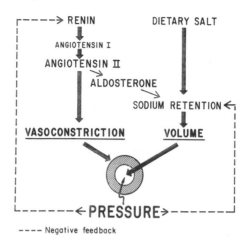

BLOOD PRESSURE=VASOCONSTRICTION X VOLUME

Figure 1. The renal-adrenal axis as a hormonal cascade involving renin, angiotensin and aldosterone for regulation of sodium and potassium balance and blood pressure. The interaction is depicted as it was first discovered in the studies of patients with malignant hypertension in whom, because of defective feedback, it is involved in causation. The syndrome is associated with massive oversecretion of aldosterone consequent to an unabated renin release. (From Laragh, 1960.)

THE RENIN AXIS AS A CONTROL SYSTEM

This research thus identified (Laragh, 1960; Laragh et al., 1960) a specific hormonal communication between the kidneys, via the bloodstream, and the adrenal cortex: the renin-angiotensin-aldosterone system. By its two-pronged stimulation of vasconstriction (the direct effect of angiotensin on the arterioles) and of volume (angiotensin's evocation of sodium-retaining aldosterone) we believed that the system was importantly involved in both the blood pressure and sodium homeostasis (Figure 1). Actually, at about the same time, but unknown to us, in Germany, Gross had postulated from rat studies a renin-aldosterone interaction for the control of sodium balance but not for blood pressure regulation (Gross, 1958).

The Renal-Adrenal Axis in Malignant Hypertension

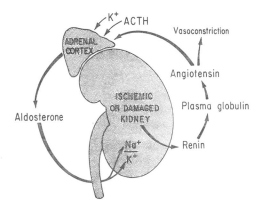

Figure 2. Renin-angiotensin-aldosterone system. Renin secreted in response to reduced arterial pressure or renal tubular sodium acts to release angiotensin II. Angiotensin II raises pressure and stimulates aldosterone secretion, leading to sodium and water retention. These pressure and volume effects turn off more renin release. Dashed line indicates negative feedback.

Further experimentation and reflection made it apparent to us that this was a self-compensating, negative feedback control system that regulates blood pressure and sodium balance simultaneously in all of us (Laragh et al., 1972). Renin is secreted (Figure 2) in response to a variety of normal or abnormal factors which reduce arterial blood pressure or renal perfusion, such as posture, shock, hemorrhage age, or heart failure, or that reduce flow in the distal renal tubule, as in sodium depletion. Correction for a flagging blood pressure and renal perfusion is provided immediately by angiotensin's vasoconstriction effect and then, more slowly, flow is restored by aldosterone's enhancement of volume via the induction of renal sodium retention. The subsequent improvement of blood pressure and renal perfusion by vasoconstriction or volume or both, shuts off, in a normally functioning kidney, the initial impulse for renin release. Baroreceptor mechanisms in the afferent renal arterioles are no doubt involved in the feedback control, together with sodium-load receptors in the macula densa of the distal renal tubules. Moreover, there is good evidence for beta-adrenergic receptor efferent modulation of the rate of renin secretion (Buehler et al., 1972).

THE HYPERALDOSTERONISM OF
MALIGNANT HYPERTENSION EXPLAINED

We put forward an explanation (Figure 1) (Laragh, 1960; Laragh et al., 1960) for the hyperaldosteronism we had observed in patients with malignant hypertension. And this process could be contrasted with what occurs in the more benign disorder of primary hyperaldosteronism. In the latter, also called Conn's syndrome, runaway autonomous production of aldosterone from an adrenocortical adenoma, in an otherwise healthy person, causes sodium retention, volume expansion, and hypertension which is usually mild and long-standing. In such patients with normally functioning kidneys, the sodium-volume induced high blood pressure and increased renal flow shuts off renin secretion — quite properly. Accordingly, a biochemical profile will show very low or absent plasma renin activity. Because of the trade-off nature of aldosterone-mediated sodium retention, there will be concurrent potassium depletion from renal potassium wastage, reflected by muscle weakness and polyuria. All of these abnormalities are entirely corrected by removing the offending adrenal cortical adenoma.

Something very different happens in malignant hypertension. Here the initiating defect is in the kidney — at the opposite pole of the renal-adrenal axis. A critical defect in the arteries of the kidneys has compromised renal blood flow. Mistaking this local perfusion and pressure defect for a systemic one, the kidneys secrete large excesses of renin in a failing attempt to restore their perfusion pressure. But this excess renin causes vasoconstriction and then volume expansion via the activation of more angiotensin and then aldosterone. However, this two-pronged elevation of systemic blood pressure is not perceived by the damaged kidneys, misinformed by underperfusion beyond vascular obstructions. Continuing to labor under the provincial impression of underperfusion (as in the Goldblatt model of the clipped renal artery), the kidney continues to pour out more renin. With greater systemic hypertension there is greater kidney vascular damage which, in turn, results in more renin release and greater hypertension still. It is a vicious, and fatal, circle. The biochemical profile includes both a high plasma renin and a high aldosterone level with attendant hypokalemia.

In comparing malignant hypertension with primary aldosteronism, we suspected that the high renin levels explained the
severe generalized vascular damage of malignant hypertension whereas the absence of renin in the bloodstream accounted for the virtual absence of vascular disease and benign
course of primary aldosteronism (Laragh, 1960; Laragh et al.,
1963). This suspicion has been reinforced by numerous published
animal experiments in which renin injections had been shown to
produce severe vascular damage especially in the kidneys, heart
and brain (Gavras et al., 1974).

These observations made it apparent to us that high blood
pressure, like high body temperature, was not necessarily the
product of a single pathophysiologic sequence. Here were two
hypertensive conditions radically different in cause, in outlook
and treatment, one with very high and the other with very low
renin, one sustained chiefly by vasoconstrictive forces and the
other by volume. Their basic pathophysiologic lesions were
located at the polar extremes of kidney-to-adrenal axis for
regulating blood pressure and electrolyte balance — one in the
service of the other.

Accordingly, it seemed eminently reasonable to pursue the
hunch that further exploration of the renin control system might
open up an understanding of the mechanisms involved in other
hypertensive forms — essential hypertension in particular — and
thereby lead us to greater diagnostic and therapeutic specificity.

The disparate biochemical derangements of the renin system
observed in the two more dramatic hypertensions — malignant
hypertension and primary aldosteronism — have been widely verified, and this knowledge has been put to useful clinical employ-
ment. Moreover, peripheral and renal vein renin assays have
been adopted worldwide as the basis for the diagnosis of surgically curable renovascular hypertension (Sealey et al., 1973;
Vaughan et al., 1981). Furthermore, oral contraceptive hypertension too (Laragh et al., 1967; Laragh et al., 1972), in which
a characterictic marked elevation of plasma renin substrate
occurs, is also now well recognized as a very common form of
secondary hypertension. However, acceptance of the renin
system's role for analyzing and treating the essential hypertension has had a much slower and stormier course.

COULD RENIN-ANGIOTENSIN II BE A VECTOR
IN ESSENTIAL HYPERTENSION?

Notwithstanding the discovery of the renin-aldosterone
system for control of blood pressure, and sodium balance and
the demonstration of its crucial participation in malignant and
subsequently, in other unusual forms of clinical hypertension,
investigators continued to doubt a role for renin in "essential"
hypertension. Perhaps this was because of a general failure in
the past to relate plasma renin levels to blood pressure levels in
this large group, and also because many such hypertensive patients were known to exhibit ostensibly "normal" renin levels.

However, because of the powerful pressor actions of angiotensin and the sodium-volume effects of aldosterone, our research group felt that the renin axis must participate in some
way, at least, in some forms of essential hypertension. A key
question was whether the so-called "normal" circulation levels
of these hormones could be sufficient to contribute to the hypertension?

Research changed traditional thought on this question. The
evidence began with studies (Ames et al., 1965) in which we
infused angiotensin or norepinephrine continuously into normal
human volunteers for up to 11 days (Figure 3). With angiotensin,
we found that, as the infusion proceeded, less and less angiotensin was needed to raise the pressure because of activaton of
aldosterone and resultant sodium retention and weight gain, so
that very small amounts of angiotensin became pressor by the
fourth or fifth day (Figure 3). Norepinephrine exhibited the
opposite features so that more and more hormone was needed
to keep the pressure elevated as sodium balance became negative. This meant to us that angiotensin fits the the model
requirements for an active pressor agent capable of mediating hypertension over the long term even in relatively small
amounts. In contrast, circulating norepinephrine levels failed
to fit the requirements of this model as a vector of long term
hypertension.

ANALYSIS OF RENIN SYSTEM PATTERNS
IN ESSENTIAL HYPERTENSION

We believed that the involvement of the renin system in
the more dramatic hypertensions demonstrates at the same
time the multiformity and coherence of hypertensive phe-

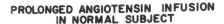

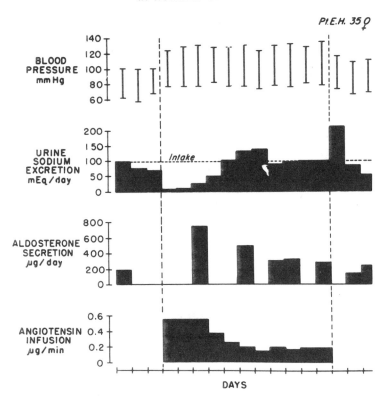

Figure 3. The prolonged continuous angiotensin infusion in a normal subject for 11 days. The dose of angiotensin was adjusted to keep a mildly pressor response. Angiotensin II induced a marked and selective increase in the adrenal corti- cal secretion of aldosterone together with consequent sodium retention. As sodium was retained, angiotensin became more pressor. Because of this increasing pressor sensitivity to angiotensin, the dose was serially reduced to a point where aldosterone secretion returned to control levels. Thus the pressor sensitivity to angiotensin increased as sodium reten- tion progressed. The results indicate that angiotensin, unlike norepinephrine, can produce and then sustain hypertension in diminishingly small amounts. (Adapted from Ames et al., 1965.)

nomena. These clinical conditions are based on widely disparate physiologic lesions, yet they share the manifestation
of high blood pressure and the inevitable reactive or primary
complicity of the renin system. Thus the renin system exhibits
different abnormal patterns associated with different types of
human hypertension. One is impelled to the hypothesis that
common essential hypertension, too, shares these disparities as
well as the coherences. Traditionally in medical research, the
physiological extravagances observed in the most severe forms
of disease has led to better understanding of subtler aberrations.

Moreover, it was clear to us that the renin-angiotensin-
aldosterone complex comprises in normal people a true control
system for regulation of blood pressure and sodium balance.
Therefore, in our analysis of essential hypertension, we proceeded on the assumption that the the patterns observed in this
group must always have meaning too because, as a true control
system for blood pressure, the renin system must either (1)
cause, (2) support, or (3) react to hypertensive phenomena in a
consistent manner.

A sizable number of investigators have studied the role of
renin in essential hypertension. Most of them, excluding us,
declared no evidence of renin involvement in essential hypertension. This was becasue they found no correlation for the
entire group between the levels of plasma renin activity and the
levels of blood pressure. Furthermore, what most nourished
their skepticism was the considerable number of patients with
"normal" renin levels.

To conclude no consistent renin involvement makes sense
only if one considers essential hypertension a single disorder
with a single cause, common course and common treatment, all
clinical evidence to the contrary. However, there are several
ways of approaching such findings. What if essential hypertension was a spectrum of disorders, in style if not in scale,
similar to the more dramatic hypertensions, i.e., high-renin
renal hypertension and low-renin adrenal hypertensions? In this
event, the renin system patterns might be a means of discriminating within such a spectrum.

Another question: was a "normal" renin level in the presence
of hypertension -- regulatory business-as-usual by the kidneys in
the face of high arterial pressures -- a healthy or a sick reaction? We know that renin falls to very low subnormal values
in normal people whose blood pressure or sodium balance is
artificially elevated. Another question: what was the best way
to standardize and evaluate the normality of a regulatory sub-

stance whose secretion fluctuated widely in quick reaction to changing physical and dietary pressor factors? And the last question: could the crude renin activity assay methods, sufficient for detecting large hormonal tides in extreme conditions, be relied on to accurately reflect the inevitably more subtle variances and smaller concentrations occurring in essential hypertension?

MEASURING PLASMA RENIN ACTIVITY

The thing to deal with first was the last question. We found that most of the renin assay method employed were insensitive or in error. In one method (Haber et al., 1969) lack of pH control and the use of incorrect angiotensinase inhibitors reduced accuracy and underestimated the true value. In another frequently used approach (Brown et al., 1964; Skinner, 1967), preliminary acid treatment of the sample inadvertently activates prorenin (Sealey and Laragh, 1975) to the more active renin and so leads to a gross overestimation, in an unpredictable way, of the truly active renin level. To solve those problems, we developed and published a reliable and accurate method that has now become a standard (Sealey and Laragh, 1980).

It is also important to standardize the conditions under which the renin sample is collected (Laragh et al., 1972). Some studies, we found, either ignored the impact on renin release of physical and dietary pressor factors or failed to establish a sufficiently sensitive relationship. Renin release, it must be kept in mind, is an act of regulation, a response to pressor events coming from outside the regulatory apparatus. Posture, ambulation, and dietary salt are the principal such events (Brunner et al., 1972; Laragh et al., 1972). We established the normal responses to varying degrees of dietary salt intake in subjects quietly seated after ambulation, and we plotted these on a continuous nomogram. We used as our measure of salt intake, and also of balance, the 24-hour urinary sodium excretion, which we found on comparison to be as sensitive an indicator as the laborious metabolism ward study and obviously was easier to obtain. We then studied patients with essential hypertension in the same way, referencing the plasma renin findings to the rate of sodium excretion as compared to a nomogram derived from normal subjects. This index we called the "renin-sodium profile" (Laragh et al., 1972).

RENIN IN ESSENTIAL HYPERTENSION

In essential hypertension we found a broader spectrum of plasma renin profile values than those which occur in normotensive people (Brunner et al., 1972). About 30% had low, 55% had "normal", and 15% had high renin values. Similar distributions have ben described around the world. Two possible conclusions from these data could be drawn: (a) either the renin level was in no way implicated, or alternatively, (b) the essential hypertension was a spectrum of hypertensive disorders classifiable by the renin profile, characterized at one extreme by excess renin production and accompanying vasoconstriction and at the other extreme by excessive sodium-volume retention resulting, appropriately enough, in depressed renin production. Based on our findings in malignant hypertension and primary aldosteronism, we chose to follow the proposition that essential hypertension was a heterogenous spectrum that could be indexed by the renin profile. We reasoned that a regulatory apparatus like the renin system, so inextricably harnessed to the control of blood pressure, simply had to either cause, react to, or be involved in some meaningful way in any abnormal pressor circumstance.

On the subject of meaning, what was the significance of a so-called "normal" renin production in a hypertensive patient? Such a level of renin activity could be called "normal" only if it maintained a normal level of blood pressure against a given level of salt intake, and consequently, blood volume. However, if that same level of renin activity supported an abnormally high blood pressure, could this be called normal or appropriate? Normal people will turn off their renin secretion when arterial pressure or blood volume is raised. Accordingly, "medium" might be a much better term than "normal" to describe patients with high blood pressure who still are secreting renin. It seemed to us that the renin system was reacting appropriately to the high pressure only in the low-renin patients. Its failure to shut down in the face of hypertension in high-renin and medium-renin patients could very well mean it was part of the problem.

All of this is hypothetical, of course, but it could be supported by evidence that the biochemical subgroups might also be differentiated by the clinical course of their disease and also by showing a reasonable predictability of their response to specific treatment — anti-renin therapy in the case of high- and medium-renin patients, and anti-volume therapy in low-renin patients.

PLASMA RENIN ACTIVITY AS AN INDICATOR OF RISK
IN ESSENTIAL HYPERTENSION

Our companion clinical data provided highly suggestive
evidence that the three renin subgroups did indeed experience
different clinical courses (Brunner et al., 1972; Brunner et al.,
1973). Low-renin patients were found to suffer fewer heart
attacks and strokes than did medium- or high-renin patients. In
219 patients studied, 14% of the high-renin patients, 11% of
medium-renin patients, and none of the 59 low-renin patients
suffered cardiovascular complications. Moreover, the low-renin
patients were older by an average of 9 years, perhaps expressing
a longer duration of disease, and this occurred even though they
were often more hypertensive than the normal renin group.

These findings, initially contested, have to a large extent
been borne out in worldwide studies. There is little doubt among
those who have charted them that there is an epidemiologic
difference, related to the renin level, among patients with essential hypertension (Laragh, 1978b). Thus, it has been generally verified that low-renin patients as a group are in fact quite
significantly older, despite higher pressures than are medium-
renin patients. Moreover, the converse has been well described.
High-renin patients such as those with renovascular hypertension tend to have the worst prognosis and the shortest survival
(Perera and Haelig, 1952; Maxwell, 1975; Davies et al., 1979).
Accordingly, low-renin patients seem to be at less risk since
they enjoy a measure of protection from cardiovascular damage. Later, I will discuss the possible reasons for this and
their implications in prognosis. For now, let these observations
stand as more evidence for the heterogeneity of essential
hypertension.

ESTABLISHING THE PHYSIOLOGIC RELEVANCE
OF THE RENIN-SODIUM PROFILE

Differential responses of the control system to different
types of antihypertensive therapies was of course the observation that could clinch the argument that the renin profile, in
metering the control system, had pathophysiologic relevance.
This had not been shown. While diuretics could be said to be
specific against sodium-sustained volume retention, there was
no agent agreed upon to be specific against renin-sustained
vasconstriction. But that, too, would come.

THE PROPRANOLOL EXPERIENCE

A breakthrough occurred in 1972. Buehler and associates reported (1972) that the hitherto inexplicable and inconsistent antihypertensive action of the beta-adrenergic receptor blocker, propranolol, could in fact be predicted with a high degree of accuracy by a properly performed renin profile. The drug was most effective in high-renin, somewhat less effective in medium-renin, and totally ineffective in low-renin patients. In the patients in whom it was effective, the fall in blood pressure was preceded by a fall in renin activity and generally to the same degree. Propranolol mono-therapy normalized most high and many medium-renin patients without the need to add any other agents (Buehler et al., 1972; Buehler et al., 1973). Equally relevant, it was consistently without effect or even acting as pressor (Drayer et al., 1976) in the low-renin forms of hypertension.

We took this as strong circumstantial evidence that propranolol's mechanism of action involved the inhibition of renin release which thereby lowered blood pressure in those patients whose hypertension was sustained by renin. Since such patients included not only those with a high but also many with medium renin levels, this supported our concept that a "normal" level in the face hypertension was indeed abnormal. Equally illuminating was the inability of propranolol to correct low-renin patients in whom diuretics were instead uniquely effective. All this appeared to vindicate the concept of a spectrum of disorders subsumed within the rubric of essential hypertension, ranging from renin-mediated vasoconstriction forms to sodium-mediated hypervolemic types.

It should be added parenthetically that, while we postulated renin blockade as the principal mechanism of the antihypertensive action of beta-receptor blockade, it by no means could be said to be the only one. The correlations were strong but not infallible. Actually, a number of alternative theories have been put forward to explain propranolol's depressor action, but none of them are well supported by clinical observation or investigative data. One theory holds that beta-blockers lower blood pressure by lowering cardiac output. This concept does not stand up too well before the observation that the beta-blocking drugs reduce cardiac output in virtually everybody -- hypertensives, normotensives, anephric patients, even patients with primary aldosteronism -- but they reduce blood pressure only in those demonstrated by the renin profile to have a renin component. In the low–renin states of essential hypertension, primary aldosteronism, and anephric humans, not only are beta-blockers without depressor effect despite the reduc tion of cardiac output, they may actually be pressor (Drayer et al., 1976), perhaps by leaving the alpha tone unopposed when there is little or no renin to suppress. Some advocates of the cardiac output theory of the antihypertensive action elicited by beta-blockers have attempted to finesse these contradictions by invoking a secondary mechanism, i.e., variable reactive changes in arteriolar tone subsequent to reduced cardiac output (Tarazi and Dustan, 1972; Hansson, 1973) but it cannot be shown that such an effect occurs independently of the reduced peripheral resistance produced by lowered angiotensin levels.

It has also been proposed that beta-blockers reduce blood pressure by an effect on the central nervous system (Lydtin and Sommerfeldt, 1972; Lewis and Haeusler, 1975), but this has not received convincing support (Ganong and Reid, 1976; Conway et al., 1978), especially since some beta-blockers with depressor action do not enter the central nervous system. Moreover, higher doses of beta blockers, as used for example in schizophrenics in whom they are more often pressor than depressor, can even induce malignant hypertension (Atsmon et al., 1972).

Other critics have rejected the propranolol-renin theory on the grounds that they could not demonstrate a similar renin-lowering effect with some of the other beta-blockers. However, it has since become apparent that these failures were usually due to the use of faulty assay methods discussed above. At least one of such claims has been retracted (Amery et al., 1976). It is now generally recognized that all beta-blockers, while they may exhibit well-known variations of $beta_1$ or $beta_2$ specificity, depress renin secretion to a generally similar extent. Extremely convincing evidence on the relevance of this anti-renin action has emerged from some more recent, rigidly controlled animal experiments in which propranolol and other beta-blockers lowered pressure proportionately to an induced renin reduction and to the pretreatment renin level, but were ineffective or even pressor in low-renin models including nephrectomized animals (Chiu and Sommer, 1979; Iaina et al., 1979; Young, 1981). Moreover, propranolol's specificity for renin secretion could be perceived from its ineffectiveness against experimental hypertension induced by angiotensin II infusion (Young and Diepstra, 1978) and from its antihypertensive action paralleling that of captopril in experimental malignant hypertension.

SARALASIN

A congruent experience was recorded in studying the depressor responses to intravenous saralasin, a pharmacologic probe that specifically competes with angiotensin II for its receptor sites, thereby blocking its vasoconstrictor action (Brunner et al., 1973; Brunner et al., 1974). This experience corresponded to that with propranolol in that saralasin was depressor mainly in high-renin patients and was completely without depressor effect in low-renin patients. However, saralasin-testing identified (Streeten et al., 1975; Case et al., 1976; MacGregor and Dawes, 1976; Marks et al., 1977) a renin-angiotensin factor in a much smaller portion of patients with essential hypertension — only 15% depressor responses as compared with about 50% for propranolol. The reason, we soon discovered, was that saralasin was itself a weaker angiotensin-like substance (Case et al., 1976), exhibiting a partial agonist or pressor actions of its own. This agonism could grossly underestimate the participation of renin in blood pressure support, particularly at medium and low renin levels, where the angiotenstin vascular receptors are partly or completely unoccupied. Accordingly, saralasin is usually pressor when given to low-renin and medium-renin patients. Saralasin only lowers pressure in such patients when they are pretreated with diuretics (Streeten et al., 1975) to produce dehydration and reactively raised renin levels. The pressure will then fall when saralasin is given because the weaker agonist numerically swamps and displaces the stronger agonist, angiotensin.

Thus, to settle the question of renin involvement in essential hypertension, we needed a pharmacologic probe with an unchallengeable anti-renin action without agonist properties that might dilute the results.

CONVERTING ENZYME INHIBITION: TEPROTIDE AND CAPTOPRIL

We found what we were looking for in SQ 20881, or teprotide, a nonapeptide isolated from snake venom (Ondetti et al., 1971) and then developed for clinical trial by Squibb. It was an answer looking for its question, which we happened to have. We began studying teprotide in 1972. For several years or more our group was the only one interested enough in its potential to even request it for the study of hypertension (Gavras et al.,

1974; Case et al., 1977). Teprotide produces a virtually complete blockade of the converting enzyme that hydrolyzes the decapeptide angiotensin I into the active II form, thereby inactivating the renin system. Moreover, it had no pressor properties of its own. Since it has to be given intravenously, its use was confined to the hospital setting.

A more specific pharmacologic probe has yet to be found; one could confidently relate most of the blood pressure effects of this drug to its disarming of the renin system. These effects, studied in 89 essential hypertension patients, thoroughly confirmed our prior approaches (Gavras et al., 1974; Case et al., 1977). The pattern of depressor reactions to teprotide -- greatest in high-renin and least in low-renin patients, as expressed by a proportional decline in blood pressure, paralleled those already shown with propranolol and with saralasin therapy -- and so verified our explanation of the antihypertensive actions of all of these drugs. Moreover, the acute depressor response to teprotide, together with a commensurate fall in angiotensin activity, could be predicted most closely by the baseline plasma renin level (Case et al., 1977). In so doing, the drug identified and quantified a renin factor that contributed to the hypertensive state of most patients with essential hypertension.

Thus teprotide administration revealed a significant-to-large renin factor in the hypertension of all high-renin patients and in 90% of medium-renin patients (Case et al., 1977). Altogether this comprises about 70% of patients with essential hypertension. Again, the low-renin patients as a group exhibited no significant depressor responses. Teprotide, as could be predicted by the vasoconstriction-volume analytical approach (see below), was, like propranolol, also ineffective in the volume-sustained, low-renin hypertensive patients including those with primary aldosteronism and those without kidneys.

CAPTOPRIL

Obviously, the practical spinoff of this research would be an orally active converting enzyme inhibitor. This became a reality with the development of captopril, a drug modeled after teprotide but which is orally active; it is indeed a triumph of modern pharmacologic engineering (Ondetti et al., 1977). As we would predict, the clinical experience so far with captopril completely retraces that observed with acute teprotide testing

(Case et al., 1978; Brunner et al., 1979). It has proven to be an extremely effective antihypertensive agent that lowers blood pressure to an extent predictable from the height of the control renin level. That it does so with fewer side effects than with other antihypertensive agents suggests that it may be more closely targeted to interrupt causal processes.

Captopril's antihypertensive effect appears to occur in stages; an immediate response is manifest about 90 minutes after the first oral dose and then a rebound, sometimes back all the way up to control levels, of several days to a week before the ultimate sustained antihypertensive benefit develops (Laragh et al., 1980). Possibly, there is a transient baroreceptor opposition to the drug. The gradual but sustained reduction of aldosterone secretion is one of the long-term benefits which reduces or obviates the need for adding a diuretic to the regimen. The delayed response pattern should restrain the clinician from prematurely prescribing adjunctive medications.

Captopril has real conceptual advantages over previous modes of therapy. It lowers blood pressure while maintaining or actually increasing blood flow to the vital organs (i.e., the heart, brain and kidneys). This is in contrast to diuretic treatment and even to beta-adrenergic blockade, in which some arterial flow to the brain, heart and kidneys is sacrificed to reduce the pressure.

Also, captopril is without the reflex tachycardia and cardiac stimulation associated with other less specific vasodilators. Yet another positive feature is that captopril's action appears merely to dampen rather than totally block the renin system, thus leaving a renin response sufficient for homeostasis in the face of such physiologic stimuli as posture and exercise. A greater order of specificity for captopril therapy is perhaps best expressed by the fact that blood pressure is lowered without a tradeoff of unwanted physiologic side effects of less specific agents. Thus, for some patients, there is no effect on mentation, sexual performance, gastrointestinal function, postural reflexes or exercise responses. Moreover, there is no dehydration, hemoconcentration or hypokalemia with increased cardiac instability. Indeed, flow to the brain, heart and kidneys is actually increased as the pressure is reduced. This, it seems to me, as will be discussed below, is a vitally important practical goal for modern antihypertensive therapy.

DISSECTION OF VASOCONSTRICTION AND
VOLUME FACTORS IN HYPERTENSION

The reciprocity between vasoconstriction and volume factors (Laragh, 1973) in blood pressure support, dramatically demonstrated in these pharmacologic studies, has broad applications. Thus, for example, when renin-vasoconstriction is opposed with vasodilator drug such as hydralazine, minoxidil, or nitroprusside, the renin system reacts and by secreting more renin induces, via aldosterone activation, salt and water retention. In the same way, diuretics, uniquely effective in low-renin patients, are likely to be ineffective or even pressor in high-renin patients, presumably by triggering of a greater reactive renin overshoot in response to more volume depletion (Baer et al., 1977). This see-saw relationship explains why diuretic-resistant patients respond to the addition of anti-renin drug (Gavras et al., 1974) and why some medium- or high-renin patients need a diuretic to cope with reactive sodium retention, consequent to vasodilator or autonomic blocking drug therapies. However, many patients will respond to a single agent providing it is the correct one for their physiologic lesion. It is therefore worthwhile to search them out. Thus, a worldwide literature has accumulated to verify the different selectivity of beta-receptor blockers and of diuretis when given to different subgroups of patients as defined by renin testing (Table 1).

This vasoconstriction-volume see-saw (Laragh, 1973) or reciprocity helps explain why many insufficiently analyzed patients do not respond to trial and error therapy: the agent prescribed may be inappropriate to deal with the factors behind their hypertension — diuretics are diminishingly effective or ineffective in vasoconstriction-dependent hypertension while, conversely, renin blockade is ineffective in volume-dependent forms of hypertension.

THE VASOCONSTRICTION-VOLUME INTERPLAY
IN EXPERIMENTAL AND CLINICAL FORMS
OF RENAL HYPERTENSION

In concurrent research in animal and human forms of renovascular hypertension, we demonstrated the same interplay between vasoconstriction and volume factors that is also apparent in essential hypertension (Laragh, 1973). The one-kidney clipped with the opposite kidney untouched hypertension model

Table 1.   The Selective Effectiveness of Antihypertensive Drugs

---

Beta Blockers are Preferentially Effective in High and Normal Renin Patients	Diuretics are Preferentially Effective in Low Renin Patients
Buehler et al., 1972	Crane et al., 1970
Buehler et al., 1973	Spark et al., 1971
Buehler et al., 1975	Crane et al., 1972
Castenfors et al., 1973	Carey et al., 1972
Pettinger et al., 1975	Aldin et al., 1972
Karlberg et al., 1976	Vaughan et al., 1973b
Hollifield et al., 1976	Castenfors et al., 1973
Weidman et al., 1976	Distler et al., 1974
Menard et al., 1976	Douglas et al., 1974
Stumpe et al., 1976	Karlberg et al., 1976
MacGregor et al., 1976	MacGregor et al., 1976
Boerth, 1976	
Bahr et al., 1976	
Zech et al., 1977	
Philipp et al., 1977	

Beta Blockers Can Actually Raise Pressure in Low Renin Patients	Diuretics Can Actually Raise Pressure in High Renin Patients
Drayer et al., 1976	Baer et al., 1977

---

is renin-dependent, and is corrected by angiotensin antibody or blockade (Brunner et al., 1971). This form resembles surgically-curable human renovascular hypertension since nephrectomy or vascular repair is curative. On the other hand, the one-kidney clipped hypertensive animal with the opposite kidney removed exhibits a low-renin level and is instead using volume to support the hypertension. But this form can be converted to renin dependency by dietary sodium depletion (Gavras et al., 1973). Only then does the blood pressure fall with anti-renin system drugs. The human counterpart of this second form is patients with bilateral kidney disease and reduced renal mass. They are similar because they exhibit medium- or low-renin levels and

THE VASOCONSTRICTION-VOLUME SPECTRUM IN HYPERTENSION

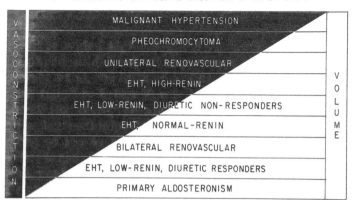

Figure 4. The vasoconstriction-volume spectrum in hypertension. (From Laragh et al., 1979.)

respond to sodium depletion but not to anti-renin drugs. These studies provide a basis for the value of the peripheral renin profile as a primary screening test for surgically curable reno-vascular hypersecretion (unilateral hypersecretion of renin) because renin hypersecretion is a characteristic of this form. Practically, this blood test often allows the physician to defer or eliminate the necessity for the more invasive tests of pyelography and arteriography until the need is definitely established by a positive renin-profile, followed then by renal-vein renin studies.

THE VASOCONSTRICTION-VOLUME ANALYTICAL MODEL

When all these research findings are put together, a construction emerges that we have come to call the Vasoconstriction-Volume Hypothesis (Laragh, 1973) (Figure 4). This serves as a useful framework for analyzing, explaining, and treating all hypertensive patients. The hypothesis sees hypertension as a bipolar spectrum ranging from a predominant excess of arterial vasoconstriction to a predominant excess of effective volume. The volume-excess form is identifiable by a low renin level and verifiable by correction of the hypertension by diuresis alone. All hypertension is characterized by vasoconstriction and an increased peripheral resistance. However, volume-dependent forms appear to have less vasoconstriction and more flow for a

given degree of blood pressure elevation. The reason for the
maintained but lesser vasoconstriction of low-renin forms remains a research problem. There is experimental evidence that
this latter vasoconstriction may be an autoregulatory response
to the volume overload hypertension.

In viewing hypertension as a spectrum, there are intermediate forms in which relative excesses of one or the other
may overlap and jointly contribute to high blood pressure
(Figure 4). Malignant hypertension and primary aldosteronism
are the polar extremes of the spectrum, and the other clinical
entities fall at intermediate points. Renin profiling can generally suggest the likelihood of the particular type of hypertension
within this spectrum. Just as important, those patients who do
not respond as expected to anti-renin or anti-volume therapy
can be set apart for further study.

PRESSURE, PLASMA RENIN LEVELS, VASCULOTOXICITY AND THE RISK OF STROKE AND HEART ATTACK

The pathophysiologic spectrum bracketed by the vasoconstriction-volume hypothesis may also be associated with a
spectrum of risk that has important clinical implications.
Earlier, I cited clinical and epidemiologic findings suggesting
that high-renin patients may be at greater risk of cardiovascular accident (i.e., stroke and heart attack) than are low-renin
patients at a comparable level of blood pressure (Brunner et al.,
1972; Brunner et al., 1973). Actually, clinicians have long
known that the risks of heart attack or stroke are not equally
distributed or necessarily related to the height of the blood
pressure. Thus the heterogeneity of renin patterns may very
well explain a longstanding clinical puzzle: why many patients
with marked hypertension can ignore all treatment with apparently unaffected health and longevity, while others with less
hypertension die prematurely.

The suggestion that renin activity, with its consequent
angiotensin-directed vasoconstriction, is in itself vasculotoxic,
producing trauma to blood vessels beyond that produced by excessive pressure per se, stems not only from our epidemiologic
study of renin-profiled patients (Brunner et al., 1972; Brunner
et al., 1973) but also from a body of laboratory and clinical
studies summarized in Table 2. Thus, in some animals, administration of renin or angiotensin with aldosterone in the presence
of available dietary sodium produces severe vasculitis, often

Table 2. *Experimental and Clinical Evidence for the
Vasculotoxic Potential of Renin System Activity*

1. In animals, renin injections cause vascular damage in the
    heart, brain and kidneys (Winternitz et al., 1939–40; Masson
    et al., 1966; Gavras et al., 1971).
    a. This is amplified by giving aldosterone (Masson et al.,
        1951; Masson et al., 1962).
    b. It is prevented by sodium deprivation (Masson et al.,
        1966).

2. Aldosterone (or DOC) excess in animals lowers renin levels
    (Goodwin et al., 1969; Gavras et et., 1975) and causes
    vascular damage which develops at a slower rate (Selye
    et al., 1943; Gavras et al., 1975;). This hypertension is
    amplified by renin or angiotensin administration (Masson
    et al., 1952; Masson et al., 1953), is prevented by sodium
    deprivation (Mulinos et al., 1941; Relman and Schwartz,
    1952) and is partially corrected by vasopressin blockade
    (Moehring et al., 1977; Crofton et al., 1979).

3. Stroke-prone SHR have markedly higher plasma renin levels
    which appear several months before the stroke (Matsunaga
    et al., 1975).

4. In human malignant hypertension total nephrectomy (Laragh
    et al., 1972) or propranolol (Buehler et al., 1972), or con-
    verting enzyme inhibitor treatment (Gavras et al., 1974;
    Case et al., 1976; Case et al., 1977; Case et al., 1978) can
    reverse the syndrome and lead to healing of vascular lesions.

5. Human (Perera and Haelig, 1952; Davis et al., 1979) or
    animal (Byrom, 1963) renovascular hypertension is more
    often associated with vascular damage and malignant
    hypertension.

6. Patients with renal artery graft closure (Laragh et al., 1972)
    or with a renin-secreting tumor (Ørjavik et al., 1975) have
    marked vascular damage affecting the brain, heart and
    kidneys.

7. Saralasin withdrawal in humans can be followed by rebound
    hyperreninemia, hypertension, acute encephalopathy, and
    coma (Keim et al., 1976).

fatal, in a few days (Gavras et al., 1974; Laragh, 1978b). Patients with malignant or renovascular hypertension and high plasma renin (Laragh et al., 1972) or with renin-secreting tumors (Ørjavik et al., 1975) have the most striking vascular damage. Acute high-renin clinical situations -- renal artery graft closure, renal trauma, or saralasin rebound (Keim et al., 1976) -- are accompanied by stroke, encephalopathy, or heart attack. The converse is also true. Also it has been recognized (Laragh et al., 1972) that total nephrectomy will reverse malignant hypertension, with biopsies showing healing of vasculitis, and a similar reversal of vasculitis occurs after nephrectomy or vascular repair in unilateral renal disease.

RENIN AS A RISK FACTOR BESIDES PRESSURE

The suggestion that plasma renin activity levels are related to cardiovascular damage has also attracted considerable criticism, the critics maintaining that hydraulic pressure is the culpable traumatic force, with no consideration given to whether it is consequent to vasoconstriction or to volume. The resulting debate is worth some comment in this discussion of the physiology of hypertension, for it has bearing on the assessment of risk and the order of treatment.

It would be unreasonable to contest the vasculo-traumatic potential of a raised hydraulic pressure. An elevated pressure, if great enough, can damage any vascular structure, and it is not surprising that experimental hypertension has described this effect (Byrom, 1969). Data from human (Garner et al., 1975; Heptinstall, 1953; Pickering, 1968) and animal studies (Byrom, 1969; Gavras et al., 1974; Okamoto et al., 1974) show that the malignant phase of hypertension may occur beyond a critically high level of pressure, after which arteriolar necrosis ensues in beds exposed to the highest pressures, followed by breakthrough of autoregulation with blowouts in the fragile distal vasculature.

Nevertheless, a number of considerations lead us to doubt that high blood pressure intrinsically is the critical or only factor in the greater vascular damage that often accompanies this condition. Actually, many acute experiments on this problem may be questioned because vasoconstrictor agents which also reduce flow and cause ischemia were used to implicate pressure as the culprit. Moreover, while acute high pressure levels can rupture critical vessels, chronic high pressure may actually bring about a hypertrophic adaptation that strengthens them (Folkow, 1971) and thus substantially raises the breakthrough threshold for autoregulation (Byrom 1969; Lassen and Agnoli, 1972; Strandgaard et al., 1973). Moreover, again, many of the acute studies cited in support of the vascular damaging effect of pressure per se have employed angiotensin or adrenergic vasoconstrictors to induce the high pressure; one could equally claim that these studies demonstrate the vasculotoxicity of vasoconstriction. Would a similar degree of hypertension induced by volume expansion alone (and therefore with better maintenance of tissue flow) produce equivalent vascular injury? That question has not been adressed by most of these older studies.

The inescapable fact remains that many hypertensive patients, and many animal models too, weather extremely high blood pressure without vascular injury while other patients suffer vascular damage at blood pressures well below what is thought to be critical. Obviously, factors other than mere pressure are at work and we should be seeking them out.

What these other factors might be are clued by several experiments suggesting that vascular damage in hypertensive, as well as in normotensive, situations may be related to hypovolemia with compromised flow and tissue ischemia. Thus, in animals (Mohring et al., 1976) and in humans (Kincaid-Smith et al., 1973) malignant hypertension due to renin excess can actually be remitted by saline infusions which, even though they can raise blood pressure further, work to improve flow and volume and relieve ischemia while also acting to suppress renin. Actu ally, in two recent animal studies (Romero et al., 1977; Seymour et al., 1980), sustained hypertension has been induced or maintained by sodium depletion and corrected by saline administration. This broadens the evidence that inordinate sodium depletion and reduced flow can be critical in inducing vasoconstriction and hypertension.

A number of animal experiments have shown that renin activity is not necessary for vascular injury to develop in the presence of hypertension (e.g., the vascular damage of DOC-salt hypertension, Gavras et al., 1975), but such research does not exclude the participation of other vasoconstrictors such as vasopressin (Moehring et al., 1977) or catechol amines. In fact the malignant syndrome of DOC-salt excess is characteristically preceded by paroxysms of natriuresis and then occurs in a setting of reduced flow and hyperviscosity (Gavras et al., 1975), a situation not unlike that occurring in experimental renovascular hypertension (Moehring et al., 1976). Accordingly, we need more research on the relative complicity of compromised flow and elevated pressure. However, the evidence so far strongly suggests that severe vasoconstriction, even in the absence of hypertension, may be an important prerequisite for vascular damage. Severe vasoconstriction leads to translocation of fluid from vascular to interstitial space, brings about hypovolemia, hemoconcentration, high blood viscosity, and ischemia with reduced tissue flow to the microcirculation. In our present state of knowledge such protracted vasoconstriction is most likely and often due to sustained action of the renin system.

This might explain why vascular damage so frequently occurs at the ostensibly subcritical levels of blood pressure. Also, it may help explain why numerous clinical trials in which diuretic therapy, successful by sphygmomanometric standards, so often fails to protect against myocardial infarction (Robinson, 1972; Steward, 1976; Smith, 1977; Jones et al.,1978; Helgeland, 1980; Morgan et al., in press). It may also explain why protection against myocardial infarction has been regularly demonstrated in clinical trials using beta-blockade alone, such as the Goteborg trial involving 7,500 subjects (Berglund et al., 1978). With the latter type of therapy, renin-induced vasoconstriction is reduced and chronic dehydration is not induced. Conversely, diuretics regularly induce dehydration and reactive renin-mediated vasoconstriction.

At any rate, all this is reason enough for serious consideration of the renin system's involvement in hypertension and its vascular sequellae, and for a program of management that is designed to protect or improve flow by going after the vasoconstriction factor whenever it can be demonstrated.

PATHOPHYSIOLOGICAL DIFFERENCES BETWEEN LOW- AND HIGH-RENIN HYPERTENSIVE PATIENTS AND THEIR RELEVANCE TO DIFFERENCES IN CARDIOVASCULAR INJURY

In view of the potentially better prognosis for low-renin as compared with high- and medium-renin patients, it is worth considering what could be a pathophysiological basis for this difference. As already indicated, the presence of an inappropriate or absolutely increased plasma renin level is now known to be accompanied by commensurate sustained vasoconstriction due to angiotensin II (Case et al., 1977). Conversely, in low-renin essential hypertension which appears significantly less prone to heart attack and stroke, there is little or no evidence for vasoconstriction due to renin activity. At the same time other evidence suggests that these patients are relatively more expanded with respect to sodium and volume. The latter evidence is derived from a tabulation (Laragh et al., 1979) of all published space measurements which reveals that, in general, low-renin hypertensive patients exhibit the highest extracellular fluid and blood volumes, while high-renin patients exhibit the lowest. Furthermore, the gamut of clinical parameters also suggest hemodilution and overfilling (Brunner et al., 1973). Moreover, numerous observations establish that the low-renin patients are the most responsive to sodium-volume depletion in terms of correction of their blood pressure (Laragh, 1978a).

The various parameters expressing likely or known physiologic differences between equally hypertensive low- and high-renin patients are summarized in Figure 5. Low-renin patients have increased peripheral resistance, to be sure, but the evidence suggests that the vasoconstriction which characterizes this form of hypertension is relatively less for a given degree of hypertension. That is to say that for a given degree of hypertension there is higher flow (i.e., higher cardiac output) and higher volume in low-renin patients. It is implied that greater vasoconstriction and greater increases in peripheral resistance, associated with renin activity, lead to poorer flow for a given level of hypertension and that this compromised flow to the microcirculation may well predispose to tissue ischemia and reduced ability to recover from vascular insult.

There is still other evidence which verifies the suggested physiologic differences among patients within the various renin subgroups, as postulated in Figure 5. In a recent computer analysis of 735 untreated patients with essential hypertension, similar significant differences in hematocrit, hemoglobin, and total protein values were again observed (Drayer et al., 1981). These data are in keeping with what the vasoconstriction-volume model predicts, i.e., that low-renin patients are relatively hemodiluted and volume expanded.

In an analysis of a smaller subgroup of high- and low-renin patients studied under metabolic ward conditions, Brunner and his colleagues (1973) demonstrated that, at three different levels of sodium intake, high-renin patients exhibit comparatively high blood urea values than do either the normal- or low-renin patients. The data showed that at the high sodium intake

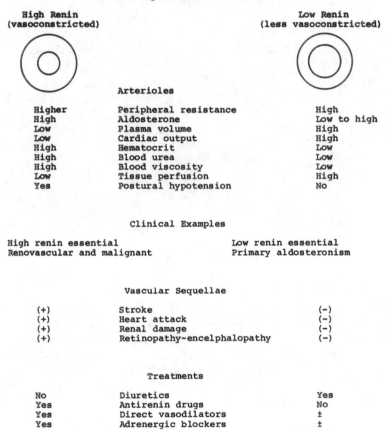

Figure 5. *High blood pressure mechanisms.* *(From Laragh, 1973.)*

BUN values of the high-renin patients never fell below 10 mg%. And for all three renin subgroups, BUN levels were inversely related to sodium intake, the lowest levels consistently seen during sodium loading and the highest during sodium depletion. It was noteworthy, however, that the low-renin patients exhibited, at all sodium intakes, the lowest mean urea levels; the difference during a normal sodium intake was statistically significant at the 5% level (Figure 2).

Recently Drayer et al. (1971) compared 27 age and sex matched untreated high- and low-renin patients with 27 normotensive people. They found that the low- and high-renin patients had similarly elevated systolic and diastolic blood pressures. However, the low-renin patients as a group had higher creatinine clearances and lower blood urea, uric acid, hemogloblin, hematocrit, as well as total protein values. These data describe once again the tendency toward hemodilution and volume expansion in low-renin patients as compared to high-renin patients, a tendency also reflected by a range of routine clinical measurements.

Complementing these observations are older findings that a high hemoglobin concentration is a risk factor for stroke: the incidence of cerebral infarction is doubled for men over 15 gm and women over 14 gm (Kannel et al., 1972). A recent study shows that cerebral blood flow and alertness is inversely related to hematocrit and plasma viscosity, even for hematocrit and viscosity values within the normal range (Willison et al., 1980)

THE TREATMENT APPROACH

The research odyssey I have just related provides the rationale for a treatment approach based on the relative contribution to a particular hypertension of vasoconstriction or of volume, that is, practically speaking, of renin activity as opposed to sodium retention. The complicity of either force is assessed by the renin profile, which then guides the choice of either an anti-renin or anti-volume agent as the first step. A surprisingly large number of patients will respond satisfactorily to such monotherapy. The particular single agent or, when necessary, a combination of the two types will normalize at least 85% of patients. The remaining 15 percent or so, testifying to the complexity and diversity of hypertensive phenomena, must still be subjected to the older empiric trial method with a battery of other agents.

For reasons I presented herein, the preferred initial therapeutic step is to pursue the renin factor rather than apply the traditional blanket of diuretics. We have described this treatment plan elsewhere in more detail (Laragh 1976; Laragh et al., 1979). I need not spend much time on it now, therefore. However, since my assignment here concerns the physiology of hypertension, I do want to emphasize that our treatment approach to hypertensive phenomena, like our analytic and re-

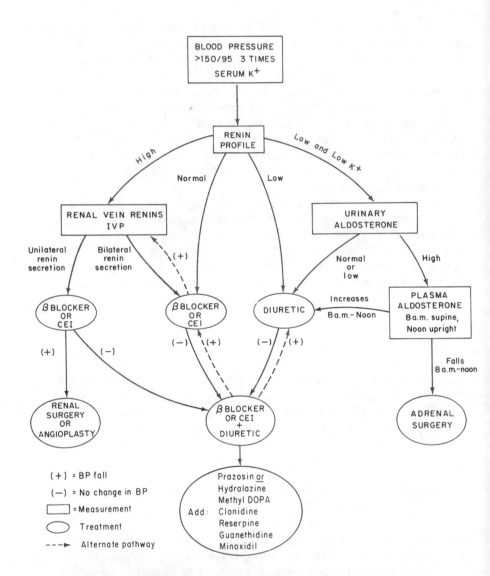

Figure 6. Flow sheet for complete diagnosis and treatment of hypertension. Low-renin patients with hypokalemia (serum K^+ <3.5) are evaluated for adrenocortical disease. Normokalemic low-renin patients receive a diuretic first. The medium-and high-renin patients are started on a beta-blocker or newer anti-renin drugs such as a converting enzyme inhibitor. Whenever either course is only partly corrective, the anti-renin agents are combined with a diuretic. Altogether this nor-

search approaches, is based on the upfront identification of degree of the dynamic reciprocity, so dramatically demonstrated in our studies, between renin-mediated vasoconstriction and sodium-volume factors.

I would also like to emphasize that the new work certainly does not refute older hard-earned empirical data on treatment. Rather, it provides a second generation of knowledge that will better inform clinical practice as it brings us closer to full understanding. Accordingly, the new research presages the onset of a new era of more predictable and selective drug treatment programs.

We have set forth in detail the methods of a complete, integrated system for the complete diagnosis and treatment of hypertension. It enables simpler, more specific, and more predictable treatment for major fractions of hypertensive patients (Laragh 1976; Laragh et al., 1979). In it (Figure 6), the renin-sodium profile and a baseline plasma-potassium measurement provide the basis for (1) definitive diagnosis of adrenocortical hypertension, (2) definitive diagnosis of surgically curable renovascular hypertension, (3) the acquisition of baseline data about the relative participation of vasoconstriction and volume factors that enables more specific therapy, (4) the evaluation of the pace, severity, and outlook of the underlying disorder, and (5) identification of patients whose hypertension cannot be explained by our current state of knowledge. The plan also

Figure 6 (cont.) malized some 85% of patients. For the residual resistant group, other less palatable drugs are superimposed in traditional trial by error fashion as indicated. Also unlike so-called "stepped care", drug subtraction and dose reduction is performed whenever pressure is normalized, to achieve the fewest drugs in the smallest dose. Those medium- or high-renin patients with a good response to a beta-blocker or captopril alone based on other clinical features too, are evaluated for surgically curable renovascular hypertension. Only if the renal vein renin study reveals hypersecretion with ischemia is angiography done for considering either angioplasty or surgery. When renin profiling is not available this basic approach can be partially applied, albeit more slowly, by serially evaluating the responses to anti-renin or anti-volume therapy, but renin profiling remains essential to diagnose curable forms. (From Laragh et al., 1979.)

defines an optional procedure for empirical use when a renin profile is not easily available.

The new system differs in concept from previous approaches such as "stepped care" in that these older systems have assumed all hypertension is alike and therefore a single additive recipe system is used for all. Thus, "stepped care" makes no provision for systematic drug substitution or dose reduction. In contrast, our new system seeks to identify those large, subgroups of different people, in whom long-term monotherapy with either an anti-vasoconstriction or anti-volume drug is possible. Among the advantages of the new system is that, for major fractions of all hypertensive patients, it enables long-term therapy with one drug instead of two, or two instead of three or more, with the attraction that the right type of drug is applied to contain the physiological lesion, i.e., anti-volume therapy with a diuretic in patients with low renin levels or anti-renin therapy with a beta-blocker in patients with high- and medium-renin levels (Figure 4 and Table 1). The new system also diagnoses or excludes surgically curable forms of hypertension, and reduces the use of and aids in the selection of patients for pyelography and arteriography.

Such an approach is centered around the renin system not because of any simplistic concept that it is the only pathogenic medium in hypertension. Rather, the approach stems from the renin system's role as central regulator of blood pressure homeostasis; it cannot help but react to any situation affecting blood pressure whether the fundamental cause is in the renin system or outside it. It is thus, to date, the most logical, convenient, and sensitive physiologic location from which to obtain a biochemical sounding. Current laboratory skills enable us to analyze such soundings and then develop and apply new pharmacologic agents which permit us to do something specific about our findings. For the control of blood pressure and perhaps more importantly, tissue flow, it is an approach whose time has come.

SUMMARY

A research journey over the past 20 years has revealed the renin-angiotensin-aldosterone system as a biochemical regulator of arterial blood pressure and sodium and potassium balance. It behaves as a control system exhibiting predictable responses to deformations in blood pressure or sodium balance.

Characteristic abnormal patterns of the system are involved in the pathogenesis of malignant hypertension, renovascular hypertension, primary aldosteronism and oral contraceptive hypertension.

Studies using a series of pharmacologic probes to block the renin system (beta-receptor blockers, saralasin, teprotide, and captopril) collectively reveal that essential hypertension is a spectrum in which absolute or relative overactivity of the renin axis actively participates in the maintenance of the hypertension of most patients. The plasma renin level itself indicates the degree of renin-mediated vasoconstriction supporting the blood pressure whereas the urinary sodium value indicates the appropriateness of the renin level to the volume status.

Renin-sodium profiling, together with determination of serum potassium levels, is basic for screening and definitive diagnosis of surgically curable forms of both renovascular and adrenocortical hypertension. For the remaining majority af patients with essential hypertension, renin profiling, used in the context of the vasoconstriction-volume analytical model, exposes the heterogeneity of what was long considered to be a single disorder. In individual patients, renin profiling reveals the participation of either excessive vasoconstriction or excessive volume. It thereby guides simpler, more direct, and more predictable treatments using either anti-renin or anti-volume agents as the first step. Renin profiling allows the physician to pick out those patients in whom it is appropriate to begin therapy with a beta-blocker or with a new anti-renin drug such as captopril (i.e., medium- and high-renin patients). Such therapy has the attractive potential for lowering pressure while improving flow. The renin profile also identifies low-renin patients where overfilling is the presumed pathophysiologic defect. In them a diuretic instead is the best first treatment.

Vasoconstriction-volume analysis as revealed by the renin profile also provides baseline information about the pace, severity, and prognosis of the disease in individual patients, and it sets apart those unusual patients whose hypertension cannot yet be explained. Accumulating evidence supports the concept that an absolute or inappropriate excess of renin-induced vasoconstriction which occurs in high- and medium-renin patients is per se a risk factor predisposing to cardiovascular damage (i.e., heart attack and stroke). Clinical studies show that high- and medium-renin hypertensive disorders exhibit more vascular damage and have a poorer prognosis than do equally hyper-

tensive low-renin patients. In animal models, too, the degree of hypertension is not necessarily related to the degree
of vascular damage. In fact, saline infusions to improve flow
can remit the malignant syndrome even as the pressure rises.
Furthermore, injections of renin will regularly induce cardiovascular damage modified by sodium balance, and stroke-
prone spontaneously hypertensive rats have higher prestroke
plasma renin levels.

There is a pathophysiologic basis for the differences in risk
of cardiovascular damage between low- and high-renin patients.
For equal degrees of hypertension, low-renin patients appear to
be less vasoconstricted: they exhibit greater plasma and extracellular volumes, they are relatively hemodiluted and they
respond best to diuretic therapy. All this implies better tissue
flow and nutrition for a given level of hypertension.

Collectively, the evidence indicates that so-called essential hypertension in fact composes a heterogenous spectrum of
inappropriate vasoconstriction-volume interactions. The participation of vasoconstriction or volume is meaningfully related
to differences in drug responsiveness, clinical course and out-
come.

For medical practice the new knowledge already provides
the basis for more specific physiologic correction enabling
long-term treatment with one drug instead of two for major
subgroups. Research suggested by this hypothetical framework
promises even better diagnosis and more specific treatments as
we near final solutions for more disorders of the hypertensive
spectrum.

REFERENCES

Adlin, E. V., Marks, A. D., and Channick, B. J. (1972). Spiro-
  lactone and hydrochlorothiazide in essential hypertension.
  Blood pressure response and plasma renin activity. Arch.
  Intern. Med. 130, 855-858.
Amery, A., Lijnen, P., Fagard, R., and Reybrouck, T. (1976).
  Plasma renin activity vs. concentration . N. Engl. J. Med.
  285, 1-198c.
Ames, R. P., Borkowski, A. J., Sicinski, A. M., and Laragh,
  J. H. (1965). Prolonged infusions of angiotensin II and
  norepinephrine and blood pressure, electrolyte balance,
  aldosterone and cortisol secretion in normal man and in
  cirrhosis with ascites. J. Clin. Invest. 44, 1171-1186.

Atsmon, A., Blum, I., Steiner, M., Latz, A., and Wijsenbeek, H. (1972). Further studies with propranolol in psychotic patients. Psychopharmacologia 27, 249.

Baer, L., Parra-Carrillo, J. Z., Radichevich, I., and Williams, G. S. (1977). Detection of renovascular hypertension with angiotensin II blockade. Ann. Intern. Med. 86, 257.

von Bahr, C., Collste, P., Frisk-Holmberg, M., Haglund, K., Jorfelt, L., Orme, M., Ostman, J., and Sjoqvist, F. (1976). Plasma levels and effects of metoprolol on blood pressure, adrenergic beta receptor blockade, and plasma renin activity in essential hypertension. Clin. Pharm. Ther. 20, 130.

Berglund, G., Sannerstedt, R., Anderson, O., Wedel, H., Wilhelmsen, L., Hansson, L., Sivertsson, R., and Wikstrant, J. (1978). Coronary heart disease after treatment of hypertension. Lancet 1, 1.

Boerth, R. C. (1976). Effect of propranolol in the treatment of hypertension in children. Pediatr. Res. 10, 328.

Brown, J. J., Davies, D. L., Lever, A. F., Robertson, J. I. S., and Tree, M. (1964). The estimation of renin in human plasma. Biochem. J. 93, 594-600.

Brunner, H. R., Kirshman, J. D., Sealey, J. E., and Laragh, J. H. (1971). Hypertension of renal origin: evidence for two different mechanisms. Science 174, 1344-1346.

Brunner, H. R., Laragh, J. H., Baer, L. Newton, M.A., Goodwin, F. T., Krakoff, L. R., Bard, R. H., and Buehler, F. R. (1972). Essential hypertension: renin and aldosterone, heart attack and stroke. N. Engl. J. Med. 286, 441-449.

Brunner, H. R., Sealy, J. E., and Laragh, J. H. (1973). Renin as a risk factor in essential hypertension: more evidence. Am. J. Med. 55, 295-302.

Brunner, H. R., Gavras, H., and Laragh, J. H. (1973). Angiotensin II blockade in man by sar^1-ala^8-angiotensin II for understanding and treatment of high blood pressure. Lancet 2, 1045.

Brunner, H. R., Gavras, H., Laragh, J. H., and Keenan, R. (1974). Hypertension in man. Exposure of the renin and sodium components using angiotensin II blockade. Circ. Res. 34 & 35 (Suppl. I), I-35-I-45.

Brunner, H. R., Gavras, H., Walker, B., Kershaw, G. R., Turini, G. A., Vukovich, R. A., McKinstry, D. N., and Gavras, I. (1979). Oral angiotensin-converting enzyme inhibitor in long-term treatment of hypertensive patients. Ann. Intern. Med. 90, 19.

Buehler, F. R., Laragh, J. H., Baer, L., Vaughan, E. D. Jr., and Brunner, H. R. (1972). Propranolol inhibition of renin secretion. A specific approach to diagnosis and treatment of renin-dependent hypertensive disease. N. Engl. J. Med. **287**, 1209-1214.

Buehler, F. R., Laragh, J. H., Vaughan, E. D. Jr., Brunner, H. R., Gavras, H., and Baer, L. (1973). The antihypertensive action of propranolol: specific anti-renin responses in high and normal renin forms of essential, renal, renovascular and malignant hypertension. Am. J. Cardiol. **32**, 511-512.

Buehler, E. R., Burkart, F., Lutold, B. E., Kuns, M., Marbet, G., and Pfisterer, M. (1975). Antihypertensive beta blocking action as related to renin and age: a pharmacological tool to identify pathogenetic mechanisms in essential hypertension. Am. J. Cardiol. **36**, 653-669.

Byrom, F. B. (1963). The nature of malignancy in hypertensive disease. Evidence from the retina of the rat. Lancet **1**, 516-520.

Byrom, F. B. (1969). The hypertensive vascular crisis: an experimental study. William Heinemann Medical Books Ltd., London.

Carey, R. M., Douglas, J. G., Schweikert, J. R., and Liddle, G. W. (1972). The syndrome of essential hypertension and suppressed plasma renin activity. Normalization of blood pressure with spironolactone. Arch. Intern. Med. **130**, 849-854.

Case, D. B., Wallace, J. M., Keim, H. J., Weber, M. A., Drayer, J. I. M., White, R. P., Sealey, J. E., and Laragh, J. H. (1976). Estimating renin participation in hypertension. Superiority of converting enzyme inhibitor over saralasin. Am. J. Med. **61**, 790-796.

Case, D. B., Wallace, J. M., Keim, H. J., Sealey, J. E., and Laragh, J. H. (1976). Usefulness and limitations of saralasin, a weak competitive agonist of angiotensin II, for evaluating the renin and sodium factors in hypertensive patients. Am. J. Med. **60**, 825.

Case, D. B., Wallace, J. M., Keim, H. J., Weber, M. A., Sealey, J. E., and Laragh J. H. (1977). Possible role of renin in hypertension as suggested by renin-sodium profiling and inhibition of converting enzyme. N. Engl. J. Med. **296**, 641-646.

Case, D. B., Atlas, S. A., Laragh, J. H., Sealey, J. E., Sullivan, P. A., and McKinstry, D. N. (1978). Clinical experience with blockade of the renin-angiotensin-aldosterone system by an oral converting–enzyme inhibitor (SQ 14,225, Captopril) in hypertensive patients. Prog. in Cardiovasc. Dis. **21,** 195–206.

Castenfors, J., Johnsson, H., and Oro, L. (1973). Effect of alprenolol on blood pressure and plasma renin activity in hypertensive patients. Acta. Med. Scan. **193,** 189–195.

Chiu, P. J. S., and Sommer, E. J. A. (1979). Effect of Na+ restriction on blood pressure responses to β-adrenoreceptor blockade in spontaneously hypertensive rats (SHR). Fed. Proc. **38,** 2372. (Abstract).

Conway, J., Greenwood, D. T., and Middlemiss, D. N. (1978). Central nervous actions of beta-adrenoreceptor antagonists. Clin. Sci. Mol. Med. **54,** 119.

Crane, M. G., and Harris, J. J. (1970). Effect of spironolactone in hypertensive patients. Am. J. Med. Sci. **260,** 311.

Crane, M. G., Harris, J. J., and Johns, V. J. Jr. (1972). Hyporeninemichypertensim. Am. J. Med. **52,** 457–466.

Crofton, J. T., Share, L., Shade, R. E., Lee-Kwon, W. J., Manning, M., and Sawyer, W. H. (1979). The importance of vasopressin in the development and maintenance of DOC-salt hypertension in the rat. Hypertension **1,** 31–38.

Davis, B. A., Crook, J. E., Vestal, R. E., and Oates, J. A. (1979). Prevalence of renovascular hypertension in patients with grade III or IV hypertensive retinopathy. N. Engl. J. Med. **301,** 1273–1276.

Distler, A., Keim, H. J., Philipp, T., Phillippi, A., Walter, U., and Werner, E. (1974). Exchangeable sodium, total-body potassium, plasma volume, and hypotensive effect of various diuretics in patients with essential hypertension and low plasma renin level. Dtsch. Med. Wochschr. **99,** 864.

Douglas, J. G., Hollifield, J. W., and Liddle, G. W. (1974). Treatment of low-renin essential hypertension, comparison of spironolactone and a hydrochlorothiazide-triamterene combination. J. Am. Med. Assoc. **227,** 518–521.

Drayer, J. I. M., Keim, H. J., Weber, M. A., Case, D. B., and Laragh, J. H. (1976). Unexpected pressor responses to propranolol in essential hypertension. Am. J. Med. **60,** 897.

Drayer, J. I. M., Weber, M. A., Sealey, J. E., and Laragh, J. H. (1981). Low and high renin essential hypertension: a comparison of clinical and biochemical characteristics. Am. J. Med. Sci. **281,** 135–142.

Folkow, B. (1971). The haemodynamic consequences of adaptive
    structural changes of the resistance vessels in hypertension.
    Clin. Sci. Mol. Med. 41, 1-12.
Ganong, W. F., and Reid, I. A. (1976). Role of the sympathetic
    nervous system and central alpha and beta receptors in
    regulation of renin secretion. In "Regulation of Blood
    Pressure by the Central Nervous System" (G. Onesti, M.
    Fernandes, and K. E. Kim eds.), pp. 261-273. Grune &
    Stratton, New York.
Garner, A., Ashton, N., Tripathi, R., Kohner, E. M., Bulpitt,
    C. J., and Dollery, C. T. (1975). Pathogenesis of hyper-
    tensive retinopathy. Br. J. Opthalmol. 59, 3-44.
Gavras, H., Brown, J. J., Lever, A. F., Macadam, R. F., and
    Robertson, J. I. S. (1971). Acute renal failure, tubular
    necrosis and myocardial infarction induced in the rabbit by
    intravenous angiotensin II. Lancet 2, 19.
Gavras, H., Brunner, H. R., Vaughan, E. D. Jr., and Laragh, J. H.
    (1973). Angiotensin-sodium interaction in blood pressure
    maintenance of renal hypertensive and normotensive rats.
    Science 180, 1369-1372.
Gavras, H., Brunner, H. R., and Laragh J. H. (1974). Renin and
    aldosterone and the pathogenesis of hypertensive vascular
    damage. Prog. Cardiovasc. Dis. 17, 39-49.
Gavras, H., Brunner, H. R., Laragh, J. H., Sealey, J. E., Gavras,
    I., and Vukovitch, R. A. (1974). An angiotensin converting
    enzyme inhibitor to identify and treat vasoconstrictor and
    volume factors in hypertensive patients. New Engl. J. Med.
    291, 817-821.
Gavras, H., Brunner, H. R., Laragh, J. H., Vaughan, E. D. Jr.,
    Koss, M., Cote, L. J., and Gavras, I. (1975). Malignant
    hypertension resulting from deoxycorticosterone acetate
    and salt excess. Circ. Res. 36, 300-309.
Goldblatt, H. J., Lynch, R. F., Hanzal, R. F., and Somerville,
    W. W. (1934). Studies on experimental hypertension. Pro-
    duction of persistent elevation of systolic blood pressure
    by means of renal ischemia. J. Exp. Med. 59, 347-379.
Goodwin, F. J., Knowlton, A. I., and Laragh, J. H. (1969).
    Absence of renin suppression by deoxycorticosterone
    acetate in rats. Am. J. Physiol. 216, 1476-1480.
Gross, F. (1958). Renin and Hypertensin, physiologische order
    pathologische Wirkstuffe? Klin. Wochenschr. 36, 693-705.
Haber, E., Koerner, T., Page, L. B., and Kliman, B. (1969).
    Application of a radioimmunoassay for angiotensin I to the

physiologic measurements of plasma renin activity in normal human subjects. J. Clin. Endocrinol. Metab. **29**, 1349-1355.

Hansson, L. (1973). Beta-adrenergic blockade in essential hypertension. Acta Med. Scand. Suppl. **550**, 1.

Helgeland, A. (1980). Treatment of mild hypertension; a 5-year controlled drug trial: the Oslo Study. Am. J. Med. **69**, 725-732.

Heptinstall, R. H. (1953). Malignant hypertension: a study of fifty-one cases. J. Pathol. and Bacteriol. **65**, 423-429.

Hollifield, J. W., Sherman, K., Zwagg, R. V., and Shand, D. G. (1976). Prepared mechanisms of propranaolol's antihypertensive effect in essential hypertension. N. Engl. J. Med. **295**, 68-73.

Iaina, A., Goldfarb, D., and Eliahou, H. E. (1979). Unexpected pressor effect of propranolol and angiotensin II in bilaterally nephrectomized rats. Life Sci. **25**, 1153.

Jones, J. V., Dunn, F. G., Fife, R., Lorimer, A. R., and Kellett, R. G. (1978). Benzothiadazine diuretics and death from myocardial infarction in hypertension. Clin. Sci. Mol. Med. **55**, 315S-317S.

Kannel, W. B., Gordon, T., Wolf, P. A., and McNamara, P. (1972). Hemoglobin and the risk of cerebral infarction: the Framingham study. Stroke **3**, 409-520.

Karberg, B. E., Kagedal, B., Tegler, L., Tolagen, K., and Bergman, B. (1976). Controlled treatment of primary hypertension with propranol and spironolactone. A crossover study with special reference to initial plasma renin activity. Am. J. Cardiol. **37**, 642-649.

Keim, H. J., Drayer, J. I. M., Case, D. B., Lopez-Ovejero, J. A., Wallace, J. M., and Laragh, J. H. (1976). A role for renin in rebound hypertension and encephalopathy after infusion of Sar^1-ala^8-angiotensin II. N. Engl. J. Med. **295**, 1175-1177.

Kincaid-Smith, P., Fang, P., and Laver, M. C. (1973). A new look at the treatment of severe hypertension. Clin. Sci. Mol. Med. **45**, 75-87.

Laragh, J. H. (1960). The role of aldosterone in man: evidence for regulation of electrolyte balance and arterial pressure by renal-adrenal system which may be involved in malignant hypertension. J. Am. Med. Assoc. **174**, 293-295.

Laragh, J. H. (1962). Hormones and pathogenesis of congestive heart failure: vasopressin, aldosterone and angiotensin II. Further evidence for renal-adrenal interaction from studies in hypertension and cirrhosis. Circulation **25**, 1015-1023.

Laragh, J. H. (1973). Vasoconstriction-volume analysis for understanding and treating hypertension: the use of renin and aldosterone profiles. Am. J. Med. 55, 261-274.

Laragh, J. H. (1976). Modern system for treating high blood pressure based on renin profiling and vasoconstriction-volume analysis: a primary role for beta blocking drugs such as propranolol. Am. J. Med. 61, 797-810.

Laragh, J. H. (1978a). The renin system in high blood pressure, from disbelief to reality: converting-enzyme blockade for analysis and treatment. Prog. in Cardiovasc. Dis. 21, 159-166.

Laragh, J. H. (1978b). Renin as a predictor of hypertensive complications: discussion. Ann. N.Y. Acad. Sci. 304, 165-177.

Laragh, J. H., and Stoerk, H. C. (1957). A study of the mechanism of secretion of the sodium-retaining hormone (aldosterone). J. Clin. Invest. 36, 383-392.

Laragh, J. H., Ulick, S., Januszewicz, V., Deming, Q. B., Kelly, W. G., and Lieberman, S. (1960). Aldosterone secretion and primary and malignant hypertension. J. Clin. Invest. 39, 1091-1106.

Laragh, J. H., Ulick, S., Januszewicz, V., Kelly, W. G., and Lieberman, S. (1960). Electrolyte metabolism and aldosterone secretion in benign and malignant hypertension. Ann. Intern. Med. 53, 259-272.

Laragh, J. H., Angers, M., Kelly, W. G., and Lieberman, S. (1960). Hypotensive agents and pressor substances. The effect of epinephrine, norepinephrine, angiotensin II and others on the secretory rate of aldosterone in man. J. Am. Med. Assoc. 174, 234-240.

Laragh, J. H., Cannon, P. J., and Ames, R. P. (1963). Aldosterone secretion and various forms of hypertensive vascular disease. Ann. Intern. Med. 59, 117-120.

Laragh, J. H., Sealey, J. E., Ledingham, J. G. G., and Newton, M. A. (1967). Oral contraceptives. Renin, aldosterone and high blood pressure. J. Am. Med. Assoc. 201, 918-922.

Laragh, J. H., Baer, L., Brunner, H. R., Buehler, F. R., Sealey, J. E., and Vaughan, E. D. Jr. (1972). Renin, angiotensin and aldosterone system in pathogenesis and management of hypertensive vascular disease. Am. J. Med. 52, 633-652.

Laragh, J. H., Letcher, R. L., and Pickering, T. G. (1979). Renin profiling for modern diagnosis and treatment of hypertension. J. Am. Med. Assoc. 241, 151-156.

Laragh, J. H., Case, D. B., Atlas, S. A., and Sealey, J. E. (1980). Captopril compared with other anti-renin system agents in hypertensive patients, its use to identify and treat the renin factor. Hypertension 2, 586-593.

Lassen, N. A., and Agnoli, A. (1972). Upper limit of autoregulation of cerebral blood flow on the pathogenesis of hypertensive encephalopathy. Scand. J. Clin. Lab. Invest. 30, 113-116.

Lewis, P. J., and Haeusler, G. (1975). Reduction in sympathetic nervous activity as a mechanism for hypotensive effect of propranolol. Nature (London) 256, 440.

Lydtin, H., and Sommerfeldt, H. (1972). The effect of d-and dl-propranolol on blood pressure and cerebral norepinephrine in rats with DOCA-hypertension. Int. J. Clin. Pharmacol. 64, 328.

MacGregor, G. A., and Dawes, P. M. (1976). Angiotensin II blockade in patients with essential hypertension. Aust. N. Z. J. Med. 6, 53.

Marks, L. S., Maxwell, M. H., and Kaufman, J. J. (1977). Renin, sodium, and vasodepressor response to saralasin in renovascular and essential hypertension. Ann. Int. Med. 87, 176.

Masson, G. M. C., Corcoran, A. C., and Page, I. H. (1951). Experimental production of a syndrome resembling toxemia of pregnancy. J. Lab. Clin. Med. 38, 213.

Masson, G. M. C., Corcoran, A. C., and Page, I. H. (1952). Renal and vascular lesions elicited by "renin" in rats with deoxycorticosterone hypertension. Arch. Pathol. 53, 217-225.

Masson, G. M. C., Corcoran, A. C., Page, I. H., and Del Greco, F. (1953). Angiotensin induction of vascular lesion in deoxycorticosterone treated rats. Proc. Soc. Exp. Biol. Med. 84, 284-287.

Masson, G. M. C., Mikasa, A., and Yasuda, H. (1962). Experimental vascular disease elicited by aldosterone and renin. Endocrinology 71, 505.

Masson, G. M. C., Aoki, K., and Deodhar, S. D. (1966). Course of hypertension during prolonged treatment with heterologous renin. Experientia 22, 531.

Matsunaga, M., Yamamoto, J., Akira, H., Yamori, Y., Ogino, K., and Okamoto, K., (1975). Plasma renin and hypertensive vascular complications: an observation in the stroke-prone spontaneously hypertensive rat. Jpn. Circ. J. 39, 1305-1310.

Maxwell, M. H. (1975). Cooperative study of renovascular
    hypertension: current status. Kidney Int. 8 (Suppl.), 163–
    160.
Menard, J., Bertagna, X., Guyen, P. T., Degoulet, P., and
    Corvol, P. (1976). Rapid identification of patients with
    essential hypertension sensitive to acebutolol (a new
    cardioselective beta-blocker). Am. J. Med. 60, 886–890.
Moehring, J., Petri, M., Szokol, M., Haack, D., and Moehring, B.
    (1976). Effects of saline drinking on malignant course of
    renal hypertension in rats. Am. J. Physiol. 230, 849–857.
Moehring, J., Moehring, B., Petri, M., and Haack, D. (1977).
    Vasopressor role in ADH in the pathogenesis of malignant
    DOC-hypertension. Am. J. Physiol. 232, F260–F269.
Morgan, T., Adam, W. R., Hodgson, M., and Gibberd, R. W. (in
    press). Failure of therapy to improve prognosis in elderly
    males with hypertension. Med. J. Aust.
Mulinos, M. G., Spingarn, C. L., and Lojkin, M. E. (1941). Dia-
    betes insipidus-like condition produced by small doses of
    desoxycorticosterone acetate in dogs. Am. J. Physiol.
    135, 102.
Okamoto, K., Yamori, Y., and Nagaoka, A. (1974). Establish-
    ment of the stroke-prone spontaneously hypertensive rat
    (SHR). Cir. Res. 34 & 35 (Suppl.), I-143 – I-153.
Ondetti, M. A., Williams, N. J., Sabo, E. F., Pluscec, J., Weaver,
    E. R., and Kocy, O. (1971). Angiotensin converting enzyme
    inhibitors from the venom of Bothrops jararaca. Isolation,
    elucidation of structure and synthesis. Biochem. 10, 4033.
Ondetti, M. A., Rubin, B., and Cushman, D. W. (1977). Design of
    specific inhibitors of angiotensin-converting enzyme: new
    class of orally active antihypertensive agents. Science 196,
    441.
Ørjavik, O. S., Aas, M., Fauchald, P., Hovig, T., Oystese, B.,
    Brodwall, E. K., and Flatmark, A. Renin secreting tumors
    with severe hypertension. Acta Med. Scand. 197, 329–336.
Perera, G. N., and Haelig, A. W. (1952). Clinical characteristics
    of hypertension associated with unilateral renal disease.
    Circulation 6, 349.
Pettinger, W. A., and Mitchell, H. C. (1975). Renin release,
    saralasin and the vasodilator-betablocker drug interaction
    in man. N. Engl. J. Med. 292, 1214–1217.
Philipp, T., Cordes, U., and Distler, A. (1977). Sympathetic
    responsiveness and antihypertensive effect of beta-receptor
    blockade in essential hypertension: the effect of atenolol.
    Dtsch. Med. Wochenschr. 102, 569–574.

Pickering, G. (1968). "High Blood Pressure." Churchill, London.

Relman, A. S., and Schwartz, W. B. (1952). Effect of DOCA on electrolyte balance in normal man and its relation to sodium chloride intake. Yale J. Biol. Med. 24, 540.

Robinson, S. K. (1972). Coronary artery disease and antihypertensive drugs. J. Clin. Pharmacol. 12, 123.

Romero, J. C., Holmes, D. R., and Strong, C. G. (1977). The effect of high sodium intake and angiotensin antagonist in rabbits with severe and moderate hypertension induced by constriction of one renal artery. Circ. Res. 40 (Suppl. I), I-17.

Sealey, J. E., and Laragh, J. H. (1975). "Prorenin" in human plasma methodological and physiological implications. Circ. Res. 36 β 37 (Suppl. I), I-10 - I-16.

Sealey, J. E., and Laragh, J. H. (1980). How to do a plasma renin assay. In "Topics in Hypertension" (J. H. Laragh ed.), pp. 224-256. Yorke Medical Publishers, New York.

Sealey, J. E., Buehler, F. R., Laragh, J. H., and Vaughan, E. D. Jr. (1973). The physiology of renin secretion in essential hypertension: estimation of renin secretion rate and renal plasma flow from peripheral and renal vein levels. Am. J. Med. 55, 391-401.

Selye, H., Hall, C. E., and Rowley, E. M. (1943). Malignant hypertension produced by treatment with desoxycorticosterone acetate and sodium chloride. Can. Med. Assoc. J. 49, 88-92.

Seymour, A. A., Davis, J. O., Freeman, R. H., Deforrest, J. M., Rowe, B. P., Stephens, G. A., and Williams, G. M. (1980). Hypertension produced by sodium depletion and unilateral nephrectomy: a new experimental model. Hypertension 2, 125-129.

Skinner, S. L. (1967). Improved assay methods for renin concentration and activity in human plasma: methods using selective denaturation of renin substrate. Circ. Res. 20, 391.

Smith, W. M. (1977). Treatment of mild hypertension: results of a ten year intervention trial. U.S. Public Health Service Hospital Cooperative Study Group. Circ. Res. 40, (Suppl. I) I-98 -I-105.

Sonnenblick, E. H., Cannon, P. J., and Laragh, J. H. (1961). The nature of the action of intravenous aldosterone: evidence for a role of the hormone in urinary dilution. J. Clin. Invest. 40, 903-913.

Spark, R. F., and Melby, J. C. (1971). Hypertension and low plasma renin activity: presumptive evidence for mineralocorticoid excess. Ann. Intern. Med. **75**, 831-836.

Stewart, I. M. G. (1971). Long-term observations on high blood pressure presenting in fit young men. Lancet **1**, 355.

Stewart, I. M. G. (1976). Compared incidence of first myocardial infarction in hypertensive patients under treatment containing propranolol or excluding β-receptor blockade. Clin. Sci. Mol. Med. **51**, 509S-511S.

Strandgaard, S., Olsen, J., Skinhoj, E., and Lassen, N. A. (1973). Autoregulation of brain circulation in severe arterial hypertension. Br. Med. J. **1**, 507-510.

Streeten, D. H. P., Anderson, G. H. Jr., Freiberg, J. M., and Dalakos, T. G. (1975). Use of an angiotensin II antagonist (saralasin) in the recognition of "angiotensinogenic" hypertension. N. Engl. J. Med. **292**, 657.

Stumpe, K. O., Kolloch, R., Vetter, H., Gramann, W., Krueck, F., Ressel, C., Higuchi, M. (1970). Acute and long-term studies of the mechanisms of action of beta-blocking drugs in lowering blood pressure. Am. J. Med. **60**, 853-865.

Tarazi, R. C., and Dustan, H. P. (1972). Beta-adrenergic blockade in hypertension. Am. J. Cardiol. **29**, 633.

The Australian therapeutic trial in mild hypertension. Report by the Management Committee. (1980). Lancet **1**, 1261-1267.

Tigerstedt, R., and Bergman, P. G. (1898). Niere und Kreislauf. Scand. Arch. Physiol. **8**, 223-271.

Ulick, S., Laragh, J. H., and Lieberman, S. (1958). The isolation of a urinary metabolite of aldosterone and its use to measure the rate of secretion of aldosterone by the adrenal cortex of man. Trans. Assoc. Am. Physicians **71**, 225-235.

Vaughan, E. D. Jr., Buehler, F. R., Laragh, J. H., Sealey, J. E., Baer, L., and Bard, R. H. (1973a). Renovascular hypertension: renin measurements to indicate hypersecretion, and contralateral suppression, estimate renal plasma flow and score for surgical curability. Am. J. Med. **55**, 402-414.

Vaughan, E. D. Jr., Laragh, J. H., Gavras, I., Buehler, F. R., Gavras, H., Bruenner, H. R., and Baer, L. (1973b). Volume factor in low and essential hypertension. Treatment with either spironolactone or chlorthalidone. Am. J. Cardiol. **32**, 523.

Vaughan, E. D. Jr., Sos, T. A., Sniderman, K. W., Pickering, T. G., Case, D. B., Sealey, J. E., and Laragh, J. H. (1981). Renal venous secretory patterns before and after percutaneous transluminal angioplasty in patients with renovascular hypertension. In "Frontiers in Hypertension Research" (J. H. Laragh, F. R. Buehler and D. W. Seldin eds.), pp. 173-176. Springer-Verlag, New York.

Veterans Administration Cooperative Study Group on Hypertensive Agents. (1970). Effects of treatment on morbidity in hypertension. II. Results in patients with diastolic blood pressure averaging 90 through 114 mmHg. J. Am. Med. Assoc. 213, 1143.

Weidman, P., Beretta-Piccoli, C., Ziegler, W., Hirsch, D., deChatel, R. D., and Reubi, F. C. (1976). Interrelations between blood pressure, blood volume plasma renin and urinary catecholamines during beta-blockade in essential hypertension. Klin. Wochenschr. 54, 765-773.

Willison, J. R., Thomas, D. J., deBoulay, G. H., Marshall, J., Paul, E. A., Pearson, T. C., Russel, R. W. R., Symon, L., and Wetherly-Mein, G. (1980). Effect of high haematocrit on alertness. Lancet 1, 846-848.

Winternitz, M. C., Mylon, E., and Waters, L. L. et al. (1939-40). Studies on the relation of the kidney to cardiovascular disease. Yale J. Biol. Med. 12, 623.

Young, D. B. (1981). Comparison of a beta-blocker and converting enzyme inhibitor in two types of experimental hypertension. In "Frontiers in Hypertension Research" (J. H. Laragh, F. R. Buehler, and D. W. Seldin, eds.), pp. 436-439. Springer-Verlag, New York.

Young, D. B., and Diepstra, G. R. (1978). Lack of antihypertensive effects of propranolol in experimental angiotensin II hypertension. Physiologist 21, 132.

Zech, P. Y., Labeeuw, M., Pozet, N., Hadj-Aissa, A., Sassard, J., and McAinsh, J. (1977). Response to atenolol in arterial hypertension in relation to renal function, pharmacokinetics and renin activity. Postgrad. Med. J. 53 (Suppl. 3), 134-141.

Hypertensive Mechanisms, with Special Emphasis on NaCl-Related Hypertensions Such as Human Essential Hypertension

Louis Tobian

Hypertension Section, Department of Medicine
University of Minnesota Hospital and School of Medicine
Minneapolis, Minnesota

Human essential hypertension is an enigmatic hypertensive model but newer knowledge is dispelling more and more of the enigma. This type of hypertension has a strong hereditary aspect. The blood presure may be only minimally elevated in the child or teenager but often becomes considerably higher during adulthood. In early human hypertension under 30 years of age, the blood pressure is elevated because of increases in both cardiac output and peripheral vascular resistance. In those over 30, cardiac output reverts to normal while peripheral vascular resistance rises still higher. The increased vascular resistance is partly due to structural narrowing and partly due to active vasconstriction. Pre-hypertensive children (both parents hypertensive) in general usually have slightly low renin levels. Obesity is associated with an increased prevalence of hypertension at all ages. Unlike some animal models of hypertension, human essential hypertension appears to have a distinct relation to sodium chloride (NaCl) in the diet and in the body. From that standpoint, the Dahl salt-sensitive (S) rat is the animal model which most closely resembles human hypertension. This model will develop virtually no hypertension if an increase of body Na balance is prevented (Tobian et al., 1979a). On regular rat chow, the Dahl S rat will

HYPERTENSION: PHYSIOLOGICAL
BASIS AND TREATMENT

95

slowly develop a mild hypertension over many months (Ganguli et al., 1981); while a 4% high NaCl diet will induce severe hypertension often above 200 mmHg (Ganguli et al., 1981). Dahl also developed a salt resistant (R) rat that does not develop any hypertension at all even on 4% or 8% high-NaCl diets.

SODIUM CHLORIDE AND HUMAN HYPERTENSION

Just as the two Dahl strains have differing responses to a high NaCl intake, human beings also appear to have differing reactions to a high NaCl diet. There are several major observations which link NaCl to hypertension:

(a) Drastic reductions of sodium intake will definitely lower the blood pressure of patients with essential hypertension (Kempner, 1944; Murphy, 1950; Watkin et al., 1950).

(b) Diuretic agents which facilitate the renal excretion of sodium, definitely reduce blood pressure in the majority of patients with essential hypertension (Dustan et al., 1959; Wilson and Freis,1959). Concomitant high salt intakes can prevent this lowering of blood pressure (Winer, 1961).

(c) Many populations in remote areas where individuals eat less than 30 mEq of sodium per day have virtually no hypertension at all and, moreover, have virtually no rise of blood pressure with advancing age (Maddocks, 1967; Prior et al., 1968; Truswell et al., 1972; Sinnet and Whyte, 1973; Page et al., 1974; Oliver et al., 1975). These same people also eat a high potassium intake of about 200 mEq/day. Furthermore, these people are not necessarily genetically resistant to hypertension since it is well-documented that they begin to have their share of hypertension whenever they migrate into towns or acculturate to the ways of western civilization. Blood pressure also begins to rise with advancing age, subsequent to the acculturation (Lowenstein, 1961; Cruz-Coke et al., 1964; Maddocks, 1967; Cruz-Coke et al., 1973; Page et al., 1974). Thus, the question naturally arises as to whether these people in remote areas have no hypertension because of their low sodium, high potassium intake, because they are lean, because of their special psychosocial situation, or because of other nutritional deficiencies and debilitating diseases.

There is good evidence that these various other factors are not responsible for the absence of hypertension. First of all, there are a few groups in widely separated areas (three continents) who have good nutrition and who lack debilitating disease, but still have no hypertension, namely, the bushmen of the

Kalahari Desert (Kaminer and Lutz, 1960), the Puka-pukans of
the Cook Islands (Prior et al., 1968), the Easter Islanders (Cruz-
Coke et al., 1964), the Solomon Islanders (Page et al., 1974), and
the Yanomamo Indians (Oliver et al., 1975). Futhermore, the
absence of obesity is apparently not the decisive factor in preventing hypertension, since the Qash'qai nomads of Iran are similarly lean and similarly unacculturated but eat about 175 mEq of
sodium per day and have a prevalence of hypertension similar to
that of Caucasians in the United States.

It is very difficult to measure psychosocial stress in primitive societies. However, one Solomon Island group cooked its
food in sea water and had a sizeable sodium intake, as well as a
10% incidence of hypertension; while another coastal Solomon
Island group, with very similar psychosocial behavior, steamed an
almost identical diet with water from freshwater streams, thereby
having a low sodium intake and a virtual absence of hypertension
(Page et al., 1974). This very important observation suggests
that psychosocial factors are not the decisive element in the
absence of hypertension among people eating the very low salt
intake. When the intake of sodium is below 30 mEq/day, there is
almost no hypertension at all. When the intake of sodium is
between 30 and 60 mEq/day, the incidence of hypertension is
still below 3%, much lower than the 9 to 20% in the United States
(Page et al., 1974).

(d) There is fairly strong evidence that a really high sodium
intake will increase the level of blood pressure. In a recent study
at the University of Indiana, 1200 mEq/day of sodium were fed
to normotensive human volunteer subjects, and they showed a
rise in blood pressure (Murray et al., 1978). The increase became
even greater when the subjects were given 1500 mEq/day.
McDonough and Wilhelmj (1954) fed one normotensive subject
600 mEq/day of sodium and produced a rise of blood pressue.
McQuarrie et al. (1936) studied a diabetic boy who had a great
craving for salt. When he was allowed to eat 700 mEq of NaCl
daily, he became hypertensive; when he was restricted to 85 mEq
of NaCl daily, he remained normotensive (McQuarrie et al.,
1936).

Takahashi et al. (1957) found a high incidence of hypertension and stroke in the Akita prefecture of Japan where people
commonly have an intake of 425 mEq of NaCl daily. When the
intake of salt exceeds 360 mEq daily, the death rate from strokes
definitely increases. When the intake reaches 400 mEq/day, the
death rate from stroke increases even more. Fodor et. al. (1973)
also noted that a very high sodium intake among people in the

coastal villages of Newfoundland was associated with a high
prevalence of hypertension, compared to inland Newfoundlanders
who did not eat as much salt fish and who had a much lower
sodium intake.

Shaper (1972) reported that when the Samburu warrior-
herdsmen were tending their herds and eating 50 mEq of sodium
daily, they had very little hypertension. However, when they
were drafted into the army of Kenya, they began eating an army
ration providing 308 mEq of NaCl daily. This sudden increase in
sodium intake did not bring on a great rise of blood pressure
during the first year. However, beginning with the second year
of high NaCl intake, blood pressure progressively rose during the
second and third year. Numerous studies have shown that human
subjects with renal parenchymal disease have a marked tendency
to a rise in blood pressure when they take in large amounts of
NaCl. This tendency is even more strikingly evident in dialysis
patients (Vertes et al., 1969; Ulvila et al., 1972).

(e) With the sodium intake usually encountered in industri-
alized western societies (100 to 200 mEq of sodium per day),
intrapopulation studies have usually failed to show a strong relationship between individual blood pressure and sodium excretion
in either white or black populations in the United States or
elsewhere. Dawber et al. (1967) found no correlation in the
Framingham population. Langford and Watson (1975) found none
in Mississippi. Miall found a negative correlation in Wales (Miall
and Oldham, 1958). Simpson et al. (1978) found only a slight
correlation in New Zealand.

Most of these studies have been based on a single 24-hr
urine collection. Langford and Watson (1975) showed that there
is wide variation in sodium excretion from day to day, but even
6-day excretions failed to correlate with blood pressure. It is
quite likely that this lack of correlation is related to the fact
that people genetically resistant to hypertension far outnumber
those that are genetically susceptible, by a ratio of 10 to 1 in
most white populations. Thus, the possible connection of sodium
to blood pressure in genetically susceptible people is "drowned
out" and diluted by the lack of a connection in the far more numerous genetically resistant people. This explanation is strongly
supported by recent observations of Langford and Watson. They
originally studied a large group of black high school girls in whom
sodium intake correlated very weakly with blood pressure. Ten
years later, they found out which of these women had become
hypertensive and hence were genetically susceptible to hypertension. They then re-examined the data during high school of just

these subjects susceptible to hypertension. In this special group of 12 genetically susceptible girls there was a very strong correlation of sodium intake with blood pressure (r = .7) (Langford and Watson, 1982). The high school girls who were not genetically predisposed to hypertension had absolutely no correlation of sodium intake with blood pressure. These observations point out very clearly that studies in a general population cannot be used to describe validly correlations that might exist only in those genetically related to hypertension. Gleibermann (1973) also found a significant positive correlation of sodium intake and blood pressure in black communities, a population with an unusually high prevalence of hypertension.

(f) Corroborating animal experiments have also been performed. Lenel et al. (1948) made chickens hypertensive by offering only 1% saline solution for drinking water. Sapirstein et al. (1950) made rats hypertensive by allowing them to drink only a 2% saline solution. In the classic experiment of Meneely and Ball (1958), various diets containing salt in very small or very large amounts and with various intermediate levels were fed to rats over a 9-month period. It was seen that each increment in salt intake brought a concomitant increase in blood pressure. The rats eating the 10% salt in the dry diet developed frank hypertension. With 2 to 5% salt in the diet, borderline or mild hypertension was observed. At the highest levels of blood pressure, obvious nephrosclerosis was encountered. In these early days, it was also clear that the full expression of deoxycorticosterone hypertension in the rat could best be obtained if a high-NaCl intake were given along with the deoxycorticosterone. Conversely, a very low-sodium intake completely prevented a rise in blood pressure after deoxycorticosterone. In the pig and in the dog, also, high-sodium feeding intensifies mineralocorticoid hypertension, while a very low-sodium intake completely prevents it. Morever, a high-sodium intake, by itself, without concomitant mineralocorticoid, will lead to hypertension in the pig and in the monkey. After removal of 70% of renal mass, the dog also can be made hypertensive by high NaCl feeding.

(g) The walls of renal arteries in hypertensive humans contain an abnormally high content of Na (Tobian and Binion, 1952). This is also true for many animal models of hypertension (Tobian, 1960). Even the veins in certain hypertensive animals have an increased Na content.

PATHOGENETIC MECHANISMS
RELATING SODIUM TO HYPERTENSION

On a moderately high–NaCl intake, some human subjects are hypertensive and others are not. As mentioned previously, on a very low-sodium intake (less than 30 mEq/day), all human subjects have normal blood pressures. Dahl et al. (1962) was aware of this situation and created through selective inbreeding two strains of rats which mimic the human situation. When his two strains are both eating a low salt diet, they both have pressure levels within the normal range through young adulthood, thus resembling people living in remote regions and eating a low–Na diet (Dahl et al., 1962). However, when the two strains are challenged with a daily high–NaCl intake, the S strain shows its susceptibility to salt hypertension by gradually becoming severely hypertensive (Dahl et al., 1962). The R strain, on the other hand, shows its great resistance to salt hypertension by having no rise in blood pressure whatsoever. Thus, the two strains again mimic civilized human subjects on a high–salt diet. A good example of this mimicking is seen in the study of Falkner and Onesti, in which normotensive teenagers with normotensive parents were fed 171 mEq of extra NaCl daily and sustained no rise in blood pressure, while normotensive teenagers with one hypertensive parent had a distinct rise in blood pressure on this same diet (Falkner et al., 1981). Studies at the University of Iowa showed similar results, with a 410 mEq Na diet causing forearm vasodilation in normotensive subjects and forearm vasoconstriction in borderline hypertensive subjects.

Thus, a good working hypothesis could be that human beings, like Dahl rats, are either genetically susceptible or resistant to hypertension. The resistant ones do not get hypertension despite the usual lifelong consumption of 200 mEq of NaCl daily. The susceptible ones also do not become hypertensive if their usual lifelong consumption is less than 60 mEq of NaCl daily. If susceptible human beings become hypertensive only when they eat generous amounts of NaCl, we likely have two links in the chain of causation. First, there must occur some initial accumulation of NaCl in the body; secondly, this initial accumulation of body Na must lead to a rise in arterial pressure. We have clinical evidence for this second link in the chain. Subjects with disease of the renal parenchyma tend to retain body Na as they come into sodium balance and, as a result, they often develop hypertension. Patients with an adenoma that puts out too much aldosterone tend to retain sodium and they frequently become hypertensive. When dialysis patients retain sodium, they usually become hypertensive. Onesti et al. (1975) purposefully raised the level of body Na in the course of dialysis treatment and most subjects had a rise in pressure. When body Na was brought down to a normal level, blood pressure returned to normal. In these studies, when an increase in body Na raised blood pressure, in 60% of cases, the rise in pressure was entirely due to an increase in peripheral resistance with no hint of even a transient increase of cardiac output. In 20% of cases, the rise in blood pressure was entirely due to a rise in cardiac output with no hint of an increase in peripheral resistance to subserve a whole body autoregulation. In the last 20% of cases, the rise in blood pressure resulted from both an increase in peripheral resistance and an increase in cardiac output. The diseased kidneys had been removed in many of these dialysis patients, so kidneys were not necessary in the Na-induced blood pressure rises. The study also indicates that "volume" hypertension in these patients is actually "vasoconstriction" hypertension, at least in 80% of these subjects, and this pressor response is not an invariable one. In six normotensive subjects with end-stage renal disease, raising body Na did not increase blood pressure at all. This probably explains why they remained normotensive as their kidneys were gradually being destroyed. Thus, Na accumulation in the body does not invariably raise blood pressure; in order to get Na-induced hypertension, this pressor response to Na accumulation must be present.

Now, regarding the first link in the chain of causal events, it would seem logical to assume that in order to get Na-induced hypertension, there would have to be some initial accumulation of sodium in the body, which would in turn bring about a rise in blood pressure. Susceptible human subjects or susceptible S rats could be different from resistant men and rats, because they initially retain more sodium when exposed to a salt challenge. However, human hypertensives do not have an increased content of sodium in the arterial walls. Similarly, Dahl S rats do not have excessive body Na levels either on high- or low-sodium diets. Moreover, when these men or rats with established hypertension are challenged with a Na load, they excrete the Na very expeditiously, actually a bit faster than the normotensive controls. Thus, they appear to have no problem in handling a sodium challenge. However, there is a consideration that perhaps makes these superficial conclusions invalid. The hypertensive kidney is perfused at an elevated pressure, while the normotensive kidney is perfused at a normal pressure. Selkurt (1951) clearly showed that high perfusion pressure in the renal artery greatly facili-

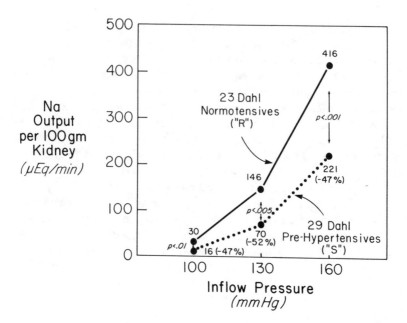

Figure 1. Sodium excretion of isolated kidneys from S and R rats at varying inflow pressures. The distance between the large black dot (the mean value) and the tip of the arrowhead represents the standard error of the mean.

tates the urinary excretion of sodium and urine volume. Thus, the intrinsic ability of kidneys to excrete sodium cannot be validly compared when one kidney is perfused at high pressure and the other at normal pressure. To get at this perplexing question Tobian et al. (1978) used isolated, blood-perfused kidneys from the two contrasting strains of Dahl rats, which are good models for human hypertension and normotension. Both strains had been eating a low-sodium diet and hence had blood pressures within the normal range.

Figure 1 gives the urinary Na excretion per 100 g of isolated kidney per minute at various inflow pressures. The top line shows the mean values of isolated kidneys from 23 hypertension-resistant R rats. As expected, the Na output markedly increases with each increment of inflow pressure. The bottom line gives the average values of isolated kidneys from 29 hypertension-prone S rats. These kidneys also show the pressure natriuresis phenomenon with more Na excreted for each increment of inflow pressure. However, it is obvious that there is a striking differ-

ence between S and R kidneys. For instance, at a normotensive
inflow pressure of 130 mmHg, the R kidneys excreted a mean of
146 µEq of Na per minute per 100 g of kidney, whereas at the
same pressure the S kidneys averaged only 70 µEq. Thus, at 130
mmHg inflow pressure, the S kidneys from hypertension-prone
rats excreted 52% less Na than comparable R kidneys. This
difference was significant (p < 0.005). At 160 mmHg infusion
pressure, we see the same phenomenon — the R kidneys averaging
416 µEq of Na excretion, whereas the S kidneys averaged only
221. This is a 47% reduction of Na excretion in S kidneys compared to R kidneys (p < 0.001). At 100 mmHg inflow pressure,
we see the same pattern, with R kidneys excreting 20 µEq/min,
while the S kidneys are excreting only 16 µEq/min. Hence, at
100 mmHg inflow pressure, the S kidneys excreted 47% less Na
than the R kidneys (p < 0.01). When compared on an equal pressure basis, the S kidneys seem to have a very pronounced natriuretic handicap at all three inflow pressures. However, raising
the inflow pressure can completely overcome this natriuretic
handicap. For instance, the S kidneys perfused at 160 mmHg
excrete about 50% more Na per minute than the normotensive R
kidneys perfused at a normal 130 mmHg pressure.

At a normal inflow pressure, the renal blood flow and glomerular filtration rates of the S and R rats were not significantly
different. These studies indicate that the isolated kidneys from
S rats excrete only half as much sodium as kidneys from R rats
when the two contrasting strains are compared at equal levels of
inflow pressure. Thus, the hypertension-prone S strain appears
to have a resetting of the pressure natriuresis curve, in that a
higher inflow pressure is required to achieve a given Na excretion. This occurs even though the S kidney had no pathological
lesions. In either strain on a very low-sodium intake, there would
be virtually no tendency for Na retention and hence little stimulus
for a rise in blood pressure beyond the normal range. However,
when the S rats begin a high-sodium intake, the resetting of the
pressure natriuresis curve could then conceivably become an
important factor. If the relative rates of natriuresis of isolated
S and R kidneys occurred in the intact rat during the high-sodium
intake, the S rat would tend to retain more sodium than the R
rat and would tend to come into sodium balance with an elevated
body Na and extracellular volume. Such high body Na and extracellular volumes frequently bring on a rise in blood pressure, as
is commonly seen in the hypertensions of renal parenchymal
disease, mineralocorticoid excess, and in dialysis patients. If the
arterial pressure did rise into the hypertensive range, the S kidney

would then increase its rate of Na excretion through the mechanism of a pressure natriuresis, and its natriuretic handicap would be overcome. With the raised arterial pressure, the kidney could then excrete sodium rapidly enough to permit attainment of sodium balance at a normal extracellular volume. The natriuretic handicap would then seem to disappear and renal excretory function would appear to be normal, and total body Na would be normal. Assuming a possible resetting of the pressure natriuresis curve for the intact S kidney in vivo, the S rat would tend to become hypertensive when on a high-sodium intake. The hypertension would thus produce natriuresis that would bring to normal its body Na content.

The experiments of Iwai et al. (1977) provide some evidence that there may indeed be an in vivo difference in pressure natriuresis curves between S and R rats. When these two contrasting strains were fed a high-NaCl intake, the feeding of chlorothiazide significantly increased urinary Na excretion in S rats but had no effect on Na excretion in R rats. Moreover, when chlorothiazide was discontinued after some weeks, the Na excretion significantly dropped in S rats while rising slightly in R rats. The findings could be interpreted as indicating that the R kidneys have a pressure natriuresis curve favoring very rapid natriuresis at relatively low inflow pressures, such that adding chlorothiazide will not make an already rapid natriuretic capacity even more rapid. However, if there existed an in vivo resetting of the pressure natriuresis curve in S rats favoring a slower rate of natriuresis, then adding chlorothiazide might have the effect of shifting the natriuresis curve of the S kidney to the left, thereby making Na excretion more rapid. The contrasting effect of chlorothiazide on Na excretion in these two strains could be accounted for by this mechanism.

This formulation could conceivably account for much of the exquisite sensitivity to NaCl-induced hypertension in the Dahl S rat. It is pertinent to wonder whether the kidneys of patients with essential hypertension might also have a resetting of the pressure natriuresis curve in favor of hypertension. Future studies wil be needed to answer this question.

The hypothesis that an intrinsic shift in the pressure natriuresis curve can lead to rat hypertension, or even human hypertension, certainly fits well with the action of diuretic drugs in reducing hypertensive pressure levels. Many diuretic agents are extremely effective in man in reducing high blood pressure. The same is true for the Dahl S rat. This would make physiological sense. If a diuretic agent were given to an S rat, it would facili-

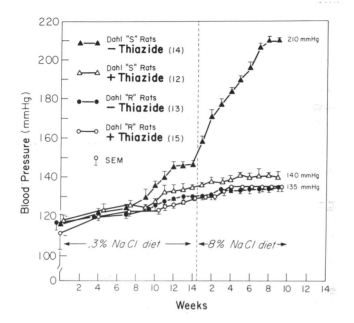

Figure 2. Blood pressure of Dahl S and R rats as influenced by high and low levels of sodium in the diet, and by treatment with a thiazide diuretic agent.

tate natriuresis and would tend to overcome the intrinsic defect in natriuresis which these rats have. Recent studies with isolated, blood-perfused S kidneys indicate that thiazides permit these kidneys to excrete 69% more sodium per minute when they are perfused at a normotensive inflow pressure (Tobian et al., 1982a). In the presence of daily diuretic therapy the body Na level comes into balance at a slightly lower than normal level. This should remove the previous Na stimulus leading to elevated pressure levels, and blood pressure should begin to drift toward normal levels. In the presence of a diuretic, an elevated pressure level would no longer be needed in S rats to facilitate natriuresis. Such a mechanism could explain the powerful antihypertensive action of diuretic agents.

In order to investigate some of these possibilities, Tobian et al. (1979a) did a study in Dahl rats using a thiazide diuretic, methyclothiazide (Figure 2) to test another facet of the sodium hypothesis. Half of the rats in each strain were given the thiazide diuretic. All rats were given low-sodium diet for the first 14 weeks. If the rat tends to retain sodium and become hypertensive on an 8% NaCl diet because of the shift in his pressure natri-

uresis curve, then a thiazide diuretic should be able to prevent
the Na retention, and the rise in blood pressure should be averted.
Where one sees the vertical line on Figure 2, all the rats began
eating the 8% NaCl diet while half of them remained on thiazide.
The group of S rats not on thiazide showed a prompt rise of blood
pressure with a steady climb to 210 mmHg by the eighth week of
the 8% NaCl diet, whereas the R rats not on thiazide had no
rise in pressure whatsoever, as expected. Moreover, the R rats
on thiazide had the same pressure as the R rats not on thiazide.
Of great interest was the observation that the S rats on thiazide
had virtually the same blood pressure as the R rats; the thiazide
had almost completely prevented any Na-induced rise in blood
pressure in the S rats, the pressure only going up 5 mmHg above
that of the R rats after 9 weeks of an 8% NaCl diet. Seemingly,
if body Na retention is prevented by thiazide, there will be no
rise in blood pressure in S rats despite the very high 8% NaCl
intake and the intrinsic limitation of natriuresis.

In an attempt to explain the reduced sodium excretion of S
kidneys, Tobian et al. (1979a) searched for sodium-retaining
hormonal agents in S rats. When the blood of S rats is perfused
through normal "neutral" isolated kidneys at 125 mmHg, the
neutral kidney excretes only half as much sodium per minute,
compared to similar perfusion of the neutral kidney with the
blood of R rats (p <0.05). Thus, S rats appear to have either a
circulating antinatriuretic hormone, or they lack a natriuretic
hormone which partially accounts for the tendency to reduced
sodium excretion of S kidneys (Tobian et al., 1979a).

In other experiments, a circulating, blood-borne vasoconstrictor effect has been found in S rats that are developing
hypertension after 4 weeks on a high salt diet (Tobian et al.,
1979b). However, this is not seen in the R rats which have remained normotensive while eating the same high salt diet.

The renal papilla in S rats even in the pre-hypertensive state
has a 60% smaller prostaglandin E_2 concentration than the R
rats (Tobian et al., 1982b). On high NaCl diets, the prostglandin
E_2 in S papillae is always half that in R papillae (Tobian et al.,
1982b), and the renal papillary interstitial cell granules are also
reduced in the S papillae (Pitcock et al., 1982). This reduction in
E_2 prostaglandin will enhance Na reabsorption in the ascending
loop of Henle, collecting tubule, and collecting duct (Stokes
et al., 1973; Stokes, 1979; Wilson et al., 1981), thereby encourag-
ing Na retention and hypertension. The reduction in renal papillary plasma flow in S rats on any NaCl diet (Ganguli, et al., 1976)
also likely promotes Na retention with its concomitant rise in

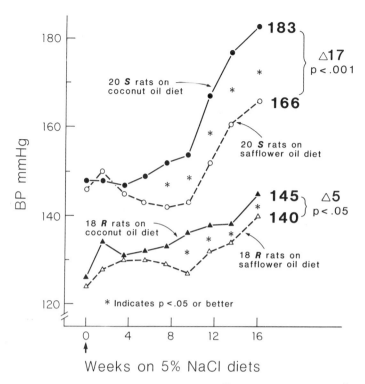

Figure 3. Blood pressure on Dahl S and R rats as influenced by 5% NaCl diets containing coconut oil (1.5% linoleic acid diet) or safflower oil (16% linoleic acid diet).

blood pressure. As shown in Figure 3, feeding a diet with 16% linoleic acid triples the E_2 prostaglandin in S papillae and also prevents about half of the rise in blood pressure after salt feeding (Tobian et al., 1982b). Diets of high linoleic acid content have also been reported to lower the blood pressure of hypertensive human subjects (Comberg et al., 1978; Stern et al., 1980; Iacono et al., 1982; Judd et al., 1982).

There are increasing lines of evidence pointing to a role of the central nervous system in NaCl-induced hypertension. Takeshita and Mark (1978) found an increased vascular resistance in Dahl S rats that had become hypertensive after one month of a high NaCl intake. When they cut the sympathetic nerves to the hindquarters of these hypertensive rats, half of the increase in vascular resistance was thereby abolished, thus pointing to a sympathetic nerve participation in the NaCl-induced increase in vascular resistance. When the peripheral sympathetic nervous in newborn Dahl S rats were destroyed (Takeshita et al., 1979), the feeding of a high-NaCl diet did not bring about a rise in blood pressure, again pointing to the participation of the sympathetic nervous system in this form of hypertension. Ikeda and Tobian (1978) induced pressor responses in normotensive Dahl S and R rats by the introduction of a hypertonic NaCl solution and the introduction of angiotensin II into the lateral ventricle of the brain. With both of these central nervous system pressor stimuli present, the rise in blood pressure was twice as great in the S rats as in the R rats, even though the baseline blood pressure was similarly normotensive for both groups. These results certainly indicate enhanced central nervous system pressor responses in the S rats, which could partially contribute to their heightened susceptibility to NaCl-induced hypertension. Ikeda and Tobian (Goto et al., 1981) introduced 6-hydroxydopamine into the lateral brain ventricle of Dahl S rats in order to cause destruction of many central adrenergic neurons. These S rats were subsequently placed on a high-NaCl diet and had only half the rise in blood pressure that the pair-fed, sham-operated control S rats experienced. Again, this would indicate the participation of central adrenergic neurons in NaCl-induced hypertension. Futhermore, either bilateral lesions of the hypothalamic paraventricular nuclei or a lesion at the anteroventral end of the third brain ventricle ("AV3V lesion") can prevent 50 to 60% of the expected NaCl-induced rise in blood pressure in S rats (Goto et al., 1981; Goto et al., 1982). Bilateral lesions of the hypothalamic suprachiasmatic nuclei, on the other hand, actually enhance the hypertension of S rats (Tobian et al., 1982c). These observations collectively point to an important role of the central nervous system in NaCl-induced hypertension.

Healthy individuals have been shown to maintain sodium balance on a sodium intake of less than 87 mEq/24 hr while sweating 9 liters/day (Conn, 1949). A variety of primitive societies in widely divergent habitats (tropical jungle, desert, arctic, etc.) subsist for generations on sodium intakes less than 43 mEq/day and show no evidence of sodium deprivation (Dahl, 1958; Page et al., 1974). Evidence from studies of ancient coproliths and tooth markings of prehistoric man indicate that he was very likely eating this same type of low-sodium, high-potassium diet. If such a diet had been biologically harmful, the world would not now be teeming with human beings. According to a report by American Academy of Pediatrics Committee on Nutrition, requirements for sodium in growing infants and children are estimated at less than 9 mEq/day (1974). It thus appears that the habitual intake of sodium in adults in the United States often exceeds body need by 10-fold or more.

SODIUM RESTRICTION AS A COMPONENT
OF THE TREATMENT OF HYPERTENSION

As mentioned above, a sodium intake under 10 mEq/day will very often reduce high blood pressure. But such a diet is very difficult to follow for most people. However, six separate studies provide evidence that modest sodium restriction alone (60 to 90 mEq/day) can be effective in producing a significant reduction of blood pressure (Parijs et al., 1973; Carney et al., 1975; Magnani et al., 1976; Morgan et al., 1978; Morgan 1981; MacGregor et al., 1982). This same modest sodium restriction enhances the anti-hypertensive effect of diuretic agents (Fallis and Ford, 1961).

Winer (1961) showed that large intakes of sodium could vitiate the antihypertensive effect of thiazide diuretics. Langford et al. (1977) have shown that diuretics increase sodium appetite and intake in man. Advice to restrict salt-intake would tend to counteract this. Owens and Brackett (1978) have shown that propranolol alone has a far more potent antihypertensive action when combined with modest sodium restriction; whereas it has a very weak antihypertensive action when combined with a high sodium intake. In the usual patient with hypertension associated with renal parenchymal disease, modest sodium restriction is especially important in antihypertensive therapy; it reduces sodium intake to match the reduced nephron population (Hunt, 1977).

Dahl et al. (1958) reported that obese hypertensives were especially benefited by a low-sodium diet in terms of blood pressure reduction. Mineralocorticoid hypertension in man is also helped by sodium restriction (Dustan et al., 1973), and Joosens found a strong correlation of sodium intake and blood pressure in the elderly. This is not unexpected since total body Na correlates quite closely with the level of blood pressure in older individuals (Baretta-Piccoli et al., 1982). Both these findings likely relate to the physiological reduction of renal function with advancing age. This reduction of renal function in the elderly thus explains why their hypertension is especially benefited by relatively modest restriction of dietary sodium intake (Morgan et al., 1978; Morgan, 1981).

It is quite likely sodium intake and calcium intake can both influence blood pressure concomitantly. It is also possible that their actions are interrelated. There is even some solid evidence that a low-sodium diet diminishes bone loss and reduces calcium excretion in elderly women (Goulding, 1981).

POTASSIUM EFFECTS ON NaCl - INDUCED HYPERTENSION

A recent study explores the protective effect of potassium salts in NaCl-induced hypertension (Ganguli et al., 1981). In this study we used males from both strains of Dahl rats (Dahl et al., 1962). On a 24-week low-salt diet with 0.3% NaCl, the Dahl R strain remained normotensive with a mean blood pressure of 131 mmHg and the Dahl S rats became mildly hypertensive with an average blood pressure of 169 mmHg. However, when the two strains of rats were on a moderately high NaCl diet with 4% NaCl for 24 weeks, the R rats continued to be normotensive with a mean blood pressure of 132 mmHg, whereas the S rats became severely hypertensive with a mean blood pressure of 208 mmHg. This 4% salt diet would be roughly equivalent to 20 g of salt/day for an adult man eating 500 g of dry food per day. Both the low- and the high-NaCl diets were tested in three variations: (1) without any potassium supplement; (2) with a 2.6% KCl supplement; (3) with a 3.8% potassium citrate supplement. The two potassium salts were added in equimolar amounts. After 24 weeks of feeding with these six different diets, the plasma flow to the renal papilla was measured with our version of the Lillienfield ^{131}I-labelled albumin method (Lillienfield et al., 1961; Ganguli and Tobian, 1974; Ganguli et al., 1976).

Figure 4 shows the results. The 14 Dahl R rats on a low (0.3%) NaCl diet had a mean plasma flow to the renal papilla of 25.7 ml/min/100 g. When 13 similar R rats ate the high-NaCl (4%) diet, the papillary plasma flow increased to 26.1 ml/min/100 g, a slight and insignificant difference. In 11 Dahl S rats eating the low-NaCl diet, the average papillary flow was 16.4 ml/min/100 g (Figure 4), 36% lower than the papillary flow in rats. Our previous work has shown that S rats, even on a low-salt diet, have significantly lower papillary flows than R rats, and we suggested that this characteristic could contribute to the greater susceptibility of the S rats to NaCl-induced hypertension (Ganguli et al., 1976). Ten other S rats were fed on the 4% high-NaCl diet and developed a mean papillary flow of 13.5 ml/min/100 g. Thus, although the high-NaCl diet slightly increased the

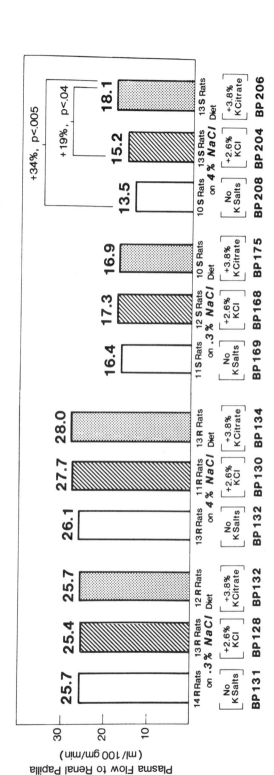

Figure 4. Renal papillary plasma flow and mean blood pressure (BP, mmHg) in Dahl R and S rats fed for 24 weeks on either low (0.3%) NaCl diets or high (4%) NaCl containing various potassium supplements: □, no added potassium salts; ▨, 2.6% potassium chloride supplement; ▨, 3.8% potassium citrate supplement. n = Number of rats.

papillary flow of the R rats, it definitely decreased the papillary
flow of the S rats by 18%, a significant reduction (p < 0.05). The
S rats consuming the high-NaCl diet had developed severe hypertension with a mean blood pressure of 208 mmHg, which in turn
produced nephrosclerosis with resulting nephron loss. We con-
templated that this nephron loss was responsible for the 18%
reduction of papillary flow on the high- NaCl diet. This reduction
of flow made a difference in the ratio of papillary flows for the
S rats and the R rats. Thus, on low- NaCl diet, the papillary flow
in S rats was 64% of that in R rats, whereas on a high-NaCl diet
the papillary flow in the S rats was only 52% of that of the R
rats.

When both of the diets were supplemented with 2.6% KCl,
the added KCl did not change the general pattern. The high-
NaCl diet increased papillary flow by 9.1% in the R rats and, as
before, it decreased papillary flow by 12% in the S rats. The S
rats on the high NaCl-2.6% KCl diet had a severely elevated
blood pressure of 204 mmHg, and the nephrosclerosis resulting
from this probably accounted for the 12% fall in papillary flow.
Apparently, KCl did not significantly prevent the hypertension or
the nephrosclerosis; again, the ratio of papillary flow in S rats to
that in R rats was 68% on a low-NaCl diet and only 55% on the
high NaCl-2.6% KCl diet.

When both of the diets were supplemented with 3.8% potassium citrate, the R rats again showed an 8.9% increase in papillary flow on the high-NaCl diet, an increase similar to that occurred on the diets with KCl. However, in the S rats, the high-
NaCl diet containing potassium citrate actually caused an increase in papillary flow by 6.5%, instead of a decrease that
was seen when the high-NaCl diet contained either KCl or no
added potassium. These S rats on the high-NaCl diet with
potassium citrate also became severly hypertensive with a blood
pressure of 206 mmHg, which was similar to the levels in S rats
on KCl or no added potassium. Nevertheless, the papillary flow
actually increased, indicating a protection against nephron loss.

Figure 4 shows the papillary flows for the R and S rats on all
six diets. The flows were in general very slightly higher in high-
NaCl diets [7% higher including all rats (p <0.05)], but potassium
citrate added to either low or high-NaCl diets did not cause any
significant increase in papillary flow.

The potassium citrate diet did not produce a rise in papillary
flow in S rats on a low (0.3%) NaCl diet. The results indicate
that potassium citrate does not ordinarily bring about a rise in
papillary flow. The S rats developed a similarly severe hyper-

tension on all three high NaCl diets. Nevertheless, papillary
flows in these rats decreased when placed on a high–NaCl diet
containing either KCl or no added potassium, whereas the flow
increased when potassium citrate was added to the high–NaCl
diet. Thus the papillary flow in the high (4%) NaCl-potassium
citrate group was 34% higher than that of the S rats on the high
(4%) NaCl diet without any added potassium. This difference
was quite significant (p <0.005). The papillary flow of the high
(4%) NaCl-potassium citrate group was 19% higher than that of
the high (4%) NaCl-KCl group (p <0.04). These differences
occurred even though the blood pressure of the rats receiving
potassium citrate was at a similar severely hypertensive level.

The most likely explanation for the higher papillary flows in
high–salt S rats fed with potassium citrate is that the potassium
citrate somehow protects against nephron loss from nephrosclerosis during severe NaCl-induced hypertension. Moreover,
feeding with KCl at an equimolar level does not provide the
same measure of protection. The reasons for this difference in
protection are obscure. However, ancient man for 3 million
years consumed a diet very high in potassium content, and this
high potassium content was combined with organic anions or
phosphate anions whereas the chloride anion was present only to
a negligible extent. Thus, substances like potassium citrate were
probably consumed in large quantities in this prehistoric human
cuisine, and it is conceivable that nephrosclerosis was somehow
retarded by this ancient ancestral diet.

In another study, potassium was shown to protect against
renal tubular lesions in NaCl fed hypertensive Dahl S rats. Focal
dilation and distortion of renal tubules are very prominent early
renal lesions in NaCl-induced hypertension of Dahl S rats, and it
has been demonstrated that extra dietary K provides significant
protection against such lesions. In one experiment the S rats (20
per group) were given 4 different Purina diets for 24 weeks: 4%
NaCl (BP 171); 4% NaCl-3.8% K citrate (BP 174); 4% NaCl-2.6%
KCl (BP 173); 0.3% NaCl (BP 158). Tubular lesions per unit area
of kidney were graded in a rigorously "blind" microscopic study
of 2 entire sections for each kidney, providing a tubular dilation
(TD) score (100, severest lesions; 0, normal). In renal cortex, the
TD score averaged 41 for rats consuming a 4% NaCl diet. However, when either 3.8% K citrate or 2.6% KCl (equimolar) were
added to the 4% NaCl diet, the TD scores dropped to 20 and
22, respectively, corresponding to a 50% reduction in lesions
(p <0.001), comparable to the TD score of 24 seen in S rats on the
0.3% NaCl diet. In renal outer medulla, an average TD score of

79 was obtained on the 4% NaCl diet verus scores of 54 and 58
when 3.8% K citrate or 2.6% KCl were added to the 4% NaCl
diet, a 30% reduction in lesions (p <0.001), making them comparable to the TD score of 53 found in S rats on 0.3% NaCl diet.
In renal papilla, TD score averaged 49 on the 4% NaCl diet verus
28 when either 3.8% K citrate or 2.6% KCl were added to the 4%
NaCl diet, a 43% reduction in lesions (p <0.001), making them
similar to the TD score of 26 seen with the 0.3% NaCl diet. Even
the glomerular lesions score was reduced by 20% after adding K
citrate or KCl to the 4% NaCl diet (29 versus 24 and 23, p <0.01),
bringing the score down to the level of 24 seen in S rats on the
0.3% NaCl diet. Since potassium did not lower blood pressure at
all, the strong protective effect of K citrate and KCl could not
be ascribed to a decrease in blood pressure. As discussed before,
the natural diet of all primitive mammals, including man, is
believed to be very high in potassium; such primitive high-K
diets appear to retard these renal lesions.

This protective effect of potassium may have at least one
possible important implication in man. When blacks become
hypertensive, they suffer an inordinate amount of renal damage
for a given degree of hypertension; frequently they developed
renal failure because of nephrosclerosis. It is also very well
known that blacks consume, on the average, approximately 40%
less potassium than whites in several different locales. It is
intriguing to speculate that this low-K diet in blacks could be
partly responsible for their heightened amount of nephrosclerosis
for a given level of hypertension.

HUMORAL FACTORS

It is interesting to bring together the bits of evidence pointing to the presence of abnormal humoral factors in salt-induced
hypertension. In the Dahl S rat, there is evidence for circulating
humoral agents which retard natriuresis in an isolated "neutral"
kidney (Tobian et al., 1979a). There is also evidence for a circulating vasoconstrictor agent in the blood of hypertensive, salt-
fed Dahl S rats (Tobian et al., 1979b). Further evidence shows
that the S rats have reduced levels of two types of humoral
agents: the ouabain-sensitive agents which retard Na-efflux in
lymphocytes and the furosemide-sensitive humoral agents which
retard Na-efflux in lymphocytes. This work was recently presented at the American Society of Nephrology meeting in De-
cember, 1982.

Furthermore, there are even more recent findings demonstrating that plasma factors in hypertensive salt-fed S rats can confer mild hypertension and a 40% increase in pressor sensitivity (to i.v. norepinephrine and angiotensin II) onto normotensive recipient Dahl S rats. Daily i.v. injections of these plasma factors into the recipient S rat can bring about the aforementioned changes which are statistically significant.

Taken together, these items constitute solid evidence that circulating humoral factors do exist in the plasma of S rats; it is likely they may play a key role in the mechanisms of NaCl-induced hypertension.

OVERVIEW

In genetically susceptible human beings as well as in genetically susceptible Dahl S rats, the eating of diets moderately high in NaCl will bring on increased arteriolar narrowing (active and passive) and development of hypertension. The first link in the chain is the tendency to sodium accumulation in the body, largely caused by the generous amounts of NaCl in the diet and the reduced ability of the kidney to excrete it rapidly. The arteriolar narrowing gradually takes place as the generous NaCl intake continues. The regulatory systems are then re-set to achieve a higer average level of arterial pressure. Increased arteriolar narrowing is usually the main change, but the cardiac output also tends to be slightly high early in the hypertension and even the veins show decreased compliance. This re-setting of the blood pressure level appears to be an integrated response and is only partially understood. However, it is very likely that control centers in the brain, in the sympathetic nervous system, in the kidney, and in the renal juxtaglomerular cells are all re-set in an integrated fashion to achieve this higher level of arterial pressure. Other components of this response may include the above mentioned circulating humoral agents and signal-receiving receptors which control the total body NaCl. Thus, it is likely that this re-setting represents an intergrated process, in which the sympathetics, renin, other circulating humoral agents as well as sodium regulators all play an integral part simultaneously. The future unraveling of this complex system which leads to hypertension will undoubtedly permit better prevention and better therapy for this life-shortening condition.

REFERENCES

American Academy of Pediatrics Committee on Nutrition
(1974). Salt intake and eating patterns of infants and
children in relation to blood pressure. Pediatrics 53,
115.

Beretta-Piccoli, C., Davies, D. L., Boddy, K. et al. (1982).
Relation of arterial pressure with body sodium, body potas-
sium and plasma potassium in essential hypertension. Clin.
Sci. 63, 257.

Carney, S., Morgan, T., Wilson, M., et al. (1975). Sodium
restriction and thiazide diuretics in the treatment of
hypertension. Med. J. Aust. 1, 803.

Comberg, H. U., Heyden, S., Hames, C. G., Vergroesen, A. J.,
and Fleischman, A. I. (1978). Hypertensive effect of dietary
prostaglandin precursor in hypertensive man. Prostaglandins
15, 193.

Conn, J. W., (1949). Mechanism of acclimatization to heat.
Adv. Intern. Med. 3, 373.

Cruz-Coke, R., Etcheverry, R., and Nagel, R. (1964). Influence
of migration on blood pressure of Easter Islanders. Lancet
1, 697.

Cruz-Coke, R., Donoso, H., and Barrera, R. (1973). Genetic
ecology of hypertension. Clin. Sci. Mol. Med. 45 (Suppl. 1),
55.

Dahl, L. K. (1958). Salt intake and salt need. N. Engl. J. Med.
258, 1152.

Dahl, L. K., Silver, L., and Christie, R. W. (1958) The role of
salt in the fall of blood pressure accompanying reduction in
obesity. N. Engl. J. Med. 258, 1186.

Dahl, L. K., Heine, M., and Tassinari, L. (1962). Effects of
chronic salt ingestion. Evidence that genetic factors play
an important role in susceptibility to experimental hypertension. J. Exp. Med. 115, 1173.

Dawber, T. R., Kannel, W. B., Kagan, A., Donabedian, R. K.,
McNamara, P. M., and Pearson, G., (1967). Environmental
factors in hypertension. In "The Epidemiology of Hypertension" (J. Stamler, R. Stamler, and T. Pullman eds.),
pp. 255. Grune and Stratton, New York.

Dustan, H. P., Cumming, G. R., Corcoran, A. C., and Page,
I. H. (1959). A mechanism of chlorothiazide enhanced
effectiveness of antihypertensive ganlioplegic drugs.
Circulation 19, 360.

Dustan, H. P., Bravo, E. L., and Tarazi, R. C., (1973). Volume-
    dependent essential and steroid hypertension. Am J.
    Cardiol. 31, 606.
Falkner, B., Onesti, G., and Hayes, P. (1981). The role of sodium
    in essential hypertension in genetically hypertensive
    adolescents. In "Hypertension in the Young and the Old" (G.
    Onesti and K. E. Kim eds.), pp. 29. Grune and Stratton,
    New York.
Fallis, N., and Ford, R. V. (1961). Electrolyte excretion and
    hypotensive response. J. Am. Med. Assoc. 176, 581.
Fodor, J. G., Abbott, E. C., and Rusted, I. E. (1973). An
    epidemiologic study of hypertension in Newfoundland. Can.
    Med. Assoc. J. 108, 1365.
Ganguli, M., and Tobian, L., (1974). Does the Kidney auto-
    regulate papillary plasma flow in chronic "post-salt"
    hypertension? Am. J. Phys. 226, 330.
Ganguli, M., Tobian, L., and Dahl, L. K. (1976). Low renal
    papillary plasma flow in both Dahl and Kyoto rats with
    spontaneous hypertension. Circ. Res. 39, 337.
Ganguli, M., Tobian, L., Iwai, J., and Johnson, M. A. (1981).
    Potassium citrate feeding protects against nephron loss in
    severe sodium chloride hypertension in rats. Clin Sci. 61,
    73.
Gleibermann, L., (1973). Blood pressure and dietary salt in
    human populations. Ecol. Food Nutri. 2, 143.
Goto, A., Ikeda, T., Tobian, L., Iwai, J., and Johnson, M. A.
    (1981). Brain lesions in the paraventricular nuclei and
    catecholaminergic neurons minimize salt hypertension in
    Dahl salt-sensitive rats. Clin. Sci. 61, 53.
Goto, A., Ganguli, M., Tobian, L., Johnson, M. A., and Iwai, J.
    (1982). Effect of an anteroventral third ventricle lesion on
    NaCl hypertension in Dahl salt-sensitive rats. Am. J.
    Physiol. 243, H614.
Goulding, A. (1981). Fasting urinary sodium/creatinine in rela-
    tion to calcium/creatinine and hydroxyproline/creatinine
    in a general population of women. N. Z. Med. J. 93, 284.
Hunt, J. (1977). Management and treatment of essential
    hypertension. In "Hypertension" (J. Genest, ed.), pp. 1068.
    McGraw-Hill, New York.
Iacono, J. M., Judd, J. T., Marshall, M. W., Canary, J. J.,
    Dougherty, R. M., Mackin, J. F., and Weinland, B. T. (1982).
    The role of dietary essential fatty acids and prostaglandins

in reducing blood pressure. In "Progress in Lipid Research; Essential Fatty Acids and Prostaglandins, Vol. 20" (R. T. Holman, ed.), pp. 349. Pergamom Press, New York.

Ikeda, T., Tobian, L., Iwai, J., and Goossens, P. (1978). Central nervous system pressor responses in rats susceptible and resistant to sodium chloride hypertension. Clin. Sci. Mol. Med. 55, 255S.

Iwai, J., Ohanian, E., and Dahl, L. K. (1977). Influence of thiazide on salt hypertension. Circ. Res. 40 (Suppl. 1), 131.

Judd, J. T., Marshall, M. W., and Canary, J. (1982). Effects of diets varying in fat and P/S ratio on blood pressure and blood lipids in adult men. In "Progress in Lipid Research; Essential Fatty Acids and Prostaglandins Vol. 20" (R. T. Holman, ed.), pp. 571. Pergamon Press, New York.

Kaminer, B., and Lutz, W. P. W. (1960). Blood pressure in Bushmen of the Kalahari Desert. Circulation 22, 289.

Kempner, W. (1944). Treatment of kidney disease and hypertensive vascular disease with rice diet. N. C. Med. J. 5, 125.

Langford, H. G., and Watson, R. L. (1975). Electrolytes and hypertension. In "Epidemiology and Control of Hypertension" (O. Paul, ed.), pp. 119. Stratton Intercontinental Medical Book Corp., New York.

Langford, H. G., and Watson, R. L. (1982). Close correlation between blood pressure and sodium excretion in hypertensives -to be. Circulation 66 (Suppl. II), 105.

Langford, H. G., Watson, R. L., and Thomas, J. G. (1977). Salt intake and treatment of hypertension. Am. Heart J. 93, 531.

Lenel, R., Katz, L. N., and Rodbard, S. (1948). Arterial hypertension in the chicken. Am. J. Physiol. 152, 557.

Lilienfield, L. S., Maganzini, H. G., and Bauer, M. H. (1961). Blood flow in the renal medulla. Circ. Res. 9, 614.

Lowenstein, F. W. (1961). Blood pressure in relation to age and sex in the tropics and subtropics. Lancet 1, 389.

MacGregor, G. A., Markandu, N. D., Best, F. E., et al. (1982). Double-blind randomised crossover trial of moderate sodium restriction in essential hypertension. Lancet 1, 351.

Maddocks, I. (1967). Blood pressure in Melanesians. Med. J. Aust. 1, 1123.

Magnani, B., Ambrosioni, E., Agosta, R., and Racco, F. (1976). Comparison of the effects of pharmacological theraphy and a low-sodium diet on mild hypertension. Clin. Sci. Mol. Med. 51, 625S.

McDonough, J., and Wilhelmj, C. M. (1954). The effect of
    excessive salt intake on human blood pressure. Am. J. Dig.
    Dis. 21, 180.

McQuarrie, I., Thompson, W. H., and Anderson, J. A. (1936).
    Effects of excessive ingestion of sodium and potassium salts
    on carbohydrate metabolism and blood pressure in diabetic
    children. J. Nutr. 11, 77.

Meneely, G. R., and Ball, C. O. T. (1958). Experimental epi-
    demiology of chronic toxicity and the protective effect
    of potassium chloride. Am. J. Med. 25, 713.

Miall, W. E., and Oldham, P. D. (1958). Factors influencing
    arterial blood pressure in the general population. Clin. Sci.
    17, 409. Morgan, T. O., Myers, J. B. (1981). Hypertension
    treated by sodium restriction. Med. J. Aust. 2, 396.

Morgan, T., Adam, W., Gillies, A. et al. (1978). Hypertension
    treated by salt restriction. Lancet 1, 227.

Murphy, R. F. J. (1950). The effect of "rice diet" on plasma
    volume and exracellular fluid space in hypertensive subjects.
    J. Clin. Invest. 29, 912.

Murray, R. H., Luft, F. C., Block, R., and Weyman, A. E. (1978).
    Blood pressure responses to extremes of sodium intake in
    normal man. Proc. Soc. Exp. Biol. Med. 159, 432.

Oliver, W. J., Cohen, E. L., and Neel, J. V. (1975). Blood
    pressure, sodium intake and sodium related hormones in the
    Yanomamo Indians, a "no-salt" culture. Circulation 52, 146.

Onesti, G., Kim, K. E., Greco, J. A., Del Guercio, E. T.,
    Fernandes, M., and Swartz, C. Blood pressure relation in
    end-stage renal disease and anephric man. Circ. Res. 36
    (Suppl. I), 37.

Owens, C. J., and Brackett, N. C. Jr. (1978). The role of sodium
    intake in the anti-hypertensive effect of propranolol. South.
    Med. J. 71, 43.

Page, L. B., Danion, A., and Moellering, R. C. Jr. (1974). Ante-
    cedents of cardiovascular disease in six Solomon Islands
    societies. Circulaton 49, 1132.

Parijs, J., Joosens, J. V., Linden, L. V., Verstreken, G., and
    Amery, A. K. P. C. (1973). Moderate sodium restriction
    and diuretics in the treatment of hypertension. Am. Heart
    J. 85, 22.

Pitcock, J. A., Brown, P. S., Righstel, W. A., Brooks, B., and
    Muirhead, E. E. (1982). Renomedullary interstitial cells of
    Dahl S and R rats differ morphologically and functionally.
    Circulation 66 (Suppl. II), 164.

Prior, I. A. M., Evans, J. G., Harvey, H. P. B., Davidson, F., and
    Lindsey, M. (1968). Sodium intake and blood pressure in two
    Polynesian populations. N. Engl. J. Med. 279, 515.
Sapirstein, L. A., Brandt, W. L., and Drury, D. R. (1950).
    Production of hypertension in the rat by substituting
    hypertonic sodium chloride solutions for drinking water.
    Proc. Soc. Exp. Biol. Med. 73, 82.
Selkurt, E. (1951). Effect of pulse pressure and mean arterial
    presure modification on renal hemodynamics and electrolyte
    and water excretion. Circulation 4, 541.
Shaper, A. G. (1972). Cardiovascular disease in the tropics. III.
    Blood pressure and hypertension. Br. Med. J. 3, 805.
Simpson, F. O., Waal-Manning, H. J., Bolli, P., Phelan, E. L., and
    Spears, G. F. (1978). Relationship of blood pressure to
    sodium excretion in a population survey. Clin. Sci. Mol.
    Med. 55 (Suppl. 4), 373S.
Sinnet, P. F., and Whyte, H. M. (1973). Epidemiological studies
    in a total highland population, Tukisenta, New Guinea.
    Cardiovascular disease and relevant clinical, electrocar-
    diographic, radiological and biochemical finds. J. Chronic
    Dis. 26, 265.
Stern, B., Heyden, S., Miller, D., Latham, G., Klimas, A., and
    Pilkington, K. (1980). Intervention study in high school
    students with elevated blood pressure: dietary experiments
    with polyunsaturated fatty acids. Nutr. Metab. 24, 137.
Stokes, J. B. (1979). Effect of prostaglandin E_2 on chloride
    transport across the rabbit thick ascending limb of Henle.
    Selective inhibitions of the medullary portion. J. Clin.
    Invest. 64, 495.
Stokes, J. B., Tisher, C. C., Kokko, J. P. (1973). Structural-
    functional heterogeneity along the rabbit collecting tubule.
    Kidney Int. 14, 585.
Takahashi, E., Sasaki, N. Takeda, J., and Ito, H. (1957). The
    geographic distribution of cerebral hemorrhage and
    hypertension in Japan. Hum. Biol. 29, 139.
Takeshita, A., and Mark, A. L. (1978). Neurogenic contribution
    to hindquarters vasoconstriction during high sodium intake
    in Dahl strain of genetically hypertensive rats. Circ. Res.
    43 (Suppl. I), 1.
Takeshita, A., Mark, A. L., and Brody, M. J. (1979). Prevention
    of salt-induced hypertension in Dahl strain by 6-hydroxy-
    dopamine. Am. J. Physiol. 236, H48.

Tobian, L. (1960). Interrelationship of electrolytes, juxtaglomerular cells and hypertension. Physiol. Rev. 40, 2.

Tobian, L., and Binion, T. (1952). Tissue cations and water in
arterial hypertension. Circulation 5, 754.

Tobian, L., Lange, J., Azar, S., Iwai, J., Koop, D., Coffee, K.,
and Johnson, M. A. (1978). Reduction of natriuretic
capacity and renin release in isolated, blood-perfused
kidneys of Dahl hypertension-prone rats. Circ. Res. 43,
I-92.

Tobian, L., Lange, J., Iwai, J., Hiller, K., Johnson, M. A., and
Goossens, P. (1979a). Prevention with thiazide of NaCl-
induced hypertension in Dahl "S" rats. Hypertension 1, 316.

Tobian, L., Pumper, M., Johnson, S., and Iwai, J. (1979b). A
Circulating humoral pressor agent in Dahl "S" rats with
NaCl hypertension. Clin. Sci. 57, 345S.

Tobian, L., Johnson, M. A., Ganguli, M., Lange, J., Kartheiser,
K., and Iwai, J. (1982a). Effect of a high linoleic diet and
thiazide on NaCl-induced hypertension. Clin. Sci. in press.

Tobian, L., Ganguli, M., Johnson, M. A., and Iwai, J. (1982b).
Influence of renal prostaglandins and dietary linoleate on
hypertension in Dahl S rats. Hypertension 4 (Suppl. II), 149.

Tobian, L., Ganguli, M., Goto, A., Ikeda, T., Johnson, M. A., and
Iwai, J. (1982c). The influence of renal prostaglandins,
central nervous system and NaCl on hypertension of Dahl S
rats. Clin. Exp. Pharm. Physiol. 9, 341.

Truswell, A. S., Kennelly, B. M., Hansen, J. D. L., and Lee, R. B.
(1972). Blood pressure of Kung bushmen in Northern
Botswana. Am. Heart J. 84, 5.

Ulvila, J. M., Kennedy, J. A., Lamberg, J. D., and Scribner, B. H.
(1972). Blood pressure in chronic renal failure: effect of
sodium intake and furosemide. J. Am. Med. Assoc. 220,
233.

Vertes, V., Cangiano, J. L., Berman, L. B., Gould A. (1969).
Hypertension in endstage renal disease. N. Engl. J. Med.
280, 978.

Watkin, D. M., Froeb, H. F., Hatch, F. T., and Gutman, A. B.
(1950). Effects of diet in essential hypertension II. Results
with unmodified Kempner rice diet in fifty hospitalized
patients. Am. J. Med. 9, 441.

Wilson, I. M., and Freis, E. D. (1959). Relationship between
plasma and extracellular fluid volume depletion and the
antihypertensive effect of chlorothiazide. Circulation 20,
1028.

Wilson, D. R., Honrath, U., and Sonnenberg, H. (1981). The role of prostaglandins in the response of medullary collecting duct (MCD) reabsorption to isotonic volume expansion (VE) (abstract). Eighth Intl. Cong. of Nephrology, Athens, pp. 175.

Winer, B. H. (1961). The antihypertensive actions of benzothiadiazines. Circulation 23, 211.

Diuretics in Hypertension: Whence and Whither

Gregory M. Shutske and Richard C. Allen

Chemical Research Department
Hoechst–Roussel Pharmaceuticals Inc.
Somerville, New Jersey

L. INTRODUCTION

For over twenty years diuretics have been the foundation of therapy in essential benign hypertension (EBH), due primarily to the proven ability of these relatively safe agents to control blood pressure in 40-70% of all patients with mild to moderate forms of this disease (Schwartz, 1977; Finnerty, 1979). Scientific and medical foundations, no matter how firm, are subject to "shaking or settling", as new knowledge and new shaping forces emerge. In this chapter we will examine the use of diuretics in EBH from the viewpoint of this knowledge and these forces. In the course of this we will reflect on current and future research needs in this area, as well as the future of diuretics in the treatment of EBH.

II. CURRENT USE PATTERNS AND TRENDS

It has been clear for a number of years that reduction of blood pressure in moderate to severe hypertensives has a profound effect on morbidity and mortality due to cardiovascular events with the exception of myocardial infarction (CHD) and sudden death (VA Cooperative Study Group on Antihypertensive Agents,

HYPERTENSION: PHYSIOLOGICAL
BASIS AND TREATMENT

123

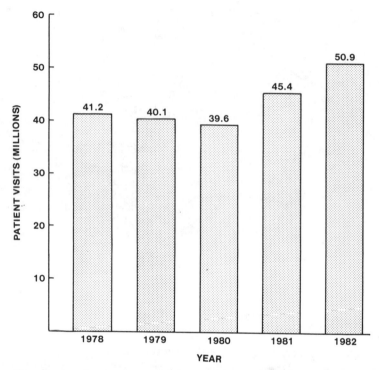

Figure 1. Patient visits for essential benign hypertension.

1967, 1970; Joint National Committee on the Detection, Evaluation and Treatment of High Blood Pressure, 1977; Freis, 1979a).
More recently, the results of the Hypertension Detection Follow-
up Program (HDFP) have suggested a benefit of treatment for individuals with diastolic blood pressure as low as 90 mmHg (Hypertension Detection Follow-up Program Cooperative Group, I and
II, 1979). Following these studies the Joint National Committee
recommended that such individuals be treated, either by dietary/
lifestyle intervention, or by pharmacologic means (The Joint
National Committee on Detection, Evaluation and Treatment of
High Blood Pressure, 1980; Krishan and Moser, 1980). The impact
of these latter studies/recommendations on the treatment of
hypertension in private practice has been to produce a compound
annual growth of 13% in the patient visits (diagnoses) over the
period 1980–82 (Figure 1).
      The effect of these events on the use of diuretics has, on
the surface, been as expected. The recommendations of the

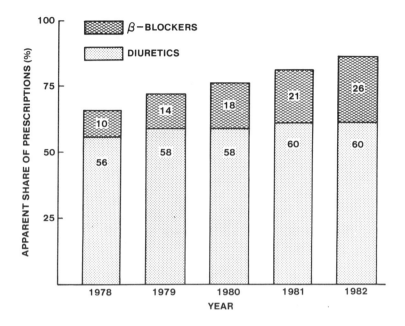

Figure 2. Treatment of essential benign hypertension in private practice.

Joint Committee involved a reaffirmation of the stepped-care approach (Finnerty, 1978), with diuretics as the first-step drug of choice in a majority of cases. Predictably, the number of diuretic prescriptions for treatment of hypertension rose by almost 19% in 1981 and by another 12% in 1982, after having been rather stable for several years.

In view of this, it could be somewhat surprising that the overall "apparent diuretic share" of the total prescriptions written for hypertension has remained almost stable (Figure 2). This appears, however, to be accounted for by the dramatically increasing use of beta-blockers either as first-step therapy, or as additive therapy. At least one authority in the U.S. has recommended that a beta-blocker be used in place of diuretics as the first-step drug of choice as in Europe (Laragh, 1976). Further, the increased promotional activity surrounding the introduction (and competition among) new beta-blockers in the last few years may have served to partially obscure the recommendations of the Joint National Committee for many general practitioners.

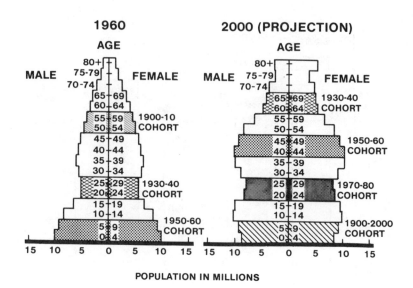

Figure 3. Age structure of U.S. population. (From Nature, 1982, with permission.)

What then does the future hold for the use of diuretics in hypertension? Contrary to some predictions, it would appear that the use of diuretics in the treatment of hypertension will continue to grow; the rate of growth is, however, less predictable. It does not appear that diuretics will lose their overall status as the first-step drug of choice, although it can be expected that other drugs, such as beta-blockers, will make significant inroads.

There are a number of factors which point to these conclusions. First, is the expanding nature of the patient population. It has been estimated (Remington, 1981) that fewer than one-half the hypertensives in U.S. communities are detected, treated and controlled. Looking further into the future, it is clear that the absolute magnitude of the potential patient population will increase as America ages (Figure 3). Acting on this expanding patient population will be a further increasing pressure to treat "mild hypertensives". A continuation publication of the HDFP studies has recently revealed specific mortality data on the 7,825 participants with diastolic blood pressures in the 90–104 mmHg range. Five-year mortality data on patients given stepped care was 20.3% lower than the control group. More significantly, a sub-group, which had no evidence of end-organ damage and were not receiving antihypertensive medication when they entered the study, showed a 28.6% mortality differential (Hypertension Detection and Follow-up Program Cooperative Group, 1982).

A number of factors point also to the continued dominance of diuretics as the first-step drug of choice alone or in combination. Two recent publications (VA Cooperative Study Group on Antihypertensive Agents, I and II, 1982) have strongly reaffirmed the recommendation of the Joint Committee that diuretics be the first-step drug of choice. Hydrochlorothiazide (HCTZ) was compared directly with propranolol in a double blind study involving 683 men. In the long term phase of the trial involving 394 of the total group, HCTZ was clearly superior to propranolol. During the 12 months of long-term treatment, hydrochlorothiazide was more effective than propranolol in controlling blood pressure (mean BP reductions of -17.5/-13.1 mm vs. -8.3/-11.3 mm). After treatment with HCTZ, a greater percentage of patients achieved the goal diastolic BP of less than 90 mmHg (65.5% compared with 52.8% taking propranolol). Also during treatment, fewer patients receiving hydrochlorothiazide required termination as compared with those receiving propranolol; comparative dosage requirements were lower, additional titration during long-term treatment was required less often, and BP remained lower with HCTZ after withdrawal of the active drugs.

The results of the VA Cooperative Group study substantiate earlier findings concerning renin profiles of the population as a whole and the aggregate responsiveness of hypertensives to mono-therapy with beta-blockers or diuretics. Thus, low renin patients (diuretic responsive) constitute 30% of the whole, while high renin patients (beta-blocker responsive) make up 15% (Laragh, 1976). Further, up to 50% of mild to moderate hypertensives are responsive to beta-blockers alone (Buehler et al., 1972; Buehler et al., 1973; Buehler et al., 1975; Hansson, 1976; Lorimer et al., 1976), while diuretics have been reported to control blood pressure in up to 70% of such patients (Schwartz, 1977; Finnerty, 1979). It would appear then that use of diuretics as first-step treatment is most logical in terms of both potential therapeutic success and minimized exposure of patients to unnecessary drugs. In certain patient populations, such as blacks, first-step use of diuretics appears strongly indicated irrespective of the renin profile of such individuals (Holland et al., 1979; VA Cooperative Study Group on Antihypertensive Agents, I, 1982).

In addition to efficacy, factors such as cost and the salt-retaining tendency of many other antihypertensives and the issues of patient-perceived side effects and compliance point to the

continuing dominance of diuretics in the step-one treatment of
hypertension (Finnerty, 1979). Diuretic therapy alone is effective
to some extent in most patients, and it enhances the efficacy of
many other agents, especially when their hypotensive effect
becomes limited by reactive salt and water retention. Further,
patient compliance with diuretics is generally excellent as their
side effects are generally benign from a perception standpoint.
It would thus appear most rational to begin treatment with diuretics and add other medications as necessary rather than vice
versa.

Despite the foregoing generally optimistic outlook for diuretics in the treatment of hypertension, there are "storm warnings"
on the horizon. With the broader and often longer term treatment
of hypertensives predicated by the 1980 Joint National Committee recommendations, there is increasing concern about the
ultimate implications of biochemical aberrations induced by
diuretics. It has been emphasized that simple reduction in elevated blood pressure may lead to little or no gain in reduction of
cardiovascular events if the patient is low risk by virtue of other
factors (Kannel, 1981). For low risk individuals, it may be necessary to treat 20-30 without benefit for one such person to benefit
(Figure 4) (Alderman, 1981). Given the biochemical abnormalities
($\uparrow$ lipoproteins, $\uparrow$ uric acid, $\downarrow$ potassium, $\uparrow$ blood glucose, etc.)
which diuretics frequently induce, decrease in the risk factor
associated with high blood pressure may be offset by an increase
in other risk factors (Ames and Hill, 1981).

No definitive studies exist on the broad scale effect on longevity of diuretic-induced biochemical changes. Two recent
studies, however, suggest a possible unfavorable response to
diuretic therapy in certain, but not all hypertensive subjects. In
an Australian study (Morgan et al., 1981a) designed to compare
the effectiveness of various forms of treatment in elderly patients, a thiazide-treated group (diastolic BP 95-109mm) showed
significantly higher mortality due to myocardial infarct and
sudden death. In a similar study involving 12,866 high-risk men
aged 35 to 57 years, participants with abnormal EKGs and receiving relatively high doses of diuretics had a 66% higher mortality
rate than expected (MRFIT Research Group, 1982). While the
unfavorable response has in neither case been attributed to diuretic-induced biochemical changes, these factors have not been
conclusively ruled out. Such findings are nonetheless cause for
some concern in view of the significant number of mild hypertensives with EKG abnormalities (~20%), elevated cholesterol
levels (~33%), elevated uric acid (~30%), and other risk elements

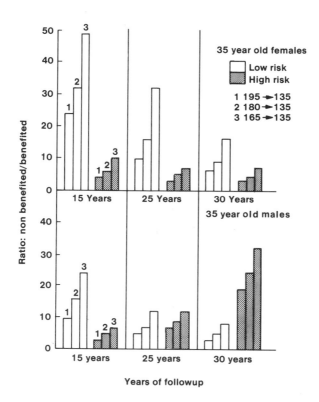

Figure 4. Relative benefit of various degrees of blood pressure reduction for three periods of follow-up and at two levels of associated risk for 35-year-old males and females. (From Alderman, 1981, with permission.)

which may be aggravated by diuretic therapy (Messerli et al., 1980; Kannel, 1981).

On the brighter side, recent years have brought a clearer basic understanding of the mechanism(s) by which diuretics lower blood pressure and the mechanisms and implications of the biochemical changes they induce. Much of the remainder of this chapter will be devoted to summarizing the current state of the art relating to these topics. Certainly it can be expected that application of this knowledge in clinical practice will lead to better patient selection for diuretic treatment, more effective use of combination therapy, and a clearer picture of the significance of diuretic-induced biochemical alterations.

III. MECHANISM OF ACTION—CURRENT CONCEPTS AND FUTURE OPPORTUNITIES

Although diuretics control blood pressure in 40-70% of all patients with mild to moderate EBH and are increasingly prescribed for this condition (see Sections I and II), the mechanism by which they exert their antihypertensive effect is still not clear. What is clear, however, is that diuretics are most effective in low-renin, volume-expanded, sodium-dependent types of EBH, and that the patient population treated most effectively by diuretics alone is roughly the same population with this type of hypertension (Laragh, 1978). Although a direct vasodilator effect of some diuretics has been postulated, the evidence is compelling that diuretics as a class exert their effect as a result of alterations in salt balance and extracellular fluid (ECF) volume. Current theories of how alterations in salt balance and ECF volume are related to the antihypertensive effect of diuretics encompass the concepts of vascular autoregulation, neurogenic and hormonal regulation of kidney and vascular function, and the concept of a circulating sodium transport inhibitor. As these theories have developed, they have led not only to an increased understanding of the mechanism by which diuretics manifest their antihypertensive effects, but also to opportunities for an increasingly rational approach to diuretic therapy.

A. Relationships Between Sodium, Kidney Function, and Diuretics

1. ROLE OF ELEVATED BODY SODIUM. The evidence regarding the role of elevated body sodium and an expanded ECF volume in the pathogenesis of essential hypertension has recently been reviewed (Freis, 1979b; Haddy, 1980; Morgan et al., 1980; Mendlowitz, 1982). In summary, body sodium may be elevated by increased intake or decreased excretion; in certain individuals these factors can lead to increased blood pressure.

Epidemiological and anthropological studies have shown that the incidence of hypertension varies between different populations and can be related to salt intake or 24 hour urinary sodium excretion (Prior et al., 1968, and references contained in Morgan et al., 1980). The validity of such studies has been criticized (Pickering, 1981), and it is indeed more difficult to show such correlations within population groups (Beevers et al., 1980; Tuomilehto et al., 1980; Simpson et al., 1982) because of the difficulties in selecting a suitable population for such studies and in finding a valid measure of dietary sodium (Watt and Foy, 1982).

The variability in such studies may well be accounted for by genetic factors that come into play. Many individuals are clearly able to excrete large salt loads (250 mmol/24 h and more) without becoming hypertensive (Ljungman et al., 1981). On the other hand, individuals with demonstrated hypertension have been shown to have higher 24 hour urinary sodium excretion than nor-motensives (Doyle et al., 1976), and hypertensive patients can be divided into salt-sensitive and nonsalt-sensitive groups based on their blood pressure response to a salt load (Kawasaki et al., 1978).

The finding that there is a subset of salt-sensitive hyperten-sive people is reminiscent of findings in rats (Tobian et al., 1977) that a genetically transmitted defect in the kidney's ability to excrete sodium is responsible for the hypertension in sensitive strains. The kidney, as the principle organ involved in maintain-ing electrolyte and fluid balance, has an implied role in salt-dependent hypertension, but studies that have tried to single out a genetic defect in the sodium-handling ability of the human kidney in salt-sensitive hypertension have been inconclusive (Luft et al., 1982). A recent study, however, has shown that essen-tial hypertension can be corrected by a renal transplant from a normotensive donor (Curtis et al., 1983). Even though the evi-dence is circumstantial, the effectiveness of low-salt diets or diuretic therapy in treating some types of hypertensive patients points to impaired kidney function.

2. REDUCING BODY SODIUM: LOW-SALT DIET AND DIURETICS. It has been known for some time that a low-salt diet is an effective form of therapy for some types of hyperten-sion (Kempner, 1948; Murphy, 1950), an observation that contin-ues to be confirmed in the current literature (Costa et al., 1981; Freis, 1981; Kawasaki et al., 1981; Langford, 1981; Parfrey et al., 1981). The fall in blood pressure seen with these diets paral-lels that seen with diuretics, both in the time course of the effect (Morgan et al., 1978) and in the magnitude of the decrease in ECF volume (Tarazi et al., 1970; Dustan et al., 1974). On the other hand, the antihypertensive effect of a diuretic may be overpowered by excessive dietary sodium (Langford, 1981; Ram et al., 1981). Such evidence suggests, in a circumstantial way, that diuretics are effective in sodium-dependent, volume-

expanded hypertension because they bring about the same kind of changes as low-salt diets, namely, decreased body sodium and reduced ECF volume.

B. Diuretics as Vasodilators?

A direct vasodilator component has been proposed to account for the antihypertensive effect of diuretics, but most of the evidence does not support this hypothesis. One can find relatively recent references suggesting a direct vasodilator action of thiazide diuretics (Nickerson and Ruedy, 1975), but newer papers (Shah et al., 1978; Freis, 1981) argue convincingly against such a direct action, citing that acute administration of the thiazide diuretics is associated with a fall in cardiac output and accompanying hemodynamic effects that are opposite to those brought about by acute administration of a bona fide vasodilator such as diazoxide. Also relevant to the argument against a direct vasodilator action is the fact that an antihypertensive effect is common to several classes of diuretics, including mercurials and loop diuretics as well as the thiazides (Dustan et al., 1974). Furthermore, patients with chronic renal failure, who are unable to respond to thiazide diuretics, show no long term antihypertensive effects with these drugs (Bennett et al., 1977).

Careful measurement shows that total peripheral resistance may actually be increased in the early stages of diuretic therapy in response to the decrease in cardiac output brought about by the above mentioned (Section III.A.2) reduction in ECF volume (Shah et al., 1978). In patients who respond to diuretics, vascular resistance is reduced, but only as part of a long-term pattern of hemodynamic adjustments subsequent to the immediate reduction in plasma ECF volume (Conway and Lauwers, 1960; Lund-Johansen, 1970; Shah et al., 1978). The results of a recent study with hydrochlorothiazide are shown in Figure 5 (van Brummelen et al., 1979). Although there is some disagreement as to whether the reduction in vascular resistance is due to decreased ECF volume or decreased cardiac output, tissue autoregulatory responses may play a role.

C. Autoregulation

Autoregulation is defined as the capability of tissues to control their own blood flows despite changes in the arterial pressure (Guyton et al., 1981). In terms of the increased peripheral resistance seen in volume expanded hypertensive states, this

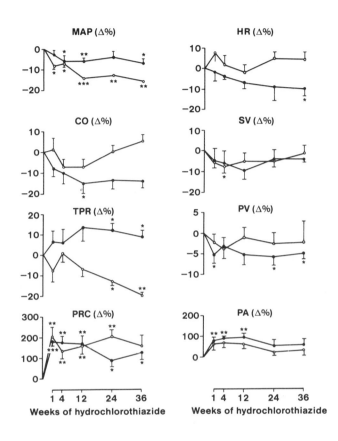

Figure 5. Effect of hydrochlorothiazide on mean arterial pressure (MAP), heart rate (HR), cardiac output (CO), stroke volume (SV), total peripheral resistance (TPR), plasma volume (PV), plasma renin concentration (PRC) and plasma aldosterone (PA) after 1, 4, 12, 24 and 36 weeks of treatment in responders of (○----○) and non-responders (●----●) to diuretic therapy. Values shown are the percentage changes (Δ%, mean ± 1 sem) from placebo values. The significances of differences from placebo values are indicated: *P < 0.05; **P < 0.01; ***P < 0.001. (From van Brummelen et al., 1979, with permission.)

concept comes into play as follows (Ledingham and Cohen, 1963): an expanded ECF volume leads to an increased blood volume and subsequent increased circulatory filling pressure and venous return to the heart, resulting in increased cardiac output (CO)

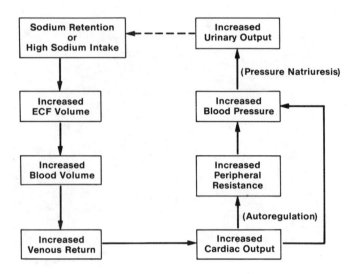

Figure 6. Relationship between the disturbance of sodium metabolism and blood pressure in essential hypertension. (The dotted line indicates a negative feedback.)

(Figure 6). The vascular beds sense this increased CO as an increase in flow; the result is an increase in vascular resistance (Granger and Guyton, 1969) which has as its result the return of local blood flows in the tissues to normal levels—hence autoregulation. The increased vascular resistance and CO combine to raise arterial pressure and also renal perfusion pressure.

In the presence of a normally functioning kidney, the increased renal perfusion pressure results in increased excretion of sodium and water (Selkurt, 1951) (pressure natriuresis), decreasing ECF volume and reversing the processes of Figure 6. In the face of an impaired ability on the part of the kidney to handle an expanded sodium (volume) load (either through a genetic defect or a pathological condition), the ECF volume remains elevated and with it, peripheral resistance. This is the phenomenon known variously as alteration of the "set-point" of the renal-blood volume-pressure control mechanism (Guyton et al., 1981) or as a shift in the pressure-natriuresis curve (Tobian, 1981). Chronic elevated peripheral resistance leads to structural adaptive change in the arterioles, contributing to the maintenance of elevated resistance (Folkow, 1978), even though cardiac output returns to near normal.

A diuretic can break this regulatory cycle by overcoming the inability of the hypertensive kidney to handle a sodium (volume) load, obviating the need for an elevated pressure, reversing the processes of Figure 6 (reverse autoregulation) (Tobian, 1974) and eventually leading to decreased blood pressure.

D. Neurogenic Mechanisms

The concept of reverse autoregulation, although providing insight into the hemodynamic events subsequent to the administration of a diuretic, does not go too far in providing details of the mechanism of action. The detailed events linking excess body sodium with increased blood pressure—and linking diuretics with decreased blood pressure—are still largely not understood. The brain and neural connections with the kidney and the peripheral vasculature are almost certainly involved, although they have been somewhat ignored until recently because of the difficulties inherent in looking at the complex interconnections involved.

Investigations have suggested that the autonomic nervous system is activated in salt-sensitive, volume-expanded hypertensive states. There are studies that show the vascular beds in rats to be hypersensitive to norepinephrine in the presence of high sodium levels (Ikeda et al., 1978), that plasma norepinephrine levels are significantly increased in salt sensitive hypertensives (Campese et al., 1982), and that there is a significant relationship between low sodium excretion and high plasma NE levels (Nicholls et al., 1980). A recent study showed that chlorthalidone lowers the exaggerated cardiovascular responsiveness to norepinephrine seen in patients with mild to moderate essential hypertension (Weidmann et al., 1983).

There is evidence that at least half of the hypertensive response to a high-salt diet in sensitive rats is mediated through the sympathetic nerves (Takeshita and Mark, 1978), perhaps through renal mechano- or chemoreceptors, which are involved in sensing changes in perfusion pressure or tubular sodium concentration by the activation of renal afferent systems (Recordati and Moss, 1978).

There is a growing body of evidence to suggest that renal tubular sodium reabsorption is directly influenced by the efferent renal sympathetic nerves (Dibona, 1983). Micropuncture experiments have shown that sodium and water reabsorption in the proximal tubule are directly controlled by autonomic neurons (Bello-Reuss et al., 1977). These connections appear to mediate the increase in tubular reabsorption of sodium and water seen upon electrical stimulation of renal sympathetic nerves in the dog (Bello-Reuss et al., 1976) and the increase in urine flow upon renal denervation in volume-expanded rats (Bello-Reuss et al., 1977). The effects of nerve stimulation are blocked by the alpha-adrenergic antagonist phenoxybenzamine (Zambraski et al., 1976). Phenoxybenzamine also mimics the effects of denervation (Gill and Casper, 1971). It has been suggested that there is a neurogenic component of pressure natriuresis (Section III.C) mediated through the baroreceptors in the carotid sinus or cardiopulmonary low-pressure receptors (Zambraski et al., 1976).

An increase in brain phenylethanolamine N-methyltransferase (PNMT) activity has been shown in Dahl S and DOC-salt rats (Saavedra et al., 1976; Saavedra et al., 1980). Recent experiments in DOC-salt rats and in rats with reduced renal mass on a high-salt diet have shown that the experimental high blood pressure was reduced by an inhibitor of PNMT that is known to cross the blood brain barrier, whereas a related peripherally acting PNMT inhibitor had no effect (Black et al., 1981; DiPette et al., 1983).

The transfer of information between the brain and the kidney may well hold the key to the relationship between sodium, kidney function, diuretics, and hypertension. Electrical activation of renal afferent nerves in rats causes vasoconstriction in the contralateral kidney (Brody and Johnson, 1980), an effect which is abolished by lesions in the AV3V region of the brainstem (see chapter by Brody et al.). An AV3V lesion also prevents at least half of the blood pressure rise induced by a high-salt diet in Dahl S rats (Goto et al., 1982). The kidney (at least in rats) may be able to sense high sodium levels or low perfusion pressure and translate this information into increased vascular resistance through renal afferent systems. The suggestion has recently been made (Blaustein and Hamyln, 1983) that an endogenous natriuretic factor, originating in the brain in response to high sodium levels, may also be an important link between the brain and the kidney (Section III.F).

E. Interactions with Humoral Regulators of the Kidney

Ever since the classic studies in genetically salt-sensitive and salt-resistant rats implicated a circulating humoral vasoconstrictor substance (Dahl et al., 1969), most of the well-characterized endogenous humoral factors affecting kidney function have been investigated for their ability to function as circulating vasoactive substances in sodium-dependent hypertension. The list includes vasopressin (ADH), the prostaglandins, the components of the renin-angiotensin-aldosterone system, the vasoactive peptides of the kallikrein-kinin system, and dopamine. A detailed description of the myriad effects of these substances on the kidney and vascular system and of their complex interrelationships with each other would be well beyond the scope of this chapter. The reader is referred to an excellent contemporary review (Smith, 1983) for a discussion of these topics. In this section we will focus on these substances as they relate to sodium-dependent volume-expanded hypertension and the antihypetensive effects of diuretics.

1. ANTIDIURETIC HORMONE (ADH). Antidiuretic hormone is secreted from the anterior pituitary in response to thirst; its main renal action is the promotion of water reabsorption in the collecting duct and the formation of a concentrated urine (Hebert et al., 1981). In high doses, it also displays vasoconstrictor activity (Wagner and Braunwald, 1956); because of this component of its action, there has been interest in its role in sodium-dependent hypertension. Urinary ADH was found to be elevated in patients with esential hypertension as compared to normotensive controls (Khokhar and Slater, 1976), and it has been concluded that it plays a role as a pressor agent in the onset and maintenance of DOC-salt hypertension in rats (Crofton et al., 1979). Other investigators could find no evidence that ADH plays a role in the maintenance of salt-induced hypertension in salt-sensitive rats (Matsuguchi et al., 1980). Plasma (as well as urinary) ADH is increased in patients with essential hypertension (Cowley et al., 1981) and is sensitive to sodium intake in these patients. No investigators have monitored plasma ADH during long-term treatment of EBH with a diuretic; intravenous infusion of furosemide or piretanide over six hours did not alter plasma ADH in normotensive volunteers (Baylis and DeBeer, 1981).

2. RENIN-ANGIOTENSIN-ALDOSTERONE. It has been suggested that the humoral vasoconstrictor in rats is probably not angiotensin II, since salt-sensitive rats have the low-renin type of hypertension (Tobian, 1981). A study from Denmark (Ibsen, 1979) in patients with mild essential hypertension concluded that angiotensin does not play a role in the maintenance of this type of hypertension; saralasin treatment of the patients did not cause a significant decrease in mean arterial pressure. Angiotensin II does play a role upon activation of the renin-angiotensin-aldosterone system by the sodium and volume depletion

brought about by diuretic treatment, tending to offset the hypotensive effect of the diuretic (Weber et al., 1977a; Vaughan et
al., 1978). In view of the fact that at least one component of
renin release is beta-receptor mediated (Ganong, 1972), it is
thought that some of the success of diuretic/beta-blocker combi-
nations (Section II) is due to the inhibition of the renin-angiotensin-aldosterone system subsequent to its activation by diuretic
treatment (Weber and Laragh, 1978). The operation of such a
mechanism probably contributes to the success of diuretics in
combination with an angiotensin II converting enzyme inhibitor
such as captopril (Brunner et al., 1980; MacGregor et al., 1982)
or enalapril (Kolloch et al., 1982).

3. KALLIKREIN-KININ SYSTEM. The kinins are potent
vasodilator peptides, causing dilatation of blood vessels in muscle,
kidney and various glands as well as coronary and cerebral vessels
(Haddy et al., 1970). Kinins are liberated from protein precursors
(kininogens) by kallikreins, a group of ubiquitous serine proteases
found in plasma, as well as in the urine, kidney, pancreas, salivary
and sweat glands, and the intestine. The two kinins produced in
the kidney are lysyl-bradykinin (L-BK or kallidin) and bradykinin
(BK) (Webster and Pierce, 1963).

Because of their function as vasodilators it is tempting to
postulate a deficiency of these peptides in volume-expanded
hypertension. The activity of the renal kallikrein-kinin system
has been shown to be decreased in patients with essential hypertension (Margolius et al., 1974; Seino et al., 1975; Levy et al.,
1977) as measured by urinary kallikrein excretion. At the same
time, kallikrein excretion increases in normotensive animals
upon the administration of diuretics, including furosemide,
bumetanide, and thiazides (Croxatto et al., 1973; Nielsen and
Arrigoni-Martelli, 1977). Furthermore, diuretics increase kallikrein excretion in hypertensive patients (O'Connor et al., 1977)
and animals (Nielsen and Arrigone-Martelli, 1977), making it
attractive to postulate a connection between the antihypertensive effect of diuretics and this increase in kallikrein activity.

There is no evidence, however, that renal kallikreins and
kinins reach the peripheral circulation where they could contribute to peripheral vasodilatation. In fact, it is probably unlikely
that they circulate to any great extent, due to the presence of
plasma protesase inhibitors (Vogel and Werle, 1970) and kininases
(Pisano, 1975). It has recently been shown that patients with
normal-renin essential hypertension have normal plasma kinin

levels even while demonstrating decreased urinary kallikrein excretion (Mersey et al., 1979).

The current state of knowledge with regard to the physiological role of the renal kinins makes it difficult to draw conclusions about them as mediators of the antihypertensive effect of diuretics. Increased renal blood flow and sodium excretion result upon the infusion of L-BK and BK into the kidney (Webster and Gilmore, 1964; Willis et al., 1969; Stein, et al., 1972) and upon the administration of kininase inhibitors (Bailie and Barbour, 1975). There is conflicting evidence regarding the relationship of kallikrein excretion in man to dietary salt (Adetayibi and Mills, 1972; Levy et al., 1978); about the only conclusion that can be drawn is that kinins help regulate renal blood flow and sodium handling and thus may contribute to the natriuretic effects of some diuretics.

The possible involvement of the renal kallikrein-kinin system in the antihypertensive action of diuretics continues to be a subject of investigation. Recent reports have suggested a role for kallikrein in the mechanism of action of HCTZ (O'Connor et al., 1981; Overlack et al., 1982) and furosemide (Olshan et al., 1981).

4. PROSTAGLANDINS. A common denominator among the previously discussed hormonal systems that have a role in regulating kidney and vascular function is the prostaglandin (PG) system. These ubiquitous arachidonic acid metabolites serve to mediate both the renal and peripheral vascular responses to the various hormonal systems and also serve to connect them at various points, either through positive or negative feedback loops or through direct effects. It is because of their wide distribution and multiplicity of function that there is only circumstantial evidence for their role in mediating the antihypertensive effects of diuretics.

Renal prostaglandins antagonize the effects of ADH, both in vitro and in vivo (Anderson et al., 1976). Prostacyclin (PGI_2) has been proposed as a mediator of the baroreceptor operated component of renin release (Frolich et al., 1978), and other PG's have been shown to be intermediate in the sequence of events initiated by renal kinins (Nasjletti and Malik, 1981). The role of renal PG's in the control of RBF, glomerular filtration rate (GFR) and sodium secretion is examined in a contemporary review (Dunn and Zumbraski, 1980).

It has been shown that patients with essential hypertension have decreased urinary excretion of PGE_2 (Abe et al., 1977; Tan et al., 1978) when compared with normotensive controls; Dahl S rats have been shown to have PGE_2 concentrations in the renal papilla as much as 50% lower than salt-resistant rats, possibly resulting in increased sodium reabsorption (Tobian et al., 1982). These observations, coupled with data showing that the natriuretic and antihypertensive effects of furosemide are attenuated by indomethacin (Patak et al., 1975; Kramer et al., 1980), make it tempting to postulate a role for PGE_2 in the antihypertensive effects of the loop diuretics. This is particularly so in light of the fact that urinary PGE_2 is increased upon administration of furosemide or ethacrynic acid to man or animals (Abe et al., 1977; Patak et al., 1979; Scherer and Weber, 1979; Brater et al., 1980). Similar findings have been reported for HCTZ, albeit in such a small sample of patients that the validity of the results could not be statistically confirmed (Kramer et al., 1980). A recent report found the natriuretic effects of HCTZ to be independent of the renal prostaglandin system (Favre et al., 1983).

These findings may only be circumstantial, however; the precise interaction between diuretics and the renal PG system remains unclear. Hypotheses have been put forward that diuretics inhibit PG-15-OH-dehydrogenase (Stone and Hart, 1976), that they inhibit PGE_2-9-ketoreductase (Abe et al., 1976; Stone and Hart, 1976), or that they enhance the release of arachidonic acid from the phospholipid pool (Weber et al., 1977b). This last hypothesis has received recent support (Craven and DeRubertis, 1982) for the loop diuretics furosemide, ethacrynic acid, bumetanide and 3-benzylamino-4-phenythio-5-sulfamoylbenzoic acid in a study in which ^{14}C arachidonic acid release was found to be Ca^{+2} dependent in vitro. This same study could not confirm the PGE-releasing properties of HCTZ.

The role of the renal prostaglandins in the expression of the hypotensive effect of diuretics is certainly not definitive. The PG's may be involved in the mechanism of action of the thiazides only to the extent that they mediate the responses of other hormonal systems, although bendrofluazide has been shown to increase circulating levels of the potent vasodilator PGI_2 in patients with EBH (Webster et al., 1980). The PG's may be more directly involved in expressing the natriuretic effects of the loop diuretics, but it is difficult to find evidence to suggest that the antihypertensive effects of compounds such as furosemide and ethacrynic acid are directly mediated by PG's instead of being secondarily related to the sodium and volume depleting effects through reverse autoregulation or neurogenic mechanisms.

5. DOPAMINE. Dopamine has come to be regarded as a substance with a significant role in the regulation of the peripheral vasculature and the kidney. The role of dopamine in kidney function and as an endogenous natriuretic substance has recently been reviewed (Lee, 1982). With regard to the role of dopamine in EBH and diuretic treatment, it has been proposed that an intrarenal deficiency of this potent natriuretic and vasodilator substance might be involved in the predisposition to EBH, manifested as the kidneys' inability to handle a sodium load (Lee, 1981). It has been shown that some patients with EBH produce inappropriately low amounts of dopamine when fed sodium chloride (Perkins et al., 1980). Intravenous furosemide increases urinary dopamine, perhaps through a chloride-dependent mechanism (Kuchel et al., 1978).

F. Circulating Sodium Transport Inhibitor (Natriuretic Hormone)

1. NATRIURETIC HORMONE HYPOTHESIS. Evidence continues to accumulate in support of the existence of a circulating sodium transport inhibitor (also called a salt-excreting hormone, natriuretic hormone, or natriuretic factor). The production of this endogenous substance would be stimulated by expansion of the ECF volume and would stimulate natriuresis, bringing ECF volume back to normal. When the existence of this putative hormone is conclusively proved or disproved, a significant step will have been taken toward understanding essential benign hypertension—its relationship to salt balance and the effectiveness of diuretics in its treatment. The data in support of the concept of a circulating inhibitor of sodium transport have been reviewed several times in recent years (Haddy, 1982; deWardener, 1982; deWardener and Clarkson, 1982). This section will attempt to outline the background of the concept and to discuss recent results, particularly those with implications for the antihypertensive effects of diuretics.

Exaggerated natriuresis has been demonstrated under conditions of volume expansion in several species, including man. In rats an exaggerated natriuresis is observed upon loading with isotonic saline (Ben-Ishay et al., 1973); upon continuous volume expansion with two-thirds blood and one-third Ringer's, as measured by an isolated kidney (Tobian et al., 1979); or upon volume expansion with homologous blood, as measured upon cross circulation with a rat of normal volume (Knock and deWardener, 1980).

In dogs, when volume is expanded with equilibrated blood, increased natriuresis can be observed in a denervated kidney (Bengele et al., 1972), while in man, increasing the intrathoracic blood volume by water immersion also leads to increased natriuresis (Epstein et al., 1978).

Experimental evidence has suggested that the natriuresis seen upon volume expansion is due to a circulating inhibitor of sodium transport acting as an endogenous inhibitor of Na,K-ATPase. The blood of volume-expanded dogs was shown to be capable of reducing the short circuit current in frog skin (Nutbourne et al., 1970) and of inhibiting net sodium and potassium transport in vitro in fragments of rabbit renal tubules (Clarkson et al., 1970). The plasma from volume-expanded rats (Gonick et al., 1977) and dogs (Gruber et al., 1980), after fraction on a G-25 Sephadex column, was found to inhibit Na,K-ATPase in various in vitro preparations. These partially purified substances are similar to the cardiac glycosides ouabain and digoxin in their ability to inhibit in vitro preparations of Na,K-ATPase. In support of their digoxin-like character, these partially purified preparations have been shown to compete for specific digoxin antibodies (Gruber et al., 1980).

Material with the properties of a sodium transport/ATPase inhibitor has also been isolated from human plasma after salt loading (Kramer, 1978) and from the fractionated, freeze-dried urine of normal (Clarkson et al., 1979) and salt loaded (Klingmuller et al., 1982) human subjects. In addition, a Na,K- ATPase inhibitor has been found in bovine hypothalamus (Haupert and Sancho, 1979), rat hypothalamus (Lichstein and Samuelov, 1980) and pig brain (Fishman, 1979).

The active substance in these preparations is described as low molecular weight (500 Daltons) because it elutes after the salts on a G-25 Sephadex column (the "post-salt" or F-IV fraction). It is heat stable (Clarkson et al., 1979), but there is some disagreement on whether or not it is a peptide (compare the preceeding reference with Gruber and Buckalew, 1978). Recently, the F-IV fraction was further purified using HPLC on cation exchange and reverse-phase columns (Licht et al., 1982). By bioassaying the fractions (isolated toad bladder), highly active material was obtained, but the quantity was too small for structure determination. From 80 l. of normal human urine the London group (de Wardener, 1982) has isolated 16 μg of a Na,K-ATPase inhibitor, which they hope to characterize. In this regard, the importance of obtaining pure material cannot be emphasized too much; extracts of guinea pig brain that inhibited Na,K-ATPase exhibited vascular effects that were probably due to contamination with vasopressin (James-Kracke et al., 1981).

Ever since it was shown that susceptibility to salt-induced hypertension could be transferred from salt-sensitive rats to resistant rats through a parabiotic connection (Dahl et al., 1969), the presence of a low molecular weight humoral factor has been implicated in salt-induced hypertension. There is evidence that the low molecular weight humoral factor is a circulating inhibitor of sodium transport. Using the technique of ouabain sensitive ^{86}Rb uptake, it has been shown that Na-K pump activity in blood vessels is reduced in low renin models of hypertension in the rat and dog (Haddy, 1982). The same reduced pump activity could be effected by volume expansion in rats; an infusion of serum from a volume expanded rat lowered ouabain sensitive ^{86}Rb uptake in the tail artery of a normal rat. In man, it is possible to show that the plasma of hypertensive patients has decreased Na,K-ATPase activity by measuring the associated increase in glucose-6-phosphate dehydrogenase (G6PD) activity (MacGregor et al., 1981). This decrease in Na,K-ATPase activity was dependent upon sodium intake, both in normotensive humans and in hypertensives. There are, as yet, no studies on the effect of diuretics on plasma G6PD activity.

The possible involvement of a circulating sodium transport inhibitor in the pathogenesis of essential hypertension has been recently reviewed (MacGregor and de Warderer, 1981). Briefly, it is postulated that the function of such an inhibitor of cellular sodium transport would be to overcome the inherited defect in the ability of the kidneys of susceptible individuals to eliminate sodium. By inhibiting Na,K-ATPase, active Na reabsorption in the kidney would be diminished, leading to increased natriuresis. Since it is a circulating factor, it may lead to a generalized inhibition of body Na,K-ATPase, one effect of which would be the retention of sodium by the cells of the resistance vessels (Figure 7). The retention of sodium would, through a sodium-calcium exchange transport system, lead to elevated intracellular calcium (Blaustein, 1977) and a concomitant increase in vascular reactivity, brought about by decreased norepinephrine reuptake, increased norepinephrine release, or increased storage of calcium in the sarcoplasmic reticulum (Blaustein and Hamyln, 1983). Alternatively, it has been postulated that calcium influx could be subsequent to the depolarization of the smooth muscle cells caused by pump suppression (Pamnani et al., 1981a). Such mechanisms could be accountable for the rise in peripheral resistance and subsequent increase in blood pressure when sodium transport

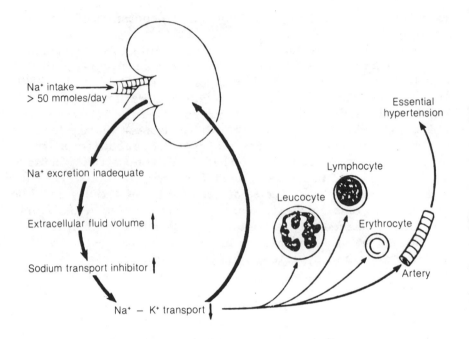

Figure 7. Hypothesis for the possible role of a circulating sodium-transport inhibitor in the etiology of essential hypertension. (From deWardener and MacGregor, 1980, with permission.)

inhibiting cardiac glycosides are administered to patients in therapeutic doses (Mason and Braunwald, 1964).

A factor that corresponds chromatographically to the putative natriuretic hormone has recently been isolated from saline-loaded dogs and found to increase the reactivity of rat cremaster arterioles to norepinephrine, arginine vasopressin, and angiotensin II (Plunkett et al., 1982).

The implications of this hypothesis in regard to the antihypertensive effect of diuretics have been recognized (Blaustein and Hamyln, 1983). A diuretic would eliminate the stimulus for the production of the natriuretic hormone by substituting for it at the kidney. The peripheral manifestations of a circulating sodium transport inhibitor would then gradually reverse themselves.

2. EVIDENCE FROM BLOOD CELLS. There is a growing body of literature that describes a wide range of abnormalities in

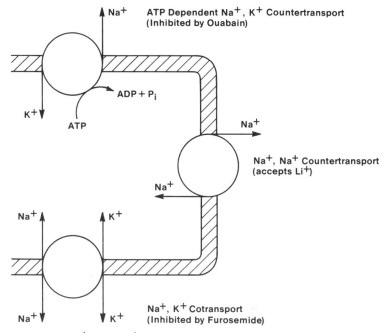

Figure 8. Na⁺ and K⁺ transport systems in blood cells.

sodium transport across the membranes of blood cells taken from patients with essential hypertension. Some of these results support the existence of a circulating sodium transport inhibitor, while others have bearing on the role of low salt diets or diuretics in the treatment of essential hypertension. This area has been recently reviewed (Swales, 1982) and we will touch on it only lightly in this section.

The subject of sodium transport in and out of blood cells is complex and sometimes confusing, partly because various investigators have looked at different systems responsible for the maintenance of appropriate concentrations of intracellular sodium and have sometimes reached different conclusions. At least part of the confusion is a result of the different types of sodium transport that have been shown to occur in blood cell membranes (Figure 8). These include the ouabain sensitive Na-K pump that exchanges internal sodium for external potassium using energy supplied by the hydrolysis of ATP (Caviares, 1977); a Na–Na countertransport system that is independent of ATP and will also exchange lithium for sodium (Haas et al., 1975); and a Na-K cotransport system that brings about the outward transport of intracellular sodium (driven by the potassium gradient) and the inward transport of extracellular potassium (driven by the sodium gradient) (Wiley and Cooper, 1974). The recent literature is summarized in Table 1 (adapted from Swales, 1982).

Numerous investigators have found increased levels of intra-cellular sodium in blood cells taken from patients with essential hypertension, including erythrocytes (Losse et al., 1960; Clegg et al., 1982), leukocytes (Edmondsen et al., 1975; Araoye et al., 1978) and lymphocytes (Ambrosioni et al., 1981a). Some have found increased sodium flux across erythrocyte membranes (Table 1), while others have pinpointed the defect as the ouabain sensi-tive pump in erythrocytes (Walter and Distler, 1982) and leuco-cytes (Edmondson et al., 1975). Sodium-potassium cotransport in erythrocytes is altered in hypertensives, but the extent of the alteration is subject to geographic variation (Table 1). Lithium-sodium countertransport in erythrocytes has been found to be uniformly increased (Canessa et al., 1980, and other references in Table 1).

Some of these results support the existence of a circulating inhibitor of sodium transport. One group (Fitzgibbon et al., 1980) found that the erythrocyte sodium efflux rate constant was in-creased only when the cells were incubated in their own plasma instead of an artificial medium. Others have found that sodium efflux in leukocytes from normotensive volunteers can be inhibited by incubating the cells in plasma obtained from patients with essential hypertension (Poston et al., 1981b). Sodium efflux in normal leukocytes has also been found to be inhibited by the "F4" fraction obtained from the urine of hypertensive patients (Clarkson et al., 1980), and plasma from hypertensive patients has been found to increase the permeability of normal erythor-cytes to the passive influx of sodium (Wessels and Zumkley, 1980). The increased rate of sodium-lithium countertransport has re-cently been attributed to a dialyzable plasma factor (Woods et al., 1983).

When essential hypertension is treated, either with low salt diets or diuretics, the sodium transport abnormalities in the blood cells—increased intracellular sodium and increased ouabain sensitive and insensitive transmembrane fluxes—are often reversed (Table 2). It is difficult to draw any conclusions concerning the mechanism of action of treatment with low salt diets or diuretics at this time, however. The removal of the stimulus for the pro-duction of natriuretic hormone is only one possibility. According to the Blaustein hypothesis (Blaustein, 1977) cellular calcium disturbances are secondary to alterations in sodium metabolism.

Table 1. *Disturbances of Cellular Sodium Metabolism in*
Essential Hypertension

Variable	Cell	Change
Intracellular sodium[a]	erythrocyte	↑
Trans-membrane sodium flux[b]	erythrocyte	↑
Sodium efflux rate constant (plasma incubated)[c]	erythrocyte	↑
Ouabain sensitive sodium efflux rate constant[d]	erythrocyte	↓
Sodium-potassium cotransport	erythrocyte	↑ (Boston)[e] ↓ (Paris)[f] ↓ (Milan)[g] ↓ (Pisa)[h]
Lithium-sodium countertransport[i]	erythrocyte	↑
Ouabain-sensitive sodium efflux rate constant[j]	leukocyte	↓
Intracellular sodium[k]	leukocyte	↑
Intracellular sodium[l]	lymphocyte	↑

a. Losse et al., 1960; Clegg et al., 1982.
b. Wessels et al., 1967; Postnov et al., 1977; Wessels
   and Zumkley, 1980; Preiss et al., 1982; and Cole, 1983.
c. Fitzgibbon et al., 1980.
d. Walter and Distler, 1982.
e. Adragna et al., 1982.
f. Garay et al., 1980.
g. Cusi et al., 1981.
h. Ghione et al., 1981.
i. Canessa et al., 1980; Adragna et al., 1982; and
   Trevisan et al., 1983.
j. Edmondson et al., 1975; and Edmondson et al., 1981.
k. Edmondson et al., 1975; and Araoye et al., 1978.
l. Ambrosioni et al., 1981a; adapted from Swales, 1982,
   with permission.

Table 2.   Influence of Salt Restriction and Diuretic Treatment
on Disturbances of Cellular Sodium Metabolism in
Essential Hypertension

Variable	Cell	Treatment	Change
Intracellular sodium[a]	erythrocyte	chlorthalidone hydrochloro- thiazide	↓ ↑ b
Ouabain sensitive sodium efflux rate constant[c]	erythrocyte	low sodium diet	↑
Trans-membrane sodium flux[d]	erythrocyte	"thiazide"	↓
Intracellular sodium[e]	leukocyte	hydrochloro- thiazide	↓
Total and Ouabain sensitive sodium efflux rate constant[f]	leukocyte	"thiazide" + amiloride + beta-blocker	↑
Intracellular sodium[g]	lymphocyte	low sodium diet	↓
Intracellular soidum[h]	lymphocyte	hydrochloro- thiazide + amiloride or fenquizone	↓

a. Gessler, 1962; Walter, 1981.
b. Performed on normotensive subjects.
c. Morgan et al., 1981b.
d. Cole, 1983.
e. Araoye et al., 1978.
f. Poston et al., 1981a.
g. Ambrosioni et al., 1982.
h. Ambrosioni et al., 1981b.

Reports of decreased calcium binding in erythrocytes from patients with essential hypertension (Postnov et al., 1977) have led to the suggestion that decreased membrane affinity for calcium is the primary pathogenic change in essential hypertension (Swales, 1982), and that diet or diuretic induced changes in sodium levels effect changes that are secondary to the defect in calcium binding.

3. IMPLICATIONS FOR DIURETIC THERAPY AND OPPORTUNITES FOR FUTURE RESEARCH. There is data to suggest that both Na-Li countertransport and Na-K cotransport are specific markers of essential, rather than secondary hypertension (Canessa et al., 1980; Garay et al., 1981). Defects in these transport systems could not be detected in hypertension secondary to nephropathy, pheochromocytoma, or renovascular disease. Furthermore, studies with the normotensive offspring of parents with essential hypertension have suggested that the defects in Na-Li countertransport and Na-K cotransport are inherited abnormalities (Canessa et al., 1980; Meyer et al., 1981). As such these transport systems have been advocated as diagnostic tools to aid in distinguishing and treating essential hypertension and to identify people at risk of developing essential hypertension because of their genetic background (Gordon, 1981).

In regard to antihypertensive therapy with diuretics, it seems to us that if these results can be confirmed, a simple test to evaluate either cotransport or countertransport function in a hypertensive patient would provide a rational alternative to the "stepped-care" approach and would allow the physician to know whether or not to expect diuretic treatment to ameliorate his patient's hypertension. In addition, if people who are pre-hypertensive because of their genetic background could be identified, they could take appropriate dietary measures in order to possibly avoid diuretic treatment in the future.

Clearly, though, many questions remain to be answered be fore any consideration of sodium transport aberrations becomes part of standard practice. The results with the different transport systems in blood cells must be put on solid footing: some investigators find no alteration of sodium transport in the cells of hypertensives (Swarts et al., 1981; Duhm et al., 1982), while others find that such alterations, while possibly inherited, are not directly associated with high blood pressure (Heagerty et al., 1982). Much would be gained if there were a unified scheme for sodium transport in and out of cells, but at this point the data are too disparate.

A step will have been taken toward a unified scheme of sodium transport when the question of the relationship of Na-Li countertransport to Na-K cotransport is settled, along with the role of each in respect to ouabain sensitive transport. It has been proposed that counter-and cotransport are systems that are different and distinct (Canessa et al., 1981; Clegg et al., 1982) although the Boston group finds them both more active in erythrocytes of patients with essential hypertension. The investigators who find increased Na-K ATPase activity in the blood cells of hypertensives have proposed that it is increased as a compensatory response to decreased Na-K cotransport (Garay and Dagher, 1980).

We must conclude that the picture is still too complex to lend itself to a unified explanation or to enable conclusions to be drawn about the mechanism of action of diuretics as antihypertensives. It seems likely to us that the sodium pumps themselves are being modified by the in vitro manipulations of the cells, giving rise to an environment which does not mirror the in vivo situation. In unmasking co- and countertansport by inhibiting Na,K-ATPase with ouabain, transport systems may be being brought into play that normally play only a small role in vivo.

If the concept of a circulating sodium transport inhibitor is valid, then the question has to be asked if the results with sodium transport in blood cells are applicable to sodium transport in the smooth muscle cells of the resistance vessels (Figure 7). There is some evidence for this in animals. As mentioned previously (section III.F.1.) Na-K pump activity has been shown to be reduced in the rat and dog in low renin states and under conditions of volume expansion. Increased cation flow rates have been observed in the vascular musculature of hypertensive rats (Jones, 1974; Altman et al., 1977), and it has been known for some time that the blood vessel walls of hypertensive rats have an abnormally high sodium content (Tobian and Binion, 1952). Some investigators have found evidence supporting increased membrane permeability in the smooth muscle cells of resistance vessels in hypertensive rats (Jandhyala et al., 1980); elevated intracellular sodium has been found in cultured aortic smooth muscle cells from spontaneously hypertensive rats (Zidek et al., 1982).

A common thread running through the literature on low-renin volume-expanded types of hypertension is the genetic predispostion to this type of hypertension and its association with an apparent defect in the sodium handling ability of the kidney, both in animal models (Tobian et al., 1977) and, less conclusively, in man (Luft et al., 1982). The evidence that the transport defect

in blood cells is inherited makes it tempting to speculate that
the genetic predispositon to essential hypertension is manifested
at the cellular level in the kidney as a defect in one or the other
of the sodium pumps, corresponding to the pumps that have been
investigated in blood cells. We know of no direct evidence for
this at the present time, however. In view of the known ability
of diuretics to influence ion transport in the kidney (Knauf, 1980),
an experiment that showed a cellular defect in sodium transport
in the kidney in essential hypertension would be a key to understanding the antihypertensive effect of diuretics. The diuretic
effect of furosemide and structurally related diuretics has recently been shown in rabbits to be related to inhibition of a
Na-K cotransport system in the cortical thick ascending limb of
Henle (Schlatter et al., 1983).

Although an understanding of the cellular mechanisms responsible for the kidney's involvement in essential hypertension
may not be immediately at hand, it seems to us that the G6PD
technique (Section III.F.1.) could be used to establish a critical
link between essential hypertension, diuretic therapy and the
putative circulating inhibitor of Na,K-ATPase. This enzyme,
whose activity is inversely related to plasma Na,K-ATPase activity, has already been shown to be elevated in hypertensives. A
key experiment will be the monitoring of G6PD activity as untreated hypertensives are begun on a diuretic regimen.

There are recent results that suggest that the AV3V region
of the rat brain is either the source of the ouabain-like humoral
factor or is intimately involved in the control of its circulating
levels (Pamnani et al., 1981b; Bealer et al., 1983). Although an
intact central nervous system has been shown to be necessary for
the maintenance of low-renin, high-volume models of hypertension
(Section III.D.), the afferent and efferent connections have not
been described. It has been suggested (deWardener and Clarkson,
1982) that intrathoracic blood volume, particularly left atrial
pressure, may be the afferent limb of this control system, with
the circulating sodium transport inhibitor being the efferent limb
(see also Dibona, 1983).

Although the natriuretic hormone hypothesis is supported by
considerable evidence, it must remain a "putative" hormone until
it can be shown to be capable of being isolated and characterized. The group from Winston-Salem (Gruber et al., 1983) has
found a heptapeptide fragment of ACTH (residues 4-10) that has
the properties of the natriuretic hormone in that it is both
pressor and natriuretic. There is as yet no evidence that any of

the purified extracts from volume expanded models of hypertension contain an identical or similar peptide.

IV. SIDE EFFECTS OF DIURETICS—PROBLEMS AND OPPORTUNITIES

The broader and earlier treatment of elevated blood pressure with drugs has brought into sharper focus the side effects of these agents and their often unknown long-term implications. Diuretics, being the first step drugs of choice, are especially subject to such concern. A better understanding of the causes and relevance of diuretic-induced side effects is providing a more rational basis for patient selection and for the design of diuretics of the future.

A. Hypokalemia

The tendency of both the thiazide and loop diuretics to cause decreases in serum potassium has been established for some time (Talso and Carballo, 1960; Bergstrom and Hultman, 1966). Within the first week of treatment, diuretics can bring about serum potassium levels less than 3.5 mEq/L (Rovner, 1972), levels that are often considered hypokalemic. In one study of 627 patients who were taking loop or thiazide diuretics for a variety of conditions including hypertension, 150 were determined to be hypokalemic (Manner et al., 1972). Serum potassium levels, however, are not necessarily related to the duration of diuretic treatment (Manner et al., 1972).

The importance of this serum electrolyte alteration, its relationship to whole body potassium, skeletal muscle potassium and cardiac muscle potassium remains uncertain. In addition the advisability of administering potassium supplements or potassium sparing diuretics remains controversial.

The ECF accounts for roughly only 2-3% of the total body potassium (Lowenstein, 1973) and there is a poor correlation between serum potassium concentration and body potassium stores (Moore et al., 1954; Healy et al., 1970). Studies on total-body potassium (TBK) using gamma-ray emission from endogenous ^{40}K have shown no significant reduction in TBK in hypertensive patients who had been treated with furosemide for one year (Dargie et al., 1974). Similar results have been shown with thiazides (Graybiel and Sode, 1971). These results have been criticized (Kassirer and Harrington, 1977), but they are substantially backed up by measurements of the potassium content of white blood cells (Edmondsen et al., 1974) and skeletal muscle cells (Bergstrom et al., 1973) from hypertensive patients who have been treated with diuretics.

These data on the incidence of hypokalemia, taken with reports of significant hyperkalemia among patients receiving diuretics and potassium chloride supplements (Lawson, 1974), have prompted recommendations that potassium not be supplemented in hypertensives being treated with diuretics as long as they remain asymptomatic (Kassirer and Harrington, 1977; Beeley, 1980; Morgan and Davidson, 1980; Sandor et al., 1982). The need for some supplementation in patients at a particular risk from hypokalemia -- those taking digoxin, those with severe liver disease, and the elderly -- continues to be recognized as important (Ibrahim et al., 1978; Krakauer and Lauritzen, 1978; Hamdy et al., 1980; McCarthy, 1982), although routine potassium prescribing in the elderly has been questioned (Henschke et al., 1981; Clark et al., 1982).

In those cases where hypokalemia is a bona-fide concern, several reports recommend potassium-sparing diuretics over potassium supplements (Kohvakka et al., 1979; Beeley, 1980; Morgan and Davidson, 1980) although the fixed combination of 50 mg HCTZ and 5 mg amiloride has been ineffective in a few instances at relieving hypokalemia (Hamdy et al., 1980; Penhall and Frewin, 1980).

Recent attention has focused on the incidence of chronic ventricular ectopic activity as a further rationale for correcting diuretic induced hypokalemia in the elderly (Caralis, 1981; McCarthy, 1982) and even in patients in the 30-60 year old group (Holland et al., 1981).

The possible adverse effects of hypokalemia should also be considered in regard to the possible hypotensive effect of diets enriched in potassium. Data in support of the beneficial effects of potassium have been in the literature for some time (Addison, 1928) and this effect continues to be investigated (Iimura et al., 1981; Parfrey et al., 1981). One recent report found that a high potassium intake improved compliance with a low salt diet, promoted sodium loss, prevented the rise in plasma catecholamines induced by the low salt diet, and increased the sensitivity of the baroreceptor reflex (Skrabal et al., 1981), while another group found that a diet containing 3.8% potassium citrate increased papillary flow in Dahl S rats on high salt diets and protected against nephrosclerosis, even though the rats became hypertensive (Ganguli et al., 1981).

The role of potassium may also be considered in terms of the various sodium and potassium pumps, although here again the picture is confused by the various membrane preparations that have been employed. Chronic potassium deficiency has been found to increase ATPase activity in erythrocytes from rats on a low potassium diet (Chan and Sanslone, 1969) and to increase the number of ^{3}H-ouabain binding sites in red cells from humans with diuretic induced hypokalemia (Erdmann et al., 1980). In addition, ouabain resistant sodium extrusion from human erythrocytes is inhibited by high external potassium concentrations (Garay and Dagher, 1980). On the other hand, potassium activates Na,K-ATPase in vitro, an effect that can lead to vasodilatation in vivo (Haddy, 1983).

B. Hyperglycemia and Glucose Intolerance

The first observations concerning the influence of thiazide diuretics on blood glucose levels came during early clinical trials with chlorothiazide (Finnerty, 1959; Freis, 1959; Wilkins, 1959). A number of subsequent studies, summarized by Dollery (1973), confirmed the hyperglycemic effects of the thiazides and numerous other diuretics (Dollery, 1968). However, the actual extent of this problem remained clouded, primarily due to inadequate control of patient selection and lack, in many cases, of pre-treatment blood sugar measurements (Dollery, 1973).

There is little question that diuretics may worsen the blood glucose picture in established diabetics (Goldner et al., 1960; Berchtold et al., 1981 and references cited therein). However, their role in inducing glucose intolerance in subjects who were previously glucose tolerant is controversial. Numerous studies in the last twelve years have sought to clarify the extent of such diuretic-induced hyperglycemia, albeit often with contradictory findings.

One prospective study of 137 hypertensives selected for normal carbohydrate metabolism and body weight failed to demonstrate a significant change in glucose tolerance during a year of diuretic therapy (Kohner et al., 1971). A follow-up study on 61 of these continued on therapy for six years, however, showed an average increase of 13% in fasting blood sugar versus pre-treatment values; although no patient developed "clinical diabetes", 22% of the patients had an abnormal glucose tolerance test (Lewis et al., 1976).

A recently published continuation of this study with 34 patients showed further deterioration; mean fasting blood glucose rose from 4.7 to 6.0 mmol/l. at fourteen years and the two-hour value from 5.5 to 8.0 mmol/l. (p<0.001) (Murphy et al., 1982). If current WHO criteria are applied, three of the 34 patients had glucose intolerance before treatment, but after fourteen years, 18% were "diabetic" and an additional 22% had glucose intolerance. Withdrawal of therapy for seven months in ten of the patients resulted in mean reductions of 10% in fasting blood glucose and 25% in the two hour value, supporting the fourteen-year changes as having been drug-induced rather than the effect of aging in a hypertensive population.

The results of the foregoing study are supported by several other contemporary studies (Amery et al., 1978; Medical Research Council Working Party on Mild to Moderate Hypertension, 1981) and would appear to be a clear indictment of diuretics in the progressive induction of hyperglycemia and glucose intolerance in otherwise normal hypertensives. Other studies, however, partially or wholly contradict these findings, suggesting that the situation is more complex than it appears. For example, in one such study, of 40 hypertensive patients who had been receiving hydrochlorothiazide therapy for a minimum of ten years, 36 had entirely normal glucose tolerance tests; those with an abnormal test had a family history of diabetes, and were in two cases obese and had a history of cardiac failure (Marks et al., 1981). Several other recently published long-term studies also suggest minimal effects of diuretics on blood glucose (Berglund and Andersson, 1981; Bengtsson et al., 1982).

The true incidence of hyperglycemia and glucose intolerance in diuretic treated hypertensives without previous personal or familial history of such disturbances thus remains open to further study. Equally elusive are the mechanism(s) by which such disturbances arise and the long term significance of these disturbances.

By far the most widely propagated explanation for diuretic-induced hyperglycemia and glucose intolerance implicates potassium and the hypokalemia induced by diuretics. Alterations in potassium-sodium ratios are postulated to lead to an increased rate of glycogenolysis mediated by inhibition of phosphodiesterase and glycogen phosphorylase phosphatase (Kaess et al., 1966; Senft et al., 1966; Senft, 1968). Enhancement of gluconeogenesis and reduction of basal cellular glucose transport and uptake have also been suggested (Bartelheimer et al., 1967). While potassium loss may be correlated with elevated blood glucose in some cases (Rapoport and Hurd, 1964; Amery et al., 1978; Nilsson, 1980), numerous other examples suggest either poor correlation (Murphy

et al., 1982) or substantial potassium depletion without significant alteration of glucose tolerance (Kaess et al., 1971). Thus,
the general implication of potassium loss in diuretic-induced
hyperglycemia apears to remain an open question.

Other proposed mechanisms of diuretic-induced elevations
in blood glucose have included suppression of insulin release
(Fajans et al., 1966) in analogy to the diabetogenic benzothiadiazine, diazoxide. This explanation lacks validity, and in fact
diuretics have been recently shown to produce elevations in
blood insulin concomitant with hyperglycemia (Ober and
Hennessey, 1978; Berchtold et al., 1981; Ames, 1983). High insulin levels in the presence of elevated blood sugar implies that
insulin resistance may be playing a role in the hyperglycemia.
Alternatively, inactive insulin may be secreted during diuretic
therapy (Ames and Hill, 1981). These findings and speculations
may lead to further studies and insight into the mechanism of
diuretic-induced hyperglycemia.

Concern over the incidence of and mechanism behind this
side effect of diuretics is derived from its unknown long term
implications. While the effects of chronic diabetes are well-
known, the relevance of long term, asymptomatic hyperglycemia
has been obscure. The findings of a recent study, however, have
suggested a correlation between even mild glucose intolerance
and CHD mortality (Fuller et al., 1979; Fuller et al., 1980). For
example it has been reported that CHD mortality increases sharp-
ly above a two hour glucose tolerance value of 5.4 mmol/l., well
below the value of 8.1 mmol/l. currently regarded as indicating
impaired glucose tolerance. In contrast to this, however, are the
inconsistent findings of a Helsinki study (Pyörälä et al., 1979)
and several Chicago studies which "do not permit a conclusion
that asymptomatic hyperglycemia is a positive coronary risk
factor" (Stamler et al., 1979, 1979a).

The uncertainty of the risk of asymptomatic hyperglycemia
not withstanding, some authorities (Ames and Hill, 1981; Ames,
1983) have recommended the replacement of diuretics as first
line therapy even though they recognize that "the changes in
serum glucose...are not sufficiently large to assure their biologic
importance" (Ames, 1983). Others have chosen a more pragmatic approach, suggesting that the situation should be monitored,
especially in patients with a personal or familial history of diabetes (Berchtold et al., 1981). This would appear to be a rational
approach in view of the incomplete data on true incidence and
cause of diuretic-induced hyperglycemia, and the fact that di-

uretic-induced glucose elevation has not yet been shown to have the same underlying risk as the genetically induced form.

C. Hyperuricemia

The hyperuricemic effect of thiazide diuretics was first recognized shortly after their introduction into clinical practice (Laragh et al., 1958). Numerous studies have since shown that 65-75% of thiazide-treated patients can be expected to show serum uric acid levels in excess of 7 mg. percent (Cannon et al., 1966; Freis and Sappington, 1966; Riddiough, 1977); similar effects occur on chronic administration of most diuretics, the incidence being somewhat lower, however, with spironolactone (Johnson and Mitch, 1981).

In most patients, except those with a personal or family history of gout or with chronic renal failure, such hyperuricemia is generally asymptomatic. In recent years, however, there has been increasing concern with asymptomatic hyperuricemia including that induced by the diuretics, especially in relation to the clear association of uric acid and hypertension and the probable association of uric acid and cardiovascular disease (Hall, 1965; Hansen, 1966; Fessel et al., 1973; Reese and Steele, 1976; Tweeddale and Fodor, 1979; Fessel, 1980). Serum uric acid levels greater than 7 mg. percent, for example, are reported to occur in 25-35% of untreated hypertensives (Cannon et al., 1966; Messerli et al., 1980).

The association of uric acid with hypertension and cardiovascular disease is somewhat controversial regarding cause/effect; nonetheless, interest has been high enough to spark the discovery of diuretics, such as tienilic acid (Thuillier et al., 1974), indacrinone (deSolms et al., 1978) and brocrynat (HP 522) (Shutske et al., 1982), which are uricosuric. Toxicity associated with one of these, tienilic acid, has caused a general reassessment of the unknown relevance of diuretic induced hyperuricemia (Johnson and Mitch, 1981).

A recent study of glomerular filtration rate, renal and systemic hemodynamics, and intravascular volume in normotensives and borderline and established hypertensives, all classified according to serum uric acid levels, could well serve to clarify this scenario (Messerli et al., 1980). A convincing correlation (p<.001) between serum uric acid and renal blood flow (inverse), renal vascular resistance, and total peripherial resistance was demonstrated. These data suggest that the heretofore unexplained hyperuricemia in patients with essential hypertension

probably reflects early nephrosclerosis. Mechanistically, decreased renal blood flow would lead to a decreased renal delivery
of urate. The resulting decrease in secretory flux could result in
substantially diminished urate delivery to post-secretory reabsorp-
tive sites, relatively greater post-secretory reabsorption, and a
sharp decrease in urinary urate (Steele and Rieselbach, 1975).

The potential diagnostic and therapeutic implications of the
Messerli studies, if they are substantiated, are intriguing. Elevated uric acid levels, when other causes have been ruled out,
may be a marker for renal vascular changes reflective of an
actual or impending hypertensive state. A prospective study of
asymptomatic hyperuricemic subjects that demonstrated an
increased incidence of raised blood pressure during follow-up is
supportive of this view (Fessel et al., 1973). Further studies are
needed to confirm these findings. Studies are also needed to
evaluate whether drugs that increase renal blood flow (ACE inhibitors, for example), might serve to prevent or retard development of hypertension in such patients if given in a prophylactic
manner. In the pretreatment work up of hypertensive patients,
it may be that plasma uric acid levels could serve as an indicator
of renal blood flow and be suggestive of a more rational therapeutic approach.

The findings of Messerli et al. (1980) also offer a plausi-
ble rationalization of the hyperuricemic effects of diuretics.
Diuretics, by virtue of their ability to inhibit sodium reuptake
(and thus facilitate excretion), obviate the "need" of the kidney
for an elevated blood pressure to maintain adequate sodium
delivery (and excretion). Initial rise in uric acid levels on
diuretic treatment is reflective of acute extracellular volume
depletion. As blood pressure drops (via mechanisms discussed
earlier), renal blood flow and perfusion pressure and delivery of
urate to the kidneys drop, resulting in decreased urate delivery,
decreased urate secretion, and gradually elevating plasma uric
acid levels.

Elevated plasma renin levels have been linearly correlated
with hyperuricemia in hypertensives receiving diuretics (Ames,
1974). Angiotensin II, when infused in amounts sufficient to
cause blood pressure to rise, produces a decrease in urate secretion in proportion to the associated reduction in renal blood flow
(Ferris and Gorden, 1968). However, in untreated hypertensives,
there appears to be no correlation between plasma renin activity
and serum uric acid (Brunner, et al., 1972). Thus, while reflex
renin secretion in response to diuretic treatment may contribute

somewhat to plasma urate elevation, it is probably secondary to the effects of the diuretics themselves on urinary blood flow.

If the foregoing evaluations are valid and if the unproven pathological effect of elevated uric acid (except in gout or pre-gouty states) is assumed negligible, there is probably little or no medical need for a uricosuric diuretic. It is, however, difficult to agree with the view (Lancet, 1981) that iatrogenic hyperuric-emia arising during antihypertensive treatment is a cause for little concern, especially when it may be reflective of a de-creased blood supply to an already compromised organ. Although a detrimental effect of diuretic-induced decreases in renal blood flow has not been shown as yet, if anything, diuretics of the future should have the ability to maintain or increase pretreat-ment renal blood flow. One approach to this may be diuretics with a renal-selective dopaminergic component (Dolak and Goldberg, 1981).

D. Hyperlipoproteinemia

Although the tendency of diuretics to elevate plasma choles-terol has been recognized for almost two decades (Schoenfeld and Goldberger, 1964), this phenomenon has been widely acknowl-edged and studied by the scientific community only in the last eight years. This interest has developed concurrent with advances in lipoprotein research (Brown et al., 1981 and references cited therein) and recognition of the strong correlations between plas-ma lipoprotein levels and mortality from cardiovascular disease (Gordon et al., 1977 and references cited therein; Hulley, 1978).

Lipoprotein synthesis, transport and catabolism in man is an extremely complex process involving both exogenenous and endo-genous cycles (Figure 9) (Brown et al., 1981). Both cycles begin with secretion into the plasma of triglyceride-rich particles (chylomycrons and very low density lipoproteins, VLDL) that are converted to cholesteryl ester-rich particles (reminants; inter-mediate density lipoproteins, IDL; and low density lipoproteins, LDL) through interaction of lipoprotein lipase (LPL). The major mechanism of clearance of these latter three atherogenic species involves a receptor mediated (LDL receptors) high affinity uptake by hepatic and extrahepatic cells wherein catabolism or transfor-mation/resecretion as non-atherogenic high density lipoproteins (HDL) or VLDL occurs. Normal lipoprotein patterns in man are illustrated in Figure 10.

A large number of studies since 1974 have, as a whole, impli-cated most diuretics in changes in plasma lipoprotein spectrum.

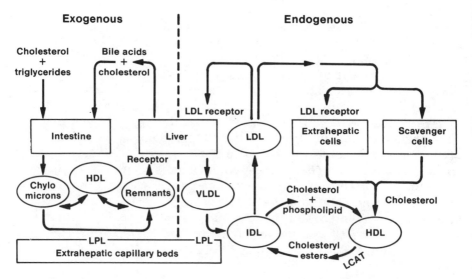

Figure 9. Lipoprotein synthesis, transport and catabolism in man. LPL=lipoprotein lipase; LCAT=lecithin-cholesterol acyltransferase. (From Brown et. al., 1981, with permission.)

In general it appears that chlorthalidone, furosemide, and thia-zides and related diuretics reversibly elevate plasma VLDL and LDL, while HDL, for the most part, remains unchanged (Goldman et al., 1980; Joos et al., 1980; Ames and Hill, 1981; Ames and Hill, 1982; Johnson, 1982; and references cited therein). The magnitude of these changes varies considerably from study to study, from several percent to more than forty percent, with most being in the 5-15% range. Such variation appears to be accounted for by the complexity of liprotein metabolism; age, sex and size of the patient population; differences in analytical methods and criteria; and the plethora of diuretics and doses employed.

    The outcome and implications of these studies with diuretics are just now beginning to reach general medical practice. Recent reviews directed at the practicing pharmacist (Am. J. Hosp. Pharm., 1975; Riddiough, 1977) do not even list hyperlipopro-teinemia as a side effect of diuretic therapy, while a more con-temporary treatment directed at physicians affords it a mere five lines of text (Ram, 1982). An editorial in the prestigious journal Lancet acknowledges the potential problem, concluding that "there is probably no case at present for a major change in prescribing habits", but that "extra vigilance is needed in hyper-

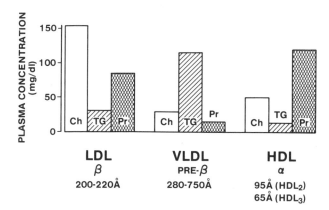

Figure 10. Normal lipoprotein spectrum in man. Ch=choles-terol; TG=triglycerides; Pr=protein.

tensive patients who are already hyperlipidaemic" (Lancet, 1980). Others (Ames, 1983), however, go so far as to suggest replacement of diuretics as first line therapy for hypertension, implying that diuretic-induced hyperlipoproteinemia may be the reason that control of blood pressure has not led to a consistent reduction in coronary heart disease (CHD).

Clearly, additional studies both at the clinical and basic research levels are necessary before such a drastic shift from accepted therapy is warranted. For example, the conclusion of Ames presupposes that the epidemiologic studies (Gordon and Kannel, 1971; Rosenman et al., 1976) linking hypertension to CHD are completely valid; it could well be that this correlation is not entirely correct and that one should not a priori expect benefit in CHD from lowering blood pressure. Additional epidemiological studies, involving patients whose blood pressure is lowered by means other than diuretics as a comparative group, would appear necessary to resolve the hypertension–CHD link and, ultimately, the question as to the long-term benefits to be expected from diuretic therapy.

The link between CHD and hypertension not withstanding, it is clear that there is a strong correlation between CHD and hyperlipoproteinemia. However, it has not been shown that diuretic-induced hyperlipoproteinemia has the same clinical risk implications as hyperlipoproteinemia of genetic or pathological origin. Yet such diuretic-induced changes technically place individuals in a statistically higher risk group, partially or fully offseting statistical morbidity and mortality gains realized from a reduction in blood pressure (Amos and Hill, 1981). A better understanding of the cause of diuretic-induced hyperlipoprotein-emia appears necessary before such statistical pooling can be considered valid.

The mechanism(s) underlying diuretic-induced hyperlipopro-teinemia remain somewhat obscure despite growing interest. Proposed mechanisms have included delayed LDL catabolism (Mordasini et al., 1980; Ames, 1983), insulin resistance resulting in accelerated synthesis (Ames, 1983), decreased blood presure (Rosenthal et al., 1980), alpha-adrenergic involvement (Joos and Kevitz, 1979; Boehringer et al., 1981) and impairment of LDL receptor activity (Ames, 1983). Some of these proposals are questionable in that other studies suggest no direct association with blood pressure, insulin, glucose, uric acid, norepinephrine or lipoprotein lipase (Glueck et al., 1978; Mordasini et al., 1980).

Of the various possibilities, the potential involvement of LDL receptors is perhaps the most intriguing. It is also perhaps the most relevant in terms of evaluating the clinical risk im-plications of diuretic-induced hyperlipoproteinemia.

The number of LDL receptors, and thus the ability of the body to clear plasma of atherogenic lipoproteins, is under multi-factorial control. A primary controlling factor is genetic, with at least six genetically determined disorders of LDL receptors having been recognized to date. The concentration of cholester-ol and related esters within hepatic and extrahepatic cells acts also, via a feedback mechanism, to regulate LDL receptor levels. High intracellular levels of such substances, resulting from ab-sorption or synthesis, act to down-regulate receptor synthesis; conversely, low intracellular levels of such compounds up-regulate LDL receptor formation.

A number of drugs and endogenous hormones also act to control LDL receptor populations. Cholestyramine, which pro-motes cholesterol excretion via bile salts, especially when com-bined with cholesterol synthesis inhibitors such as compactin or mevinolin, acts via such feedback mechanisms to up-regulate LDL receptor synthesis. Hormones, including insulin, thyroxin, and platelet derived growth factors can also increase LDL re-ceptors.

Increased knowledge of LDL receptors appears to have pro-vided those who are interested in the mechanisms of diuretic-induced plasma lipoprotein elevation with hypotheses and tools to further study this phenomenon. Speculatively, it is possible that diuretics block such receptors, leading to LDL elevation. Alternatively, diuretics, through their effects on secondary messengers (insulin, K^+, etc.?) may promote a down-regulation of such receptors, or an alteration in lipoprotein apoproteins (and thus their ability to be recognized and cleared by receptors). Countless other possibilities also abound.

A recently developed double isotope method (Mahley et al., 1977) offers the exciting possibility to measure the effects of diuretics on the number of LDL receptors in intact humans. Cyclohexanedione treatment of LDL has been shown to block its ability to bind to receptors, and thus, simultaneous administration of ^{125}I-labeled LDL and ^{131}I-labeled cyclohexnedione-treated LDL (Shepherd et al., 1979), with measurement of differential clearance rates, can provide an indication of the LDL receptor population.

Use of such techniques, along with other biochemical measurements in carefully controlled studies, may provide the answer to the mechanism(s) involved in diuretic-induced hyperlipoproteinemia. From a purely pragmatic point of view, however, the underlying cause and clinical relevance of lipoprotein changes induced by diuretics may be moot subjects, since it appears that such changes may easily be reversed by simple dietary measures (Grimm et al., 1981) or co-administration of beta-blockers (Meier et al., 1982; Schiffl et al., 1982).

V. CONCLUSION

From the foregoing discussions it is evident that a considerable body of knowledge has accumulated over the past 25 years on the use of diuretics in the treatment of EBH. We are closer than ever to understanding how these agents produce their antihypertensive effects, and to an appreciation of the mechanisms behind and significance of the side effects that accompany their use. Yet, controversy continues to exist on all of these fronts, both from basic and practical standpoints. This controversy will catalyze continuing research in these areas, producing, hopefully, in time, an even clearer picture than we have today.

Although there is general agreement on the value of treatment of moderate to severe EBH, there continues to be considerable debate on the value of treatment of the mild or borderline forms this disease (McAlister, 1983). The decision to treat such patients will, for the immediate future, be highly individualized, taking into consideration each patient's lifestyle, cardiovascular risk factors and likelihood of compliance with therapy.

It is generally accepted, however, that in the treatment of EBH, "blood pressure reduction should be planned as a gentle seduction rather than acute battle" (Lancet, 1977). Among other factors, "quality of life" and patient compliance are important considerations behind such philosophy, especially as it relates to the treatment of the milder forms of the disease. All factors considered, it appears that diuretics remain the most appropriate "seductress" with which to begin therapy of EBH. Further advances in our understanding of EBH and the effects and side effects of diuretics, as well as the development of diuretics with improved profiles, will likely further solidify this position in the future.

REFERENCES

Abe, K., Otsuka, Y., Yasujima, M., Chiba, S., Seino, M., Irokawa, N., and Yoshinaga, K. (1976). Metabolism of PG in man: effect of furosemide on the excretion of the main metabolite of PG $F_{2\alpha}$. Prostaglandins 12, 843-848.

Abe, K., Yasujima, M., Chiba, S., Irokawa, N., Ito, T., and Yoshinaga, K. (1977). Effect of furosemide on urinary excretion of prostaglandin E in normal volunteers and patients with essential hypertension. Prostaglandins 14, 513-521.

Addison, W. L. T. (1928). The use of sodium chloride, potassium chloride, sodium bromide and potassium bromide in cases of arterial hypertension which are amenable to potassium chloride. Can. Med. J. 18, 281-285.

Adetuyibi, A., and Mills, I. H. (1972). Relation between urinary kallikrein and renal function, hypertension, and excretion of sodium and water in man. Lancet 2, 203-207.

Adragna, N. C., Canessa, M. L., Solomon, H., Slater, E., and Tosteson, D. C. (1982). Red cell lithium-sodium countertransport and sodium-potassium cotransport in patients with essential hypertenison. Hypertension 4, 795-804.

Alderman, M. H. (1981). Position Paper: the variation in risk among hypertensive patients: is broad scale therapy to help only a few justifiable? What pressure levels should be treated? In "Frontiers in Hypertension Research" (J. H. Laragh, F. R. Buehler and D. W. Seldin, eds.), pp. 9-14.

Springer-Verlag, New York.

Altman, J., Garay, R., Papadimitriou, A., and Worcel, M. (1977). Alterations in ^{22}Na fluxes of arterial smooth muscles of spontaneously hypertensive rats. Br. J. Pharmacol. **59**, 496P.

Ambrosioni, E., Costa, F. V., Montebugnoli, L., Tartagni, F., and Magnani, B. (1981a). Increased intralymphocytic sodium content in essential hypertension: an index of impaired Na^+ cellular metabolism. Clin. Sci. **61**, 181-186.

Ambrosioni, E., Costa, F. V., Montebugnoli, L., Cavallini, C., and Magnani, B. (1981b). Effects of antihypertensive therapy on intralymphocytic sodium content. Drugs Exptl. Clin. Res. **7**, 757-762.

Ambrosioni, E., Costa, F. V., Borghi, C., Montebugnoli, L., Giordani, M. F., and Magnani, B. (1982). Effects of moderate salt restriction on intralymphocytic sodium and pressor response to stress in borderline hypertension. Hypertension **4**, 789-794.

American Journal Hospital Pharm. (1975). Current drug therapy-- thiazide diuretics. **32**, 473-480.

Amery, A., Bulpitt, C., deSchaepdryver, A., Fagard, R., Hellemans, J., Mutsers, A., Berthaux, P., Deruyttere, M., Dollery, C., Forette, F., Lund-Johansen, P., and Tuomilehto, J. (1978). Glucose intolerance during diuretic therapy. Results of trial by the European working party on hypertension in the elderly. Lancet **1**, 681-683.

Ames, R. P. (1974). Relation of serum uric acid to plasma renin activity and the response of primary hypertension to treatment. Am. Soc. Neph. Abst. **7**, 2.

Ames, R. P. (1983). Negative effects of diuretic drugs on metabolic risk factors for coronary heart disease: possible alternative drug therapies. Am. J. Cardiol. **51**, 632-638.

Ames, R. P., and Hill, P. (1981). Metabolic risks of diuretic therapy. In "Frontiers in Hypertension Research" (J. H. Laragh, F. R. Buehler and D. W. Seldin, eds.), pp. 49-53. Springer-Verlag, New York.

Ames, R. P., and Hill, P. (1982). Antihypertensive therapy and risk of coronary heart disesase. J. Cardiovasc. Pharmacol. **4**, S206-S212.

Anderson, R. J., Berl, T., McDonald, K. M., and Schrier, R. W. (1976). Prostaglandins: effects on blood pressure, renal blood flow, sodium, and water excretion. Kidney Int. **10**

(Suppl. 2), 205-215.

Araoye, M. A., Khatri, I. M., Yao, L. L., and Freis, E. D. (1978). Leukocyte intracellular cations in hypertension: effect of antihypertensive drugs. Am. Heart J. 96, 731-738.

Bailie, M. D., and Barbour, J. A. (1975). Effect of inhibition of peptidase activity on distribution of intrarenal blood flow. Am. J. Physiol. 228, 850-853.

Bartelheimer, H. K., Losert, W., Senft, G., and Sitt, R. (1967). Stoerungen des kohlenhydratstoffwechsels im kaliummangel. Naunyn-Schmiedeberg's Arch. Pharmakol. Exp. Pathol. 258, 391-408.

Baylis, P. H. and DeBeer, F. C. (1981). Human plasma vaso-pression response to potent loop-diuretic drugs. Eur. J. Clin. Pharmacol. 20, 343-346.

Bealer, S. L., Haywood, J. R., Gruber, K. A., Buckalew, V. M., Jr., Fink, G. D., Brody, M. J., and Johnson, A. K. (1983). Preoptic-hypothalamic periventricular lesions reduce na-triuresis to volume expansion. Am. J. Physiol. 244, R51-R57.

Beeley, L. (1980). Errors and misconceptions in drug prescribing. J. Royal Coll. Phy. London 14, 58-64.

Beevers, D. G., Hawthorne, V. M., and Padfield, P. L. (1980). Salt and blood pressure in Scotland. Br. Med. J. 281, 641-642.

Bello-Reuss, E., Trevino, D. L., and Gottschalk, C. W. (1976). Effect of renal sympathetic nerve stimulation on proximal water and sodium reabsorption. J. Clin. Invest. 57, 1104-1107.

Bello-Reuss, E., Pastoriza-Munoz, E., and Colindres, R. E. (1977). Acute unilateral renal denervation in rats with extracellular volume expansion. Am. J. Physiol. 232, F26-F32.

Bengele, H. H., Houttuin, E., and Pearce, J. W. (1972). Volume natriuresis without renal nerves and renal vascular pressure rise in the dog. Am. J. Physiol. 223, 68-73.

Bengtsson, C., Lennartsson, J., Lindquist, O., Lindstedt, G., Lundberg, P. A., Noppa, H., Sigurdsson, J. A., and Tibblin, E. (1982). On metabolic effects of diuretics and β-blockers. Acta Med. Scand. 212, 57-64.

Ben-Ishay, D., Knudsen, K. D., and Dahl, L. K. (1973). Exagger-ated response to isotonic saline loading in genetically hypertension-prone rats. J. Lab. Clin. Med. 82, 597-604.

Bennett, W. M., McDonald, W. J., Kuehnel, E., Harnett, M. N., and Porter, G. A. (1977). Do diuretics have antihypertensive properties independent of natriuresis? Clin. Pharmacol.

Ther. **22**, 499-504.

Berchtold, P., Cueppers, H. J., and Berger, M. (1981). Diuretika, serum-glucose und diabetes mellitus. Dtsch. Med. Wschr. **106**, 1712-1714.

Berglund, G., and Andersson, O. (1981). Beta-blockers or diuretics in hypertension? A six year follow-up of blood pressure and metabolic side effects. Lancet **1**, 744-747.

Bergstrom, J., and Hultman, E. (1966). The effect of thiazides, chlorthalidone, and furosemide on muscle electrolytes and muscle glycogen in normal subjects. Acta Med. Scand. **180**, 363-376.

Bergstrom, J., Hultman, E., and Solheim, S. B. (1973). The effect of mefruside on plasma and muscle electrolytes in normal subjects and in patients with essential hypertension. Acta Med. Scand. **194**, 427-433.

Black, J., Waeber, B., Bresnahan, M. R., Gavras, I., and Gavras, H. (1981). Blood pressure response to central and/or peripheral inhibition of phenylethanolamine N-methyltransferase in normotensive and hypertensive rats. Circ. Res. **49**, 518-524.

Blaustein, M. P. (1977). Sodium ions, calcium ions, blood pressure regulation, and hypertension: a reassessment and a hypothesis. Am. J. Physiol. 232, C165-C173.

Blaustein, M. P., and Hamlyn, J. M. (1983). Role of a natriuretic factor in essential hypertension: an hypothesis. Ann. Intern. Med. **98** (Part 2), 785-792.

Boehringer, K., Meier, A., Weidmann, P., Schiffl, H., Mordasini, R., and Riesen, W. (1981). Einfluss von hydrochlorothiazid/amilorid allein oder in kombination mit α-methyldopa auf die serumlipoproteine. Schweiz. Med. Wschr. **111**, 525-530.

Brater, D. C., Beck, J. M., Adams, B. V., and Campbell, W. B. (1980). Effects of indomethacin on furosemide-stimulated urinary PGE_2 excretion in man. Eur. J. Pharmacol. **65**, 213-219.

Brody, M. J., and Johnson, A. K. (1980). Role of the anteroventral third ventricle region in fluid and electrolyte balance, arterial pressure regulation and hypertension. In "Frontiers in Neuroendocrinology" (L. Martini and W. F. Ganong, eds.), pp. 249-292. Raven Press, New York.

Brown, M. S., Kovanen, P. T., and Goldstein, J. L. (1981). Regulation of plasma cholesterol by lipoprotein receptors. Science 212, 628-635.

Brunner, H. R., Gavras, H., and Waeber, B. (1980). Enhancement by diuretics of the antihypertensive action of long-term angiotensin converting enzyme blockade. Clin. Exp. Hypertension 2, 639-657.

Brunner, H. R., Laragh, J. H., Baer, L., Newton, M. A., Goodwin, F. T., Krakoff, L. R., Bard, R. H., and Buehler, F. R. (1972). Essential Hypertension: renin and aldosterone, heart attack and stroke. N. Engl. J. Med. 286, 441-449.

Buehler, F. R., Burkart, F., Luetold, B. E., Kung, M., Marbet, G., and Pfisterer, M. (1975). Antihypertensive beta blocking action as related to renin and age: A pharmacologic tool to identify pathogenetic mechanisms in essential hypertension. Am. J. Cardiol. 36, 653-669.

Buehler, F. R., Laragh, J. H., Vaughan, E. D., Jr., Brunner, H. R., Gavras, H., and Baer, L. (1973). Antihypertensive action of propranolol. Specific antirenin responses in high and normal renin forms of essential renal, renovascular and malignant hypertension. Am. J. Cardiol. 32, 511-522.

Buehler, F. R., Laragh, J. H., Baer, L., Vaughan, E. D., Jr., and Brunner, H. R. (1972). Propranolol inhibition of renin secretion. N. Engl. J. Med. 287, 1209-1214.

Campese, V. M., Romoff, M. S., Levitan, D., Saglikes, Y., Friedler, R. M., and Massry, S. G. (1982). Abnormal relationship between sodium intake and sympathetic nervous system activity in salt-sensitive patients with essential hypertension. Kidney Int. 21, 371-378.

Canessa, M., Adragna, N., Solomen, H. S., Connolly, T. M., and Tosteson, D. C. (1980). Increased sodium-lithium countertransport in red cells of patients with essential hypertension. N. Engl. J. Med. 302, 772-776.

Canessa, M., Bize, I., Solomon, H., Adragna, N., Tosteson, D. C., Dagher, G., Garay, R., and Meyer, P. (1981). Na countertransport and cotransport in human red cells: function, dysfunction, and genes in essential hypertension. Clin. Exp. Hypertension 3, 783-795.

Cannon, P. J., Stason, W. B., Demartini, F. E., Sommers, S. C., and Laragh, J. H. (1966). Hyperuricemia in primary and renal hypertension. N. Engl. J. Med. 275, 457-464.

Caralis, P., Perez-Stable, E., Materson, B., and Rozanski, J. (1981). Ventricular ectopy and diuretic-induced hypokalemia in hypertensive patients. Clin. Res. 29, 832A.

Caviares, J. D. (1977). The sodium pump in human red cells. In "Membrane transport in red cells" (J. C. Ellory and V. L. Lew, eds.), pp. 1-37. Academic Press, London.

Chan, P. C., and Sanslone, W. R. (1969). The influence of a low-potassium diet on rat-erythrocyte membrane adenosine triphosphatase. Arch. Biochem. Biophys. **134**, 48-52.

Clark, B. G., Wheatley, R., Rawlings, J. L., and Vestal, R. E. (1982). Female preponderance in diuretic-associated hypokalemia: a retrospective study in seven long-term care facilities. J. Am. Geriatr. Soc. **30**, 316-321.

Clarkson, E. M., Talner, L. B., and deWardener, H. E. (1970). The effect of plasma from blood volume expanded dogs on sodium, potassium and PAH transport of renal tubule fragments. Clin. Sci. **38**, 617-627.

Clarkson, E. M., Raw, S.M., and deWardener, H. E. (1979). Further observations on a low-molecular-weight natriuretic substance in the urine of normal man. Kidney Int. **16**, 710-721.

Clarkson, E. M., MacGregor, G. A., and deWardener, H. E. (1980). Observations using red cells, on the natriferic properties of plasma from normotensive and hypertensive individuals, and of the low molecular weight natriuretic substance obtained from human urine. In "Intracellular Electrolytes and Arterial Hypertension" (H. Zumkley and H. Losse, eds.), pp. 95-97. Theime-Stratton, New York.

Clegg, G., Morgan, D. B., and Davidson, C, (1982). The heterogeneity of essential hypertension: relation between lithium efflux and sodium content of erythrocytes and a family history of hypertension. Lancet **2**, 891-894.

Cole, C. H. (1983). Erythrocyte membrane sodium transport in patients with treated and untreated essential hypertension. Circulation **68**, 17-22.

Conway, J., and Lauwers, P. (1960). Hemodynamic and hypotensive effects of long term therapy with chlorothiazide. Circulation **21**, 21-27.

Costa, F. V., Ambrosioni, E., Montebugnoli, L., Paccaloni, L., Vasconi, L., and Magnani, B. (1981). Effects of a low-salt diet and of acute salt loading on blood pressure and intra-lymphocytic sodium concentration in young subjects with borderline hypertension. Clin. Sci. **61**, 21S-23S.

Cowley, A. W., Jr., Cushman, W. C., Quillen, E. W., Jr., Skelton, M. M., and Langford, H. G. (1981). Vasopressin elevation in essential hypertension and increased responsiveness to sodium intake. Hypertension **3**, (Suppl. I), I-93--I-100.

Craven, P. A., and DeRubertis, F. R. (1982). Calcium-dependent stimulation of renal medullary prostaglandin synthesis by furosemide. J. Pharmacol. Exp. Ther. 222, 306–314.

Crofton, J. T., Share, L., Shade, R. E., Lee-Kwon, W. J., Manning, M., and Sawyer, W. H. (1979). The importance of vasopressin in the development and maintenance of DOC-salt hypertension in the rat. Hypertension 1, 31–38.

Croxatto, H. R., Roblero, J., Garcia, R., Corthorn, J., and San Martin, A. L. (1973). Effect of furosemide upon urinary kallikiein excretion. Agents and Actions 3, 267–274.

Curtis, J. J., Luke, R. G., Dustan, H. P., Kashgarian, M., Whelchel, J. D., Jones, P., and Diethelm, A. G. (1983). Remission of essential hypertension after renal transplantation. N. Engl. J. Med. 17, 1009–1015.

Cusi, D., Barlassina, C., Ferrandi, M., Palazzi, P., Celega, E., and Bianchi, G. (1981). Relationship between altered Na^+- K^+ cotransport and Na^+-Li^+countertransport in the erythrocytes of 'essential' hypertensive patients. Clin. Sci. 61, 33S–36S.

Dahl, L. K., Knudsen, K. D., and Iwai, J. (1969). Humoral transmission of hypertension: evidence from parabiosis. Circ. Res. 24 (Suppl. I), 21–33.

Dargie, H. J., Boddy, K., Kennedy, A. C., King, P. C., Read, P. R., and Ward, D. M. (1974). Total body potassium in long-term frusemide therapy: is potassium supplementation necessary? Br. Med. J. 4, 316–319.

Dawber, T. R., Kannel, W. B., Kagan, A., Donabedian, R. K., and McNamara, P. M. (1967). Environmental factors in Hypertension. In "Epidemiology of hypertension" (J. Stamler, R. Stamler, and R. B. Pulliman, eds.), pp. 255– 288. Grune and Stratton, New York.

deSolms, S. J., Woltersdorf, O. W., Jr., and Cragoe, E. J., Jr. (1978). (Acylaryloxy)acetic acid diuretics. 2. (2-Alkyl-2-aryl-1-oxo-5-indanyloxy)acetic acids. J. Med. Chem. 21, 437–443.

deWardener, H. E. (1982). The natriuretic hormone. Ann. Clin. Biochem. 19, 137–140.

deWardener, H. E., and Clarkson, E. M. (1982). The natriuretic hormone: recent developments. Clin. Sci. 63, 415–420.

deWardener, H.E., and Macgregor, G. A. (1980). Dahl's hypothesis that a saluretic substance may be responsible for a sustained rise in arterial pressure: Its possible role in essential hypertension. Kidney Int. 18, 1–9.

DiBona, G. F. (1983). Neural mechanisms of volume regulation. Ann. Intern. Med. 98 (Part 2), 750–752.

DiPette, D., Waeber, B., Volicer, L., Chao, P., Gavras, I., Gavras, H., and Brunner, H. (1983). Salt-induced hypertension in chronic renal failure: evidence for a neurogenic mechanism. Life Sci. 32, 733-740.

Dolak, T. M., and Goldberg, L. I. (1981). Renal blood flow and dopaminergic agonists. Annu. Rep. Med. Chem. 16, 103-111.

Dollery, C. T. (1968). Changes in carbohydrate metabolism after the use of diuretics. In "Drug Induced Diseases, Vol. 3" (L. Meyler and H. M. Peck, eds.), pp. 95-102. Excerpta Medica, Amsterdam.

Dollery, C. T. (1973). Diabetogenic effect of long-term diuretic therapy. In "Modern Diuretic Therapy in the Treatment of Cardiovascular and Renal Disease" (A. F. Lant and G. M. Wilson, eds.), pp. 320-330. Excerpta Medica, Amsterdam.

Doyle, A. E., Chua, K. G., and Duffy, S. (1976). Urinary sodium potassium and creatinine excretion in hypertensive and normotensive Australians. Med. J. Aust. 2, 898-890.

Duhm, J., Gobel, B. O., Lorenz, R., and Weber, P. C. (1982). Sodium-lithium exchange and sodium-potassium cotransport in human erythrocytes. Hypertension 4, 477-482.

Dunn, M. J., and Zambraski, E. J. (1980). Renal effects of drugs that inhibit prostaglandin synthesis. Kidney Int. 18, 609-622.

Dustan, H. P., Tarazi, R. C., and Bravo, E. L. (1974). Diuretic and diet treatment of hypertension. Arch. Intern. Med. 133, 1007-1013.

Edmondson, R. P. S., Thomas, R. D., Hilton, P. J., Patrick, J., and Jones, N. F. (1974). Leucocyte electrolytes in cardiac and non-cardiac patients receiving diuretics. Lancet 1, 12-14.

Edmondson, R. P. S., Thomas, R. D., Hilton, P. J., Patrick, J., and Jones, N. F. (1975). Abnormal leucocyte composition and sodium transport in essential hypertension. Lancet 1, 1003-1005.

Edmondson, R. P. S., and MacGregor, G. A. (1981). Leucocyte cation transport in essential hypertension: its relation to the renin-angiotensin system. Br. Med. J. 282, 1267-1269.

Epstein, M., Bricker, N. S., and Bourgoignie, J. J. (1978). Presence of a natriuretic factor in urine of normal men undergoing water immersion. Kidney Int. 13, 152-158.

Erdmann, E., Werdan, K., Hegelberger, R., Pruchniewski, M., and Christl, St. (1980). Determination of the number of (Na^++K^+)-ATPase molecules, their enzymatic activity and

the active Na⁺/K⁺-transport of human erythrocytes in
hypokalaemia and in hypertension. In "Intracellular Elec-
trolytes and Arterial Hypertension" (H. Zumkley and H.
Losse, eds.), pp. 164-170. Thieme-Stratton, New York.
Fajans, S. S., Floyd, J. C., Jr., Knopf, R. F., Rull, J., Guntsche,
E. M., and Conn, J. W. (1966). Benzothiadiazine suppression
of insulin release from normal and abnormal islet tissue in
man. J. Clin. Invest. 45, 481-492.
Favre, L., Glasson, P., Riondel, A., and Vallotton, M. B. (1983).
Interaction of diuretics and nonsteroidal antiinflammatory
drugs in man. Clin. Sci. 64, 407-415.
Ferris, T. F., and Gorden, P. (1968). Effect of angiotensin and
norepinephrine upon urate clearance in man. Am. J. Med.
44, 359-365.
Fessel, W. J., Siegelaub, A. B., and Johnson, E. S. (1973). Correlates and consequences of asymptomatic hyperuricemia.
Arch. Intern. Med. 132, 44-54.
Fessel, W. J. (1980). High uric acid as an indicator of cardiovascular disease. Independence from obesity. Am. J. Med.
68, 401-404.
Finnerty, F. A. (1959). Special problems in therapy of hypertension. Discussion. In "Hypertension: First Hahneman
Symposium on Hypertensive Disease" (J. H. Moyer, ed.), pp.
653-654. W. B. Saunders Co., Philadelphia.
Finnerty, F. A., Jr. (1978). Hypertension: current management.
Part 2. Therapy—the stepped care approach. Consultant,
126-139.
Finnerty, F. A., Jr. (1979). Diuretics as initial treatment for
essential hypertension. Br. J. Clin. Pharmacol., 185S-
187S.
Fishman, M. C. (1979). Endogenous digitalis-like activity in
mammalian brain. Proc. Nat. Acad. Sci. 76, 4661-4663.
Fitzgibbon, W. R., Morgan, T. O., and Myers, J. B. (1980).
Erythrocyte ²²Na efflux and urinary sodium excretion in
essential hypertension. Clin. Sci. 59 (Suppl. 6), 195S-197S.
Folkow, B. (1978). Cardiovascular structural adaptation: its role
in the initiation and maintenance of primary hypertension.
Clin. Sci. Mol. Med. 55, 3S-22S.
Freis, E. D. (1959). Clinical pharmacology and use of chloro-
thiazide in the treatment of hypertension. In "Hyper-
tension: First Hahneman Symposium on Hypertensive
Disease" (J. H. Moyer, ed.), pp. 545-549. W. B. Saunders Co,
Philadelphia.

Freis, E. D. (1979a). Treatment of hypertension: state of the art in 1979. Clin. Sci. **57**, 349S-353S.

Freis, E. D. (1979b). Salt in hypertension and the effects of diuretics. Annu. Rev. Pharmacol. Toxicol. **19**, 13-23.

Freis, E. D. (1981). Sodium in hypertension: clinical aspects and dietary management. Curr. Concepts Nutr. **10**, 127-130.

Freis, E. D. and Sappington, R. F. (1966). Long-term effect of Probenecid on diuretic-induced hyperuricemia. J. Am. Med. Assoc. **198**, 127-129.

Frolich, J. C., Whorton, A. R., Walker, L., Smigel, M., Oates, J. A., France, R., Hollifield, J. W., Data, J. L., Gerber, J. G., Nies, A. S., Williams, W., and Robertson, G. L. (1978). Renal prostaglandins: regional differences in synthesis and role in renin release and ADH action. Proc. Int. Congr. Nephrol. **7**, 107-114.

Fuller, J. H., McCartney, P., Jarrett, R. J., Keen, H., Rose, G., Shipley, M. J., and Hamilton, P. J. S. (1979). Hyperglycaemia and coronary heart disease: the Whitehall study. J. Chronic Dis. **32**, 721-728.

Fuller, J. H., Shipley, M. J., Rose, G., Jarrett, R. J., and Keen, H. (1980). Coronary-heart-disease risk and impaired glucose tolerance. The Whitehall study. Lancet **1**, 1373-1376.

Ganguli, M., Tobian, L., Iwai, J., and Johnson, M. A. (1981). Potassium citrate feeding protects against nephron loss in severe sodium chloride hypertension in rats. Clin. Sci. **61**, 73S-75S.

Ganong, W. F. (1972). Sympathetic effects on renin secretion: mechanism and physiological role. In "Control of Renin Excretion" (T. A. Assaykeen, ed.), pp. 17-32. Plenum Press, New York.

Garay, R. P., and Dagher, G. (1980). Erythrocyte Na^+ and K^+ transport systems in essential hypertension. In "Intracellular Electrolytes and Arterial Hypertension" (H. Zumkley and H. Losse, eds.), pp. 69-76. Thieme-Stratton New York.

Garay, R. P., Dagher, G., Pernollet, M. G., Devynck, M. A., and Meyer, P. (1980). Inherited defect in a Na^+-K^+-co-transport system in erythrocytes from essential hypertensive patients. Nature **284**, 281-283.

Garay, R. P., Hannaert, P., Dagher, G., Nazaret, C., Maridonneau, I., and Meyer, P. (1981). Abnormal erythrocyte Na^+-K^+ cotransport system, a proposed genetic marker of essential hypertension. Clin. Exp. Hypertension **3**, 851-859.

Gessler, U. (1962). Intra- und extrazellulare electrolyt-veranderungen bei essentieller hypertonie vor und nach behandlung. Z. Kreislaufforsch. **51**, 177-183.

Ghione, S., Buzzigoli, G., Bartolini, V., Balzan, S., and Donato, L. (1981). Comparison of outward and inward Na^+/K^+ cotransport-mediated fluxes in erythrocytes of essential hypertensive patients. Preliminary results. Clin. Exp. Hypertension 3, 809-814.

Gill, J. R., Jr., and Casper, A. G. T. (1971). Depression of proximal tubular sodium reabsorption in the dog in response to renal beta adrenergic stimulation by isoproterenol. J. Clin. Invest. **50**, 112-118.

Glueck, Z., Baumgartner, G., Weidmann, P., Peheim, E., Bachmann, C., Mordasini, R., Flammer, J., and Keusch, G. (1978). Increased ratio between serum alpha-and beta-1 ipoproteins during diuretic therapy: an adverse effect? Clin. Sci. Mol. Med. **55**, 325s-328s.

Goldman, A. I., Steele, B. W., Schnaper, H. W., Fitz, A. E., Frohlich, E. D., and Perry, H. M., Jr. (1980). Serum lipoprotein levels during chlorthalidone therapy. A Veterans Administration-National Heart, Lung, and Blood Institute cooperative study on antihypertensive therapy: mild hypertension. J. Am Med. Assoc. **244**, 1691-1695.

Goldner, M. G., Zarowitz, H., and Akgun, S. (1960). Hyperglycemia and glycosuria due to thiazide derivatives administred in diabetes mellitus. N. Engl. J. Med. **262**, 403-405.

Gonick, H. C., Kramer, H. J., Paul, W., and Lu, E. (1977). Circulating inhibitor of sodium-potassium activated adenosine triphosphatase after expansion of extracellular fluid volume in rats. Clin. Sci. **53**, 329-334.

Gordon, R. S. (1981). Sodium transport as diagnostic tool for secondary hypertension. J. Am. Med. Assoc. **245**, 1404.

Gordon, T., and Kannel, W. B. (1971). Premature mortality from coronary heart disease. The Framingham Study. J. Am. Med. Assoc. **215**, 1617-1625.

Gordon, T., Castelli, W. P., Hjortland, M. C., Kannel, W. B., and Dawber, T. R. (1977). High density lipoprotein as a protective factor against coronary heart disease. The Framingham study. Am. J. Med. **62**, 707-714.

Goto, A., Ganguli, M., Tobian, L., Johnson, M. A., and Iwai, J. (1982). Effect of an anteroventral third ventricle lesion on NaCl hypertension in Dahl salt-sensitive rats. Am. J.

Physiol. **243**, H614-H618.

Granger, H. J., and Guyton, A. C. (1969). Autoregulation of the total systemic circulation following destruction of the central nervous system in the dog. Circ. Res. **25**, 379-388.

Graybiel, A. L., and Sode, J. (1971). Diuretics, potassium depletion and carbohydrate intolerance. Lancet **2**, 265.

Grimm, R. H. Jr., Leon, A. S., Hunninghake, D. B., Lenz, K., Hannan, P., and Blackburn, H. (1981). Effects of thiazide diuretics on plasma lipids and lipoproteins in mildly hypertensive patients. Ann. Intern. Med. **94**, 7-11.

Gruber, K. A., and Buckalew, V. M., Jr. (1978). Further characterization and evidence for a precursor in the formation of plasma antinatriferic factor. Proc. Soc. Exp. Biol. Med. **159**, 463-467.

Gruber, K. A., Hennessy, J. F., Buckalew, V. M. Jr., and Lymangrover J. R. (1983). Identification of a heptapeptide with digitalis and natriuretic hormone like properties. Kidney Int. **23**, 170.

Gruber, K. A., Whitaker, J. M., and Buckalew, V. M., Jr. (1980). Endogenous digitalis-like substance in plasma of volume-expanded dogs. Nature **287**, 743-745.

Guyton, A. C., Hall, J. E., Lohmeier, T. E., Jackson, T. E., and Kastner, P. R. (1981). Blood pressure regulation: basic concepts. Fed. Proc. **40**, 2252-2256.

Haas, M., Schooler, J., and Tosteson, D. C. (1975). Coupling of lithium to sodium transport in human red cells. Nature **258**, 425-427.

Haddy, F. J., Emerson, T. E., Jr., Scott, J. B., and Daugherty, R. M., Jr. (1970). The effect of the kinins on the cardiovascular system. In "Handbook of Experimental Pharmacology" **25** (E. G. Erdos, ed.), pp. 362-384. Springer-Verlag, New York.

Haddy, F. J. (1980). Mechanism, prevention and therapy of sodium-dependent hypertension. Am. J. Med. **69**, 746-758.

Haddy, F. J. (1982). Humoral factors and the sodium-potassium pump in low renin hypertension. Klin. Wochenschr. **60**, 1254-1257.

Haddy, F. J. (1983). Sodium-potassium pump in low-renin hypertension. Ann. Int. Med. **93** (Part 2), 781-784.

Hall, A. P. (1965). Correlations among hyperuricemia, hypercholesterolemia, coronary disease and hypertension. Arthritis and Rheumat. **8**, 846-852.

Hamdy, R. C., Tovey, J., and Perera, N. (1980). Hypokalaemia and diuretics. Br. Med. J. **280**, 1187.

Hansen, O. E. (1966). Hyperuricemia, gout, and atherosclerosis. Am. Heart J. **72**, 570-573.

Hansson, L. (1976). The use of propranolol in hypertension: a review. Postgrad. Med. J. **52** (Suppl. 4), 77-80.

Haupert, G. T., Jr., and Sancho, J. M. (1979). Sodium transport inhibitor from bovine hypothalamus. Proc. Nat. Acad. Sci. **76**, 4658-4660.

Heagerty, A. M., Bing, R. F., Milner, M., Thurston, H., and Swales, J. D. (1982). Leucocyte membrane sodium transport in normotensive populations: dissociation of abnormalities of sodium efflux from raised blood-pressure. Lancet **2**, 894-896.

Healy, J. J., McKenna, T. J., Canning, B. St. J., Brien, T. G., Duffy, G. J., and Muldowney, F. P. (1970). Body composition changes in hypertensive subjects on long-term oral diuretic therapy. Br. Med. J. **1**, 716-719.

Hebert, S. C., Schafer, J. A., and Andreoli, T. E. (1981). The effects of antidiuretic hormone (ADH) on solute and water transport in the mammalian nephron. J. Membr. Biol. **58**, 1-19.

Henschke, P. J., Spence, J. D., and Cape, R. D. T. (1981). Diuretics and the institutional elderly: a case against routine potassium prescribing. J. Am. Geriatr. Soc. **29**, 145-150.

Holland, O. B., Gomez-Sanchez, C., Fairchild, C., and Kaplan, N. M. (1979). Role of renin classification for diuretic treatment of black hypertensive patients. Arch. Intern. Med. **139**, 1365-1370.

Holland, O. B., Nixon, J. V., and Kuhnert, L. (1981). Diuretic-induced ventricular ectopic activity. Am. J. Med. **70**, 762-768.

Hulley, S. B. (1978). The high-density lipoproteins: epidemiological and practical considerations. Pract. Cardiol. **4**, 70-82.

Hypertension Detection and Follow-up Program Cooperative Group (1979). Five-year findings of the hypertension detection and follow-up program. I. Reduction in mortality of persons with high blood pressure, including mild hypertension. J. Am. Med. Assoc. **242**, 2562-2571.

Hypertension Detection and Follow-up Program Cooperative Group (1979). Five-year findings of the hypertension detection and follow-up program. II. Mortality by Race-Sex and Age. J. Am. Med. Assoc. **242**, 2572-2577.

Hypertension Detection and Follow-up Program Cooperative Group (1982). The effect of treatment on mortality in "mild" hypertension. Results of the hypertension detection and follow-up program. N. Engl. J. Med. **307**, 976-980.

Ibrahim, I. K., Ritch, A. E. S., MacLennan, W. J., and May, T. (1978). Are potassium supplements for the elderly necessary? Age and Ageing **7**, 165-170.

Ibsen, H., Leth, A., Hollnagel, H., Kappelgaard, A. M., Nielsen, M. D., Christensen, N. J., and Giese, J. (1979). Renin-angiotensin system in mild essential hypertension. Acta Med. Scand. **205**, 547-555.

Iimura, O., Kijima, T., Kikuchi, K., Miyama, A., Ando, T., Nakao, T., and Takigami, Y. (1981). Studies on the hypotensive effect of high potassium intake in patients with essential hypertension. Clin. Sci. **61**, 77S-80S.

Ikeda, T., Tobian, L., Iwai, J., and Goossens, P. (1978). Central nervous system pressor responses in rats susceptible and resistant to sodium chloride hypertension. Clin. Sci. Mol. Med. **55** (Suppl. 4), 225S-227S.

James-Kracke, M. R., Kracke, G. R., and Lang, S. (1981). Identification of a vasoactive substance (vasopressin) in a brain extract containing an unknown inhibitor of Na,K-ATPase. Clin. Exp. Hypertension **3**, 523-538.

Jandhyala, B., Gothberg, G., and Folkow, B. (1980). Resistance vessel responsiveness in the Okamoto-Aoki spontaneously hypertensive rat (SHR) compared with Wistar-Kyoto (WKY) and ordinary Wistar normotensive controls (NCR) before and after ouabain inhibition of the membrane sodium and potassium pump. In "Intracellular Electrolytes and Arterial Hypertension" (H. Zumkley and H. Losse, eds.), pp. 127-134. Thieme-Stratton, New York.

Johnson, M. W., and Mitch, W. E. (1981). The risks of asymptomatic hyperuricaemia and the use of uricosuric diuretics. Drugs **21**, 220-225.

Joint National Committee on Detection, Evaluation, and Treatment of High Blood Pressure (1977). Report of the Joint National Commiteee on detection, evaluation and treatment of high blood pressure. A cooperative study. J. Am. Med. Assoc. **237**, 255-261.

Joint National Committee on Detection, Evaluation, and Treatment of High Blood Pressure (1980). The 1980 report of the Joint National Commiteee on detection, evaluation and treatment of high blood pressure. Arch. Intern. Med. **140**, 1280–1285.

Jones, A. W. (1974). Altered ion transport in large and small arteries from spontaneously hypertensive rats and the influence of calcium. Circ. Res. **34** (Suppl. I), 117–122.

Joos, C., and Kewitz, H. (1979). Erhohung der "very low density lipoproteine" (VLDL) im plasma gesunder manner wahrend der behandlung mit diuretica. Verh. Dtsch. Ges. Inn. Med. **85**, 604–607.

Joos, C., Kewitz, H., and Reinhold-Kourniati, D. (1980). Effects of diuretics on plasma lipoproteins in healthy men. Eur. J. Clin. Pharmacol. **17**, 251–257.

Johnson, B. F. (1982). The emerging problem of plasma lipid changes during antihypertensive therapy. J. Cardiovasc. Pharmacol. **4** (Suppl. 2), S213–S221.

Kaess, H., Schlierf, G., Ehlers, W., von Mikulicz-Radecki, J.-G., Hassenstein, P., Walter, K., Brech, W., and Hengstmann, J. (1971). The carbohydrate metabolism of normal subjects during potassium depletion. Diabetologia **7**, 82–86.

Kaess, H., Senft, G., Losert, W., Sitt, R., and Schultz, G. (1966). Mechanismus der gesteigerten glykogenolytischen wirkung des diazoxids im kaliummangel. Naunyn-Schmiedebergs Arch. Exp. Pathol. Pharmakol. **253**, 395–401.

Kannel, W. B. (1981). Implications of Framingham study data for treatment of hypertension: impact of other risk factors. In "Frontiers in Hypertension Research" (J. H. Laragh, F. R. Buehler, and D. W. Seldin, eds.), pp. 17–21. Springer-Verlag, New York.

Kassirer, J. P., and Harrington, J. T. (1979). Diuretics and potassium metabolism: a reassessment of the need, effectiveness and safety of potassium therapy. Kidney Int. **11**, 505–515.

Kawasaki, T., Delea, C. S., Bartter, F. C., and Smith, H. (1978). The effect of high-sodium and low-sodium intakes on blood pressure and other related variables in human subjects with idiopathic hypertension. Am. J. Med. **64**, 193–198.

Kawasaki, T., Ueno, M., Uezono, K., Abe, I., Kawano, Y., Ogata, M., Omae, T., and Fukiyama, K. (1981). Salt intake and hypertension. Jpn. Circ. J. **45**, 810–816.

Kempner, W. (1948). Treatment of hypertensive vascular disease with rice diet. Am. J. Med. **4**, 545–577.

Khokhar, A. M., and Slater, J. D. H. (1976). Increased renal excretion of arginine-vasopressin during mild hydropenia in young men with mild essential hypertension. Clin. Sci. Mol. Med. **51**, 691S-694S.

Klingmuller, D., Weiler, E., and Kramer, H. J. (1982). Digoxin-like natriuretic activity in the urine of salt loaded healthy subjects. Klin. Wochenscrift, **60**, 1249-1253.

Knauf, H. (1980). Effects of diuretics on ion transport in the kidney. In "Intracellular Electrolytes and Arterial Hypertension" (H. Zumkley and H. Losse, eds.), pp. 197-204. Theime-Stratton, New York.

Knock, C. A., and deWardener, H. E. (1980). Evidence in vivo for a circulating natriuretic substance in rats after expanding the blood volume. Clin. Sci. **59**, 411-421.

Kohner, E. M., Dollery, C. T., Lowy, C., and Schumer, B. (1971). Effect of diuretic therapy on glucose tolerance in hypertensive patients. Lancet **1**, 986-990.

Kohvakka, A., Eisalo, A., and Manninen, V. (1979). Maintenance of potassium balance during diuretic therapy. Acta Med. Scand. **205**, 319-324.

Kolloch, R., Stumpe, K. O., Bahner, U., and Kruck, F. (1982). Effect of the new angiotensin converting enzyme inhibitor MK-421 on blood pressure and the renin angiotensin system in hypertensive patients. Clin. Pharmacol. Ther. **31**, 239.

Krakauer, R., and Lauritzen, M. (1978). Diuretic therapy and hypokalemia in geriatric out-patients. Danish Medical Bulletin **25**, 126-129.

Kramer, H. J. (1978). Antinatriferic and natriuretic activities in human plasma following acute and chronic salt loading. In "Natriuretic hormone" (H. J. Kramer and F. Kruck, eds.), pp. 24-33. Springer-Verlag, New York.

Kramer, H. J., Dusing, R., Stinnesbeck, B., Prior, W., Backer, A., Eden, J., Kipnowski, J., Glanzer, K., and Kruck, F. (1980). Interaction of conventional and antikaliuretic diuretics with the renal prostaglandin system. Clin. Sci. **59**, 67-70.

Krishan, I., and Moser, M. (1980). 1980 Recommendations of the joint national committee on detection, evaluation, and treatment of high blood pressure. Hypertension **2**, 821-822.

Kuchel, O., Buu, N. T., and Unger, T. (1978). Dopamine—sodium transport: is dopamine a part of the endogenous natriuretic system? Contributions to Nephrology **13**, 27-36.

Lancet (1977). Hypertension in the elderly. **1**, 684-685.

Lancet (1980). Antihypertensive drugs, plasma lipids, and coronary disease. **2**, 19-20.

Lancet (1981). Hypertension and uric acid. **1,** 365–366.

Langford, H. G. (1981). Electrolyte intake, electrolyte excretion, and hypertension. Heart Lung **10,** 269–274.

Laragh, J. H. (1976). Modern system for treating high blood pressure based on renin profiling and vasoconstriction-volume analysis: a primary role for beta blocking drugs such as propranolol. Am. J. Med. **61,** 797–810.

Laragh, J. H. (1978). The renin system in high blood pressure, from disbelief to reality: converting enzyme blockade for analysis and treatment. Prog. Cardiovasc. Dis. **21,** 159–166.

Laragh, J. H., Heinemann, H. O., and Demartini, F. E. (1958). Effect of chlorothiazide on electrolyte transport in man. Its use in the treatment of edema of congestive heart failure, nephrosis, and cirrhosis. J. Am. Med. Assoc. **166,** 145–152.

Lawson, D. H. (1974). Adverse reaction to potassium chloride. Q. J. Med. **43,** 433–440.

Ledingham, J. M., and Cohen, R. D. (1963). The role of the heart in the pathogenesis of renal hypertension. Lancet **2,** 979–981.

Lee, M. R. (1981). The kidney fault in essential hypertension may be a failure to mobolize renal dopamine when dietary sodium chloride is increased. Cardiovasc. Rev. Rept. **2,** 785–789.

Lee, M. R. (1982). Dopamine and the kidney. Clin. Sci. **62,** 439–448.

Levy, S. B., Lilley, J. J., Frigon, R. P., and Stone, R. A. (1977). Urinary kallikrein and plasma renin activity as determinants of renal blood flow. The influence of race and dietary sodium intake. J. Clin. Invest. **60,** 129–138.

Levy, S. B., Frigon, R. P., and Stone, R. A. (1978). The relationship of urinary kallikrein activity to renal salt and water excretion. Clin. Sci. Mol. Med. **54,** 39–45.

Lewis, P. J., Kohner, E. M., Petrie, A., and Dollery, C. T. (1976). Deterioration of glucose tolerance in hypertensive patients on prolonged diuretic treatment. Lancet **1,** 564–566.

Lichstein, D., and Samuelov, S. (1980). Endogenous "ouabain like' activity in rat brain. Biochem. Biophys. Res. Commun. **96,** 1518–1523.

Licht, A., Stein, S., McGregor, C. W., Bourgoignie, J. J., and Bricker, N. S. (1982). Progress in isolation and purification of an inhibitor of sodium transport obtained from dog urine. Kidney Int. **21,** 339–344.

Ljungman, S., Aurell, M., Hartford, M., Wikstrand, J., Wilhelm-sen, L., and Berglund, G. (1981). Sodium excretion and blood pressure. Hypertension 3, 318–326.

Lorimer, A. R., Dunn, F. G., Jones, J. V., and Lawrie, T. D. V. (1976). Beta-adrenoreceptor blockade in hypertension. Am. J. Med. 60, 877–885.

Losse, H., Wehmeyer, H., and Wessels, F. (1960). The water and electrolyte content of erythrocytes in arterial hypertension. Klin. Wochenschr. 38, 393–395.

Lowenstein, J. (1973). Hypokalemia and hyperkalemia. Med. Clin. North Am. 57, 1435–1439.

Luft, F. C., Weinberger, M. H., and Grim, C. E. (1982). Sodium sensitivity and resistance in normotensive humans. Am. J. Med. 72, 726–736.

Lund-Johansen, P. (1970). Hemodynamic changes in long-term diuretic therapy of essential hypertension. Acta Med. Scand. 187, 509–518.

MacGregor, G. A., and deWardener, H. E. (1981). Is a circulating sodium transport inhibitor involved in the pathogenesis of essential hypertension? Clin. Exp. Hypertension 3, 815–830.

MacGregor, G. A., Fenton, S., Alaghband-Zadeh, J., Markandu, N., Roulston, J. E., and deWardener, H. E. (1981). Evidence for a raised concentration of a circulating sodium transport inhibitor in essential hypertension. Br. Med. J. 283, 1355–1357.

MacGregor, G. A., Markandu, N. D., Banks, R. A., Bayliss, J., Roulston, J. E., and Jones, J. C. (1982). Captopril in essential hypertension: contrasting effects of adding hydrochlorothiazide or propranolol. Br. Med. J. 284, 693–696.

Mahley, R. W., Innerarity, T. L., Pitas, R. E., Weisgraber, K. H., Brown, J. H., and Gross, E. (1977). Inhibition of lipoprotein binding to cell surface receptors of fibroblasts following selective modification of arginyl residues in arginine-rich and B apoproteins. J. Biol. Chem. 252, 7279–7287.

Manner, R. J., Brechbill, D. O., and DeWitt, K. (1972). Prevalence of hypokalemia in diuretic therapy. Clin. Med. 79, 15–18.

Margolius, H. S., Horwitz, D., Pisano, J. J., and Keiser, H. R. (1974). Urinary kallikrein excretion in hypertensive man. Relationships to sodium intake and sodium-retaining steroids. Circ. Res. 35, 820–825.

Marks, P., Nimalasuriya, A., and Anderson, J. (1981). The glucose tolerance test in hypertensive patients treated long term with thiazide diuretics. Practitioner 225, 392–393.

Mason, D. T., and Braunwald, E. (1964). Studies on digitalis: X. Effects of ouabain on forearm vascular resistance and venous tone in normal subjects and in patients in heart failure. J. Clin. Invest. 43, 532–543.

Matsuguchi, H., Schmid, P. G., Van Orden, D., and Mark, A. L. (1980). Does vasopressin contribute to salt-induced hypertension in the Dahl strain? Hypertension 3, 174–181.

McAlister, N. H. (1983). Should we treat "mild" hypertension? J. Am. Med. Assoc. 249, 379–382.

McCarthy, S. T. (1982). Body fluid, electrolytes and diuretics. Curr. Med. Res. Opin. 7 (Suppl. 1), 87–95.

Meier, A., Weidmann, P., Mordasini, R., Riesen, W., and Bachmann, C. (1982). Reversal or prevention of diuretic-induced alteration in serum lipoproteins with betablockers. Atherosclerosis 41, 415–419.

Mendlowitz, M. (1982). Sodium and human hypertension. Clin. and Exper. Hyper.-Theory and Practice A4, 333–340.

Mersey, J. H., Williams, G. H., Emanuel, R., Dluhy, R. G., Wong, P., and Moore, T. J. (1979). Plasma bradykinin levels and urinary kallikrein excretion in normal renin essential hypertension. J. Clin. Endocrinol. Metab. 48, 642–647.

Messerli, F. H., Frohlich, E. D., Dreslinski, G. R., Suarez, D. H., and Aristimuno, G. G. (1980). Serum uric acid in essential hypertension: an indicator of renal vascular involvement. Ann. Intern. Med. 93, 817–821.

Meyer, P., Garay, R. P., Nazaret, C., Dagher, G., Bellet, M., Broyer, M., and Feingold, J. (1981). Inheritance of abnormal erythrocyte cation transport in essential hypertension. Br. Med. J. 282, 1114–1117.

Moore, F. D., Edelman, I. S., Olney, J. M., James, A. H., Brooks, L., and Wilson, G. M. (1954). Body sodium and potassium. III. Inter-related trends in alimentary, renal and cardio-vascular disease; lack of correlation between body stores and plasma concentration. Metabolism 3, 334–350.

Mordasini, R., Glueck, Z., Weidmann, P., Keusch, G., Meyer, A., and Riesen, W. (1980). Zur pathogenese der diuretika-induzierten hyperlipoproteinamie. Klin. Wochenschr. 58, 359–363.

Morgan, D. B., and Davidson, C. (1980). Hypokalaemia and diuretics: an analysis of publications. Br. Med. J. 280, 905–908.

Morgan, T., Adam, W., Gillies, A., Wilson, M., Morgan, G., and

Carney, S. (1978). Hypertension treated by salt restriction. Lancet 1, 227-230.

Morgan, T., Carney, S., and Myers, J. (1980). Sodium and hypertension. A review of the role of sodium in pathogenesis and the action of diuretic drugs. Pharmac. Ther. 9, 395-418.

Morgan, T., Myers, J., and Adam, W. (1981a). Adverse effects of diuretic therapy. In "Frontiers in Hypertension Research" (J. H. Laragh, F. R. Buehler and D. W. Seldin, eds.), pp. 62-64. Springer-Verlag, New York.

Morgan, T., Myers, J., and Fitzgibbon, W. (1981b). Sodium intake, blood pressure, and red cell sodium efflux. Clin. Exp. Hypertension 3, 641-653.

Multiple Risk Factor Intervention Trial Research Group (1982). Multiple risk factor intervention trial. Risk factor changes and mortality results. J. Am. Med. Assoc. 248, 1465-1477.

Murphy, M. B., Lewis, P. J., Kohner, E., Schumer, B., and Dollery, C. T. (1982). Glucose intolerance in hypertensive patients treated with diuretics; a fourteen-year follow-up. Lancet 2, 1293-1295.

Murphy, R. J. F. (1950). The effect of "rice diet" on plasma volume and extracellular fluid space in hypertensive subjects. J. Clin. Invest. 29, 912-917.

Nasjletti, A., and Malik, K. U. (1981). Interrelationships among prostaglandins and vasoactive substances. Med. Clin. North Am. 65, 881-889.

Nature (1982). Life as a wonderful one-hoss shay. 298, 779-780.

Nicholls, M. G., Kiowski, W., Zweifler, A. J., Julius, S., Schork, M. A., and Greenhouse, J. (1980). Plasma norepinephrine variations with dietary sodium intake. Hypertension 2, 29-32.

Nickerson, M., and Ruedy, J. (1975). Antihypertensive agents and the drug therapy of hypertension. In "The Pharmacological Basis of Therapeutics" (L. S. Goodman and A. Gilman, eds.), p. 712. McMillan Publishing Co., Inc., New York.

Nielsen, C. K., and Arrigoni-Martelli, E. (1977). Effects on rat urinary kallikrein excretion of bumetanide, bendroflumethiazide and hydralazine. Acta Pharmacol. Toxicol. 40, 267-272.

Nilsson, G. (1980). Symptomatic diabetes mellitus cured by potassium and withdrawal of polythiazide in a hypokalemic hypertensive woman. Acta Med. Scand. 208, 129-131.

Nutbourne, D. M., Howse, J. D., Schrier, R. W., Talner, L. B.,

Ventom, M. G., Verroust, P. J., and deWardener, H. E. (1970). The effect of expanding the blood volume of a dog on the short-ciurcuit current across an isolated frog skin incorporated in the dog's circulation. Clin. Sci. **38**, 629–648.

Ober, K. P., and Hennessy, J. F. (1978). Glucose tolerance and insulin response: effect of thiazide diuretics. Clin. Res. **26**, 775A.

O'Connor, D. T., Eurman, G., Frigon, R. P., and Stone, R. A. (1977). Antihypertensive mechanisms of chronic diuretic and propanalol therapy. Kidney Int. **12**, 471.

O'Connor, D. T., Preston, R. A., Mitas, J. A., Frigon, R. P., and Stone, R. A. (1981). Urinary kallikrein activity and renal vascular resistance in the antihypertensive response to thiazide diuretics. Hypertension **3**, 139–147.

Olshan, A. R., O'Connor, D. T., Preston, R. A., Frigon, R. P., and Stone, R. A. (1981). Involvement of kallikrein in the antihypertensive response of furosemide in essential hypertension. J. Cardiovasc. Pharmacol. **3**, 161–167.

Overlack, A., Stumpe, K. O., Muller, H.-M., Kollock, R., and Higuchi, M. (1982). Interactions of diuretics with the renal kallikrein-kinin and prostaglandin systems. Klin. Wochenschr. **60**, 1223–1228.

Pamnani, M. B., Harder, D. R., Huot, S. J., Bryant, H. J., Kutyna, F. A., and Haddy, F. J. (1981a). Vascular smooth muscle membrane potentials and the influence of a ouabainlike humoral factor in rats with one-kidney, one clip hypertension. Physiologist **24**, 6.

Pamnani, M. B., Buggy, J., Huot, S. J., and Haddy, F. J. (1981b). Studies on the role of a humoral sodium-transport inhibitor and the anteroventral third ventricle (AV3V) in experimental low renin hypertension. Clin. Sci. **61**, 57S–60S.

Parfrey, P. S., Vandenburg, M. J., Wright, P., Holly, J. M. P., Goodwin, F. J., Evans, S. J. W., and Ledingham, J. M. (1981). Blood pressure and hormonal changes following alteration in dietary sodium and potassium in mild essential hypertension. Lancet **1**, 59–63.

Patak, R. V., Mookerjee, B. K., Bentzel, C. J., Hysert, P. E., Babej, M., and Lee, J. B. (1975). Antagonism of the effects of furosemide by indomethacin in normal and hypertensive man. Prostaglandins **10**, 649–659.

Patak, R. V., Fadem, S. Z., Rosenblatt, S. G., Lifschitz, M. D., and Stein, J. H. (1979). Diuretic-induced changes in renal blood flow and prostaglandin E excretion in the dog. Am. J.

Physiol. **236**, F494-F500.

Penhall, R. K., and Frewin, D. B. (1980). Plasma potassium levels in hypertensive patients receiving fixed-combination diuretic therapy. Med. J. Aust. **1**, 376-378.

Perkins, C. M., Casson, I. F., Cope, G. F., and Lee, M. R. (1980). Failure of salt to mobilise renal dopamine in essential hypertension. Lancet **2**, 1370.

Pickering, G. W. (1981). Dietary sodium and human hypertension. In "Frontiers in Hypertension Research" (J. H. Laragh, F. R. Buehler and D. W. Seldin, eds.), pp. 37-42. Springer-Verlag, New York.

Pisano, J. J. (1975). Chemistry and biology of the kallikrein-kinin system. In "Proteases and Biological Control", Cold Spring Harbor Conference on Cell Proliferation, **2**, 199-222.

Plunkett, W. C., Hutchins, P. M., Gruber, K. A., and Buckalew, V. M., Jr. (1982). Evidence for a vascular sensitizing factor in plasma of saline-loaded dogs. Hypertension **4**, 581-589.

Postnov, Y. V., Orlov, S. N., Shevchenko, A., and Adler, A. M. (1977). Altered sodium permeability, calcium binding and Na,K-ATPase activity in the red cell membrane in essential hypertension. Pfluegers Arch. **371**, 263-269.

Poston, L., Jones, R. B., Richardson, P. J., and Hilton, P. J. (1981a). The effect of antihypertensive therapy on abnormal leucocyte sodium transport in essential hypertension. Clin. Exp. Hypertension **3**, 693-701.

Poston, L., Sewell, R. B., Wilkinson, S. P., Richardson, P. J., Williams, R., Clarkson, E. M., MacGregor, G. A., and deWardener, H. E. (1981b). Evidence for a circulating sodium transport inhibitor in essential hypertension. Br. Med. J. **282**, 847-849.

Preiss, R., Prumke, H.-J., Sohr, R., Muller, E., Schmeck, G., Schmidt, J., and Banaschak, H. (1982). Sodium flux and lipid spectrum in the erythrocyte membrane in essential hypertension. Int. J. Clin. Pharmacol. Ther. Toxicol. **20**, 105-112.

Prior, I. A. M., Evans, J. G., Harvey, H. P. B., Davidson, F., and Lindsey, M. (1968). Sodium intake and blood pressure in two Polynesian populations. N. Engl. J. Med. **279**, 515-520.

Pyorala, K., Savolainen, E., Lehtovirta, E., Punsar, S., and Siltanen, P. (1979). Glucose tolerance and coronary heart disease: Helsinki policemen study. J. Chron. Dis. **32**, 729-745.

Ram, C. V. (1982). Diuretics in the management of hypertension. Postgrad. Med. **71**, 155-168.

Ram, C. V., Garrett, B. N., and Kaplan, N. M. (1981). Moderate sodium restriction and various diuretics in the treatment of hypertension. Arch. Intern. Med. **141**, 1015-1019.

Rapoport, M. I., and Hurd, H. F. (1964). Thiazide-induced glucose intolerance treated with potassium. Arch. Intern. Med. **113**, 405-408.

Recordati, G. M., and Moss, N. G. (1978). Electrophysiological study of renal mechano- and chemoreceptors in the rat. Proc. VII Int. Cong. Nephrol., 559-563.

Reese, O. G., Jr., and Steele, T. H. (1976). Uric acid and the kidney in hypertension. In "New Antihypertensive Drugs", (A. Scriabine and C. S. Sweet, eds.) pp. 13-24. Spectrum Publications, New York.

Remington, R. D. (1981). Interpretation of the hypertension detection and follow-up program. In "Frontiers in Hypertension Research" (J. H. Laragh, F. R. Buehler and D. W. Seldin, eds.), pp. 15-16. Springer-Verlag, New York.

Report of Medical Research Council Working Party on Mild to Moderate Hypertension (1981). Adverse reactions to bendrofluazide and propranolol for the treatment of mild hypertension. Lancet **2**, 539-543.

Riddiough, M. A. (1977). Preventing, detecting and managing adverse reactions of antihypertensive agents in the ambulant patient with essential hypertension. Am. J. Hosp. Pharm. **34**, 465-479.

Rosenman, R. H., Brand, R. J., Sholtz, R. I., and Friedman, M. (1976). Multivariate prediction of coronary heart disease during 8.5 year follow-up in the Western Collaborative Group Study. Am. J. Cardiol. **37**, 903-910.

Rosenthal, T., Holtzman, E., and Segal, P. (1980). The effect of chlorthalidone on serum lipids and lipoproteins. Atherosclerosis **36**, 111-115.

Rovner, D. R. (1972). Use of pharmacologic agents in treatment of hypokalemia and hyperkalemia. Ration. Drug Ther. **6**, 1-6.

Saavedra, J. M., Correa, F. M., and Iwai, J. (1980). Discrete changes in adrenaline-forming enzyme activity in brain stem areas of genetic salt-sensitive hypertensive (Dahl) rats. Brain Res., **193**, 199-303.

Saavedra, J. M., Grobecker, H., and Axelrod, J. (1976). Adrenaline-forming enzyme in brainstem: elevation in genetic and experimental hypertension. Science **191**, 483-484.

Sandor, F. F., Pickens, P. T., and Crallan, J. (1982). Variations of plasma potassium concentrations during long-term treatment of hypertension with diuretics without potassium supplements. Br. Med. J. **284**, 711-715.

Scherer, B., and Weber, P. C. (1979). Time-dependent changes in prostaglandin excretion in response to frusemide in man. Clin. Sci. **56**, 77-81.

Schiffl, H., Weidmann, P., Mordasini, R., Riesen, W., and Bachmann, C. (1982). Reversal of diuretic-induced increases in serum low-density-lipoprotein cholesterol by the beta-blocker pindolol. Metabolism **31**, 411-415.

Schlatter, E., Greger, R., and Weidtke, C. (1983). Effect of 'high ceiling' diuretics on active salt transport in the cortical thick ascending limb of Henle's loop of rabbit kidney. Pfluegers Arch. **396**, 210-217.

Schoenfeld, M. R., and Goldberger, E. (1964). Hypercholesterolemia induced by thiazides: a pilot study. Curr. Ther. Res. **6**, 180-184.

Schwartz, A. B. (1977). Diuretics in the treatment of hypertension. Drug Ther. **7**, 158-161.

Seino, M., Abe, K., Otsuka, Y., Saito, T., Irokawa, N., Yasujima, M., Chiba, S., and Yoshinaga, K. (1975). Urinary kallikrein excretion and sodium metabolism in hypertensive patients. Tohoku J. Exp. Med. **116**, 359-367.

Selkurt, E. E. (1951). Effect of pulse pressure and mean arterial pressure modification on renal hemodynamics and electrolyte and water excretion. Circulation **4**, 541-551.

Senft, G. (1968). Hormonal control of carbohydrate and lipid metabolism and drug induced alterations. Naunyn Schmiedebergs Arch. Pharmakol. Exp. Pathol. **259**, 117-148.

Senft, G., Losert, W., Schultz, G., Sitt, R., and Bartelheimer, H. K. (1966). Ursachen der storungen im kohlenhydratstoffwechsel unter dem einfluss sulfonamidierter diuretica. Naunyn-Schmiedebergs Arch. Pharmakol. Exp. Patho. **255**, 369-382.

Shah, S., Khatri, I., and Freis, E. D. (1978). Mechanism of antihypertensive effect of thiazide diuretics. Am. Heart J. **95**, 611-618.

Shepherd, J., Bicker, S., Lorimer, A. R., and Packard, C. J. (1979). Receptor-mediated low density lipoprotein catabolism in man. J. Lipid Res. **20**, 999-1006.

Shutske, G. M., Setescak, L. L., Allen, R. C., Davis, L., Effland, R. C., Ranbom, K., Kitzen, J. M., Wilker, J. C., and Novick,

W. J. Jr. (1982). [(3-Aryl-1,2-benzisoxazol-6-yl)oxy]acetic acids. A new diuretic series. J. Med. Chem. **25**, 36-44.

Simpson, F. O., Paulin, J. M., Phelan, E. L., Thaler, B. I., Waal-Manning, H. J., Nye, E. R., and Herbison, G. P. (1982). Further surveys in Milton, 1978 and 1981: blood pressure, height, weight and 24-hour excretion of sodium and potassium. N. Z. Med. J. **95**, 873-876.

Skrabal, F., Aubock, J., and Hortnagl, H. (1981). Low sodium/high potassium diet for prevention of hypertension: probable mechanism of action. Lancet **2**, 895-900.

Smith, R. L. (1983). Endogenous agents affecting kidney function: their interrelationships, modulation, and control. In "Diuretics. Chemistry, Pharmacology and Medicine" (E. J. Cragoe, Jr., ed.), pp. 571-651. John Wiley & Sons, New York.

Stamler, R., Stamler, J., Lindberg, H. A., Marquardt, J., Berkson, D. M., Paul, O., Lepper, M., Dyer, A., and Stevens, E. (1979). Asymptomatic hyperglycemia and coronary heart disease in middle-aged men in two employed populations in Chicago. J. Chronic Dis. **32**, 805-815.

Stamler, R., Stamler, J., Schoenberger, J. A., Shekelle, R. B., Collette, P., Shekelle, S., Dyer, A., Garside, D., and Wannamaker, J. (1979a). Relationship of glucose tolerance to prevalence of ECG abnormalities and to 5-year mortality from cardiovascular disease: findings of the Chicago heart association detection project in industry. J. Chronic Dis. **32**, 817-828.

Steele, T. H., and Rieselbach, R. E. (1975). Renal urate excretion in normal man. Nephron **14**, 21-32.

Stein, J. H., Congbalay, R. C., Karsh, D. L., Osgood, R. W., and Ferris, T. F. (1972). The effect of bradykinin on proximal tubular sodium reabsorption in the dog. Evidence for functional nephron heterogeneity. J. Clin. Invest. **51**, 1709-1721.

Stone, K. J., and Hart, M. (1976). Inhibition of renal PGE_2-9-ketoreductase by diuretics. Prostaglandins **12**, 197-207.

Swales, J. D. (1982). Ion transport in hypertension. Bioscience Reports **2**, 967-990.

Swarts, H. G. P., Bonting, S. L., DePont, J. J. H. H. M., Schuurmans-Stekhoven, F. M. A. H., Thien, T. A., and Van't Laar, A. (1981). Cation fluxes and (Na^++K^+)-activated ATPase activity in erythrocytes of patients with essential hypertension. Clin. Exper. Hypertension **3**, 831-849.

Takeshita, A., and Mark, A. L. (1978). Neurogenic contribution to hindquarter vasoconstriction during high sodium intake in

Dahl strain of genetically hypertensive rat. Circ. Res. **43**, 86-91.

Talso, P. J., and Carballo, A. J. (1960). Effects of benzothia-diazines on serum and total body electrolytes. Ann. N.Y. Acad. Sci. **82**, 822-840.

Tan, S. Y., Sweet, P., and Mulrow, P. J. (1978). Impaired renal production of prostaglandin E_2: a newly identified lesion in human essential hypertension. Prostaglandins **15**, 139-150.

Tarazi, R. C., Dustan, H. P., and Frohlich, E. D. (1970). Long-term thiazide therapy in essential hypertension. Circulation **41**, 709-717.

Thuillier, G., Laforest, J., Cariou, B., Bessin, P., Bonet, J., and Thuillier, J. (1974). Derives heterocycliques d'acides phenoxyacetiques, synthese et etude preliminaire de leurs activites diuretique et uricosurique. Eur. J. Med. Chem. **9**, 625-633.

Tobian, L., and Binion, J. T. (1952). Tissue cations and water in arterial hypertension. Circulation **5**, 754-758.

Tobian, L. (1974). How sodium and the kidney relate to the hypertensive arteriole. Fed. Proc. **33**, 138-142.

Tobian, L., Lange, J., Azar, S., Iwai, J., Koop, D., and Coffee, K. (1977). Reduction of intrinsic natriuretic capacity in kidneys of Dahl hypertension-prone rats. Circulation **55**, (Suppl. III), 240.

Tobian, L., Lange, J., Iwai, J., Hiller, K., Johnson, M. A., and Goossens, P. (1979). Prevention with thiazide of NaCl-induced hypertension in Dahl "S" rats. Hypertension **1**, 316-323.

Tobian, L. (1981). Hypertension Mechanisms in Experimental Animals and their relevance to humans. In "Frontiers in Hypertension Research" (J. H. Laragh, F. R. Buehler and D. W. Seldin, eds.), pp. 355-366. Springer-Verlag, New York.

Tobian, L., Ganguli, M., Johnson, M. A., and Iwai, J. (1982). Influence of renal prostaglandins and dietary linoleate on hypertension in Dahl S rats. Hypertension **4** (Suppl. II), 149-153.

Trevisan, M., Ostrow, D., Cooper, R., Liu, K., Sparks, S., Okonek, A., Stevens, E., Marquardt, J., and Stamler, J. (1983). Abnormal red blood cell ion transport and hyper-tension. The people's gas company study. Hypertension **5**, 363-367.

Tuomilehto, J., Karppanen, H., Tanskanen, A., Tikkanen, J., and Vuori, J. (1980). Sodium and potassium excretion in a

sample of normotensive and hypertensive persons in eastern
Finland. J. Epidemiol. Comm. Health **34**, 174-178.

Tweeddale, M. G., and Fodor, J. G. (1979). Elevated serum uric
acid. A cardiovascular risk factor? Nephron **23** (Suppl. 1),
3-6.

van Brummelen, P., Man in 't Veld, A., and Schalekamp, M. A. D.
H. (1979). Haemodynamics during long-term thiazide
treatment in essential hypertension: differences between
responders and non-responders. Clin. Sci. **57**, 359S-362S.

Vaughan, E. D., Carey, R. M., Peach, M. J., Ackerly, J. A., and
Ayers, C. R. (1978). The renin response to diuretic therapy.
A limitation of antihypertensive potential. Circ. Res. **42**,
376-381.

Veterans Administration Cooperative Study Group on Antihypertensive Agents (1967). Effects of treatment on morbidity in hypertension. Results in patients with diastolic blood pressure averaging 115 through 129 mmHg. J. Am.
Med. Assoc. **202**, 1028-1034.

Veterans Administration Cooperative Study Group on Antihypertensive Agents (1970). Effects of treatment on morbidity in hypertension. II. Results in patients with diastolic blood pressures averaging 90 through 114 mmHg. J. Am.
Med. Assoc. **213**, 1143-1152.

Veterans Administration Cooperative Study Group on Antihypertensive Agents (1982). Comparison of propranolol and
hydrochlorothiazide for the initial treatment of hypertension. I. Results of short-term titration with emphasis
on racial differences in response. J. Am. Med. Assoc. **248**,
1996-2003.

Veterans Administration Cooperative Study Group on Antihypertensive Agents (1982). Comparison of propranolol and
hydrochlorothiazide for the initial treatment of hypertension. II. Results of long-term therapy. J. Am. Med. Assoc.
248, 2004-2011.

Vogel, R., and Werle, E. (1970). Kallikrein inhibitors. In "Handbook of Experimental Pharmacology" (E. G. Erdos, ed.),
25, pp. 213-249. Springer-Verlag, New York.

Wagner, H. N., Jr., and Braunwald, E. (1956). The pressor effect
of the antidiuretic principle of the posterior pituitary in
orthostatic hypotension. J. Clin. Invest. **35**, 1412-1418.

Walter, U. (1981). Red blood cell sodium and potassium after
hydrochlorothiazide. Clin. Pharmacol. Ther. **30**, 373-377.

Walter, U., and Distler, A. (1982). Abnormal sodium efflux in

erythrocytes of patients with essential hypertension.
Hypertension **4**, 205-210.

Watt, G. C. M., and Foy, C. J. W. (1982). Dietary sodium and
arterial pressure: problems of studies within a single
population. J. Epidemiol. Comm. Health **36**, 197-201.

Weber, M. A., Lopez-Ovejero, J. A., Drayer, J. I., Case, D. B.,
and Laragh, J. H. (1977a). Renin reactivity as a determinant of responsiveness to antihypertensive treatment.
Arch. Intern. Med. **137**, 284-289.

Weber, P. C., Scherer, B., and Larsson, C. (1977b). Increase of
free arachidonic acid by furosemide in man as the cause of
prostaglandin and renin release. Eur. J. Pharmacol. **41**,
329-332.

Weber, M. A., and Laragh, J. H. (1978). A physiological basis
for the treatment of essential hypertension. Bull. N.Y.
Acad. Med. **54**, 931-943.

Webster, J., Dollery, C. T., and Hensby, C. N. (1980). Circulating
prostacyclin levels may be increased by bendrofluazide in
patients with essential hypertension. Clin. Sci. **59**, p. 125S-
128S.

Webster, M. E., and Gilmore, J. P. (1964). Influence of kallidin-
10 on renal function. Am. J. Physiol. **206**, 714-718.

Webster, M. E., and Pierce, J. V. (1963). The nature of kallidins
released from human plasma by kallikreins and other enzymes. Ann. N.Y. Acad. Sci. **104**, 91-107.

Weidmann, P., Beretta-Piccoli, C., Meier, A., Keusch, G., Gluck,
Z., and Ziegler, W. H. (1983). Antihypertensive mechanism
of diuretic treatment with chlorthalidone. Complementary
roles of sympathetic axis and sodium. Kidney Int. **23**, 320-
326.

Wessels, V. F., Junge-Husling, G., and Losse, H. (1967). Untersuchungen zur natrium permeabilitat der erythrozyten
bei hyptertonikern and normotonikern mit familiarer hoch-
druckbelasturn. Z. Kreislaufforsch. **56**, 374-380.

Wessels, F., and Zumkley, H. (1980). Sodium metabolism of red
blood cells in hypertensive patients. In "Intracellular
Electrolytes and Arterial Hypertension" (H. Zumkley and H.
Losse, eds.), pp. 59-68. Thieme-Stratton, New York.

Wiley, J. S., and Cooper, R. A. (1974). A furosemide-sensitive
cotransport of sodium plus potassium in the human red cell.
J. Clin. Invest. **53**, 745-755.

Wilkins, R. W. (1959). New drugs for the treatment of hypertension. Ann. Intern. Med. **50**, 1-10.

Willis, L. R., Ludens, J. H., Hook, J. B., and Williamson, H. E. (1969). Mechanism of natriuretic action of bradykinin. Am. J. Physiol. **217**, 1–5.

Woods, J. W., Parker, J. C., and Watson, B. S. (1983). Perturbation of sodium–lithium countertransport in red cells. N. Engl. J. Med. **308**, 1258–1261.

Zambraski, E. J., Dibona, G. F., and Kaloyanides, G. J. (1976). Effect of sympathetic blocking agents on the antinatriuresis of reflex renal nerve stimulation. J. Pharmacol. Exp. Ther. **198**, 464–472.

Zidek, W., Losse, H., Grunwald, J., Zumkley, H., and Vetter, H. (1982). Intracellular Na^+ and Ca^{2+} activities in aortic smooth muscle cells from spontaneously hypertensive rats. Res. Exp. Med. **181**, 221–224.

Vasodilators in Hypertension

Alexander Scriabine and Catherine E. Johnson[1]

Miles Institute for Preclinical Pharmacology
Miles Laboratories, Inc.
New Haven, Connecticut

I. INTRODUCTION

Interest in vasodilators was recently renewed with the development of Ca^{2+} antagonists and discovery of their activity in the control of arterial pressure. It is likely that in the future, vasodilators in general, and Ca^{2+} antagonists in particular, will partially replace diuretics and β-adrenoceptor antagonists as the initial and/or sole therapy of hypertension. This expectation is based on the recognition by the medical community of the effectiveness and relative safety of new vasodilator drugs, on the advances in our understanding of causes of hypertension and on the possible relationship between the mechanisms of action of these drugs and mechanisms underlying hypertensive disease.

Although many antihypertensive vasodilators are presently available, their usefulness is limited by side effects. The development of new and superior vasodilators is being actively pursued and continues to represent a challenge to the pharmaceutical industry. This chapter reassesses present status, recent developments and future perspectives in the field of vasodilator therapy.

[1]*Present address: E. I. duPont de Nemours and Co., Stine Laboratory, Newark, Delaware 19711.*

HYPERTENSION: PHYSIOLOGICAL
BASIS AND TREATMENT

II. GENERAL PHARMACOLOGY OF VASODILATOR DRUGS

A. Classification of Vasodilator Drugs

There is no general agreement in the literature on nomen-
clature for vasodilators. A rather misleading term "peripheral
vasodilator" is commonly used for drugs which dilate blood vessels by a mechanism unrelated to the autonomic nervous system
or to interaction with endogenous vasoactive substances. Drugs
known to interact with specific receptors for neurotransmitters,
e.g., α_1-adrenoceptors, are not considered "peripheral vasodilators" although their receptors are located in the plasma membrane of vascular smooth muscle cells.

In accordance with terminology introduced by van Nueten
(1978), the term "directly acting smooth muscle relaxant" includes drugs acting at specific receptors for neurotransmitters
at the level of the vascular smooth muscle cell, but excludes
drugs which modify the release or formation of endogenous vasoactive substances, e.g., converting enzyme inhibitors, or drugs
acting at sympathetic nerve endings. According to another recently proposed classification (Packer, 1982), vasodilator drugs
are either "direct acting agonists" or "neurohumoral antagonists." Hydralazine and minoxidil belong to the first and prazosin
and captopril to the second category. This classification recog-
nizes α-adrenoceptor antagonists as vasodilators, but fails to differentiate between many mechanisms of vasodilation which do
not involve autonomic receptors.

Our own modification of previously attempted classifications for vasodilator drugs is shown in Figure 1. Packer's term
"neurohumoral antagonists" is retained. Acetylcholine, isoproterenol and vasodilator prostaglandins are classified as "neurohumoral agonists" while Ca^{2+} antagonists are viewed as a subdi-
vision of "directly acting vasodilators."

Calcium antagonists can be defined as drugs which interfere
with either the intracellular availability or the effect of Ca^{2+} at
doses lower than needed for other pharmacological effects
(Janis, 1981). In accordance with this definition, the term Ca^{2+}
antagonists encompasses Ca^{2+} channel inhibitors (verapamil,
nifedipine or diltiazem) as well as calmodulin antagonists (trifluoperazine). With the eventual recognition of new mechanisms of vasodilation and further elucidation of the sites of

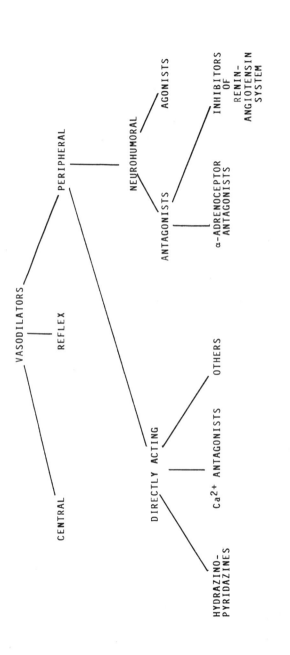

Figure 1. Classification of vasodilator drugs.

action of vasodilator drugs, new classifications will be proposed;
they hopefully will reflect a better understanding of the mechanisms involved.

B. Place for Vasodilators in the Therapy of Hypertension

Many clinical investigators found the "stepped care approach" (Report of Joint National Committee, 1977) convenient
because of its simplicity. In the United States the first step is a
diuretic. If no satisfactory effect is obtained, a β-adrenoceptor
antagonist is used as a second step. Vasodilators, e.g., hydralazine
or prazosin, are used as step 3 drugs, while adrenergic neuron
blocking agents, e.g., guanethidine, are considered step 4 drugs.
In Europe β-adrenoceptor antagonists are often used as the initial therapy, particularly in younger patients; diuretics are added
as a second step.

There is a growing tendency to use vasodilators as the initial
and even sole therapy of hypertension. This approach is possible
with the new vasodilators, e.g., Ca^{2+} antagonists, which produce
less or no tachycardia and do not cause retention of salt and
water.

C. Hemodynamic Effects of Vasodilator Drugs

To understand the hemodynamic effects of antihypertensive
vasodilator drugs, it is important to differentiate arterial versus
venous sites of vasodilator action. The currently used vasodilator drugs differ significantly in their effects on arterial versus
venous circulation (Table 1). Because of reduction in afterload
and reflex sympathetic stimulation of the heart, arterial vasodilation leads to an increase in cardiac output (Figure 2) while reflex vasoconstriction, which occurs concurrently, tends to reduce
cardiac output. Drugs with pure venous vasodilator action reduce venous return and cardiac output, and drugs which dilate
arteries and veins will increase cardiac output to a lesser extent
than pure arterial vasodilators (Figure 3).

Alpha$_1$-adrenoceptor antagonists, e.g., prazosin, differ in
their hemodynamic effects from direct acting vasodilator drugs
in their ability to block reflex vasoconstriction. By virtue of this
effect they will tend to increase cardiac output.

Table 1. *Differential Effects of Antihypertensive Vasodilator Drugs on Arteries Versus Veins*

Drug	Arterial Dilation	Venous Dilation
hydralazine	+ + +	+
diazoxie	+ +	+
prazosin	+ + +	+ +
Na^+ nitroprusside	+ + +	+ + +

D. Advantages and Disadvantages of Vasodilator Drugs in the Therapy of Hypertention

One of the important advantages of vasodilator drugs is their ability to decrease peripheral vascular resistance. The decrease in resistance is expected to be associated with an increase in blood flow to vital organs: heart, kidney and brain. Not all vasodilators, however, increase blood flow to vital organs; diazoxide may decrease renal blood flow. Although diazoxide consistently increases coronary blood flow, this increase may not be sufficient for the increased oxygen demand, and hypoxia may result.

Another important advantage of vasodilator drugs in the therapy of hypertension is the absence of central side effects, e.g., depression or sedation, and of effects associated with the blockade of the autonomic nervous system, such as dry mouth or impotency.

The major advantage is, however, the effectiveness of some vasodilator drugs in patients in which other drugs fail. Minoxidil, for example, was found to be effective in severe cases of malignant hypertension where other antihypertensive drugs produced no benefit.

The disadvantages of vasodilator drugs are determined by their side effects: salt retention, headache, flushing and tachy-

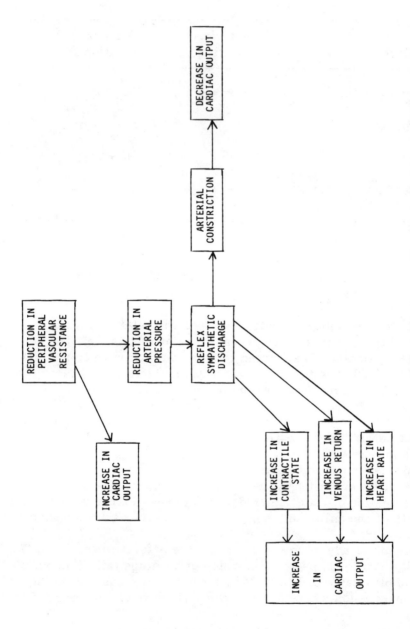

Figure 2. Effect of drugs with arterial vasodilator action on cardiac output. Factors which tend to increase cardiac output predominate.

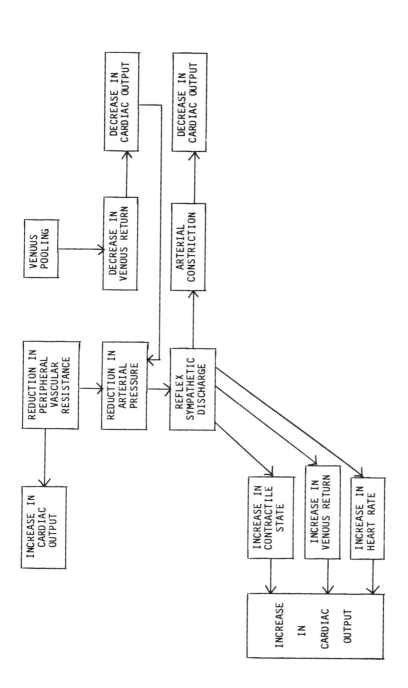

Figure 3. Effect of drugs with arterial and venous vasodilator action on cardiac output. There is a greater tendency for cardiac output to decrease.

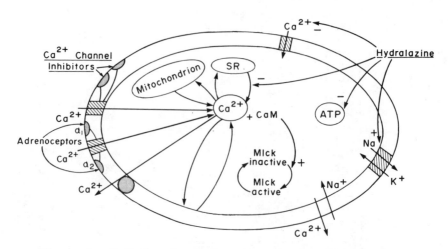

Figure 4. Cellular sites of action of vasodilator drugs. Interference with Ca^{2+} entry or release as the mechanisms of action of drugs. Sites of hydralazine action. SR, sarcoplasmic reticulum; Mlck, myosin light chain kinase; CaM, calmodulin.

cardia. Because of different mechanisms of vasodilator action and differences in the distribution of blood flow after various vasodilator drugs, their side effects also differ. The side effect profile of Ca^{2+} antagonists appears to be more acceptable; salt and water retention and/or tachycardia are usually absent. Nitrendipine (Meyer et al., 1981; Stoepel et al., 1981) has been described to have diuretic and saluretic effects in saline loaded rats (Garthoff et al., 1982). Minoxidil or hydralazine, but not nifedipine, are known to produce cardiac hypertrophy in rats (Kazda et al., 1982).

In acute experiments, vasodilator drugs tend to elevate blood glucose. This can be either a transient phenomenon due to reflex stimulation of epinephrine release from adrenal medulla or a sustained diabetogenic effect known to occur with diazoxide and associated with the inhibition of insulin release and of glucose uptake (Barnett and Whitney, 1966; Loubatieres et al., 1968).

An increase in plasma renin activity (PRA) is a common property of vasodilators. It can lead to an increased formation of aldosterone, to salt and water retention and to the development of tolerance. Minoxidil and diazoxide produce pronounced elevation of PRA whereas Ca^{2+} antagonists cause only a slight

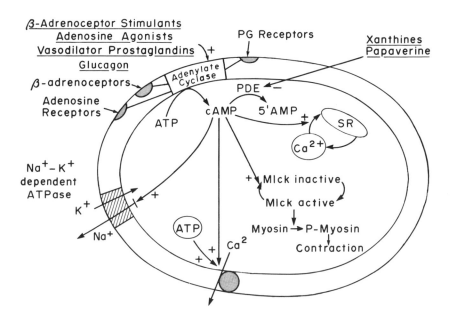

Figure 5. Cellular sites of action of vasodilator drugs. Role of cAMP in the mediation of vasodilator response. Stimulation of adenylate cyclase and inhibition of phosphodiesterase as sites of action of drugs. PDE, phosphodiesterase; PG, prostaglandins.

or moderate increase in PRA for a similar blood pressure lowering effect. Prazosin either has no effect or lowers PRA in man (Hayes et al., 1976).

Many vasodilators, e.g., hydralazine or diazoxide, are known to produce myocardial necrosis in animals primarily in the left ventricular papillary muscles. The lesions can be found in the hearts of rats or dogs after chronic administration of vasodilator drugs at relatively high dose levels. Myocardial necrosis can be prevented by β-adrenoceptor antagonists and is assumed to be caused by reflex sympathetic activation of the heart. At doses producing only a slight to moderate decrease in blood pressure, no myocardial necrosis is usually seen.

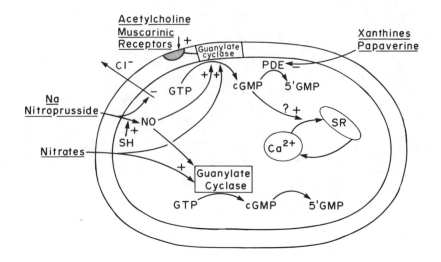

Figure 6. Cellular sites of action of vasodilator drugs. Possible role of cGMP in the mediation of vasodilator response. NO, nitroso-group; SH, sulfhydryl group.

E. Cellular Sites of Action of Vasodilator Drugs

The mechanisms of contraction in vascular smooth muscle has not yet been precisely defined (Adelstein et al., 1982; Ebashi et al., 1982) and the cellular sites of action of vasodilators are even more controversial. Many vasodilator drugs are thought to act at the membrane of the vascular smooth muscle cell modifying ion transport or on various cytosolic enzymes. Figures 4-6 illustrate some of the proposed cellular mechanims. The sites of action of Ca^{2+} antagonists at specific receptors, which are Ca^{2+} channels or channel-associated proteins, are shown on Figure 4. Their mechanism of action is more extensively discussed in other chapters of this volume. Hydralazine is thought to interfere with Ca^{2+} entry as well as Ca^{2+} release from sarcoplasmic reticulum (McLean et al., 1978). It was also reported to decrease ATP levels (Diamond and Reichert, 1982) and to stimulate Na^+,K^+-ATPase (Kreye et al., 1980). Alpha-adrenoceptors are thought to mediate Ca^{2+} entry; α-adrenoceptor antagonists tend to reduce Ca^{2+} entry mediated by α-adrenoceptors. Contrary to some claims in the literature (De Mey and Vanhoutte, 1981; Van Zwieten et al., 1981), both types of adrenoceptors (α_1 and α_2) are probably involved in the control of Ca^{2+} entry into vascular smooth muscle cell. At 10^{-6} M, Ca^{2+} ions occupy four binding sites of calmodulin; the Ca^{2+}-calmodulin complex binds to and activates myosin kinase, which then phosphorylates myosin, converting it to a form which can be activated by actin (Adelstein, 1982). In Figure 5, β-adrenoceptor stimulants, adenosine agonists, and vasodilator prostaglandins are shown to stimulate adenylate cyclase. cAMP is likely to promote relaxation by inactivating myosin light chain kinase, by increasing Ca^{2+} binding to sarcoplasmic reticulum, by enhancing Ca^{2+} efflux or by stimulating Na^+-K^+ dependent ATPase (Diamond, 1978; Kukovetz et al., 1981; Webb et al., 1981; Hardman, 1981).

As shown in Figure 6, acetylcholine stimulates muscarinic receptors associated with guanylate cyclase. This leads to elevation of cGMP. Guanylate cyclase is also stimulated by Na nitroprusside as well as by nitrates (Gruetter et al., 1980). Xanthines and papaverine inhibit cGMP phosphodiesterase as well as cAMP phosphodiesterase. It is presently unclear how and whether cGMP produces relaxation (Janis and Diamond, 1979). It was suggested that cGMP may decrease cytosolic Ca^{2+} either by increasing its uptake into storage sites or by enhancing its efflux (Kukovetz et al., 1981). Sodium nitroprusside, independently of cGMP, was proposed to stimulate the uptake of Ca^{2+} into sarcoplasmic reticulum (Klinner et al., 1977), stimulate Ca^{2+} efflux or inhibit Cl efflux through the cell membrane (Kreye, 1980). Still another proposed mechansim of vasodilator action of sodium nitroprusside is inhibition of norepinephrine-stimulated Ca^{2+} uptake (Karaki et al., 1980).

It is apparent from the above discussion that the mechanisms of drug-induced vasodilatation are not yet established and remain highly speculative. It is also apparent that Ca^{2+} plays a major role in the maintenance of the contractile state of vascular smooth muscle and drugs can influence free cytosolic Ca^{2+} levels by various mechanisms.

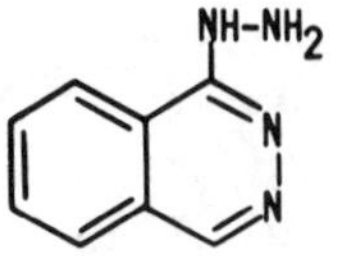

HYDRALAZINE

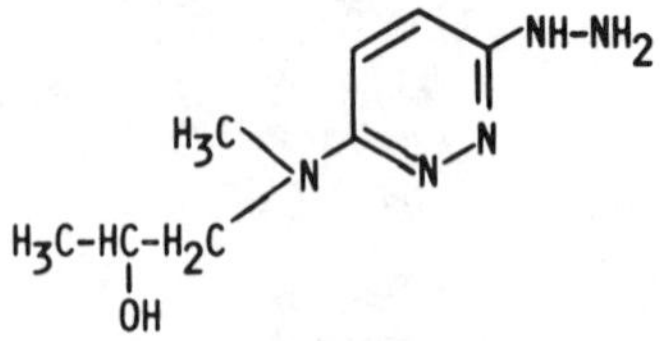

PROPILDAZINE

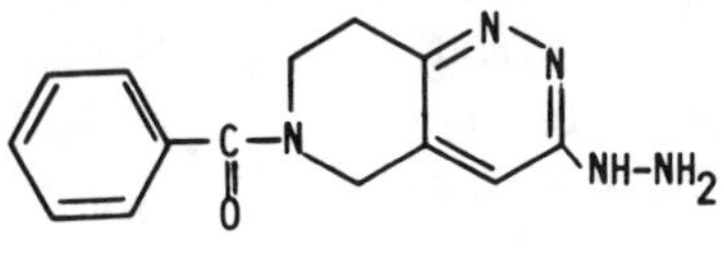

ENDRALAZINE

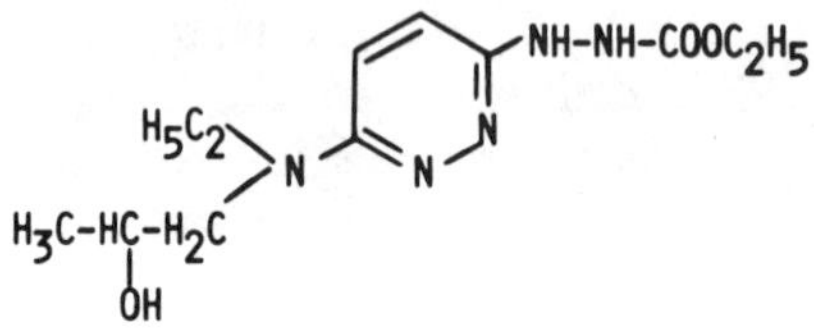

CADRALAZINE

Figure 7. Chemical structures of hydralazine and closely related hydrazinopyridazines.

III. REVIEW OF MAJOR VASODILATOR DRUGS USED IN THE TREATMENT OF HYPERTENSION

A. Hydralazine and Hydrazinopyridazines

The chemical structures of hydralazine and closely related hydrazinopyridazines are shown in Figure 7. Hydralazine was discovered by Gross et al. (1950) and was previously thought to lower arterial pressure by a central action. Most investigators today agree that the site of action of hydralazine is peripheral, but the precise mode of action should still be considered largely unknown. In addition to the proposed mechanisms of cellular action of hydralazine shown on Figure 4, hydralazine was thought to lower arterial pressure by chelation of Ca^{2+} (Perry, 1953), stimulation of adenylate cyclase (Anderson, 1973), inhibition of dopamine-β-hydroxylase (Liu et al., 1974), inhibition of thromboxane synthetase and/or release of PGI_2 (Greenwald et al.,

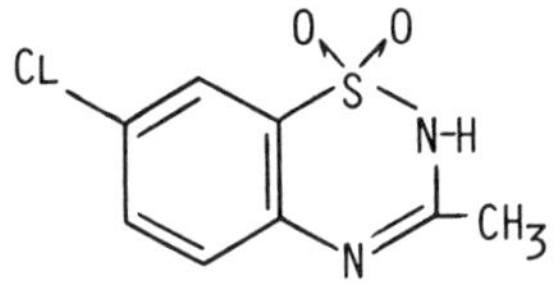

Figure 8. Chemical structure of diazoxide.

1980), inhibition or norepinephrine release (Chevillard et al., 1980), and more recently, by release of endothelial factor (Spokas et al., 1982). The hemodynamic effects of hydralazine are those of a typical arterial vasodilator; its hypotensive effect is associated with an increase in cardiac output, tachycardia, salt and water retention, and an increase in plasma renin activity.

The most characteristic side effect and the limiting factor in hydralazine therapy is its tendency to produce lupus erythematosus. This syndrome occurs more often in females and is usually reversible on discontinuation of the therapy.

One of the advantages of hydralazine is its renal vasodilator effect (Reubi, 1950), although the renal fraction of cardiac output is not changed by hydralazine. For more extensive reviews of pharmacology of hydralazine see Gross (1977), Taylor (1980) and Reece (1981).

New hydralazine derivatives, e.g., endralazine (Salzmann et al., 1979; Oates and Stokes, 1981), propildazine (Carpi and Dorigotti, 1974; Worcel, 1978), and cadralazine (Semeraro et al., 1981), were claimed either to be less toxic, to produce less tachycardia or to be better adsorbed orally than hydralazine. There is no evidence yet that these new hydralazine derivatives are less likely to produce lupus erythematosus.

B. Diazoxide

The discovery of acute hypotensive effects of diazoxide (Rubin et al., 1961) was used as supportive evidence for vascular effects of thiazide diuretics, to which diazoxide is closely related. In spite of its chemical similarity, the pharmacological effects of diazoxide bear no relation to those of chlorothiazide or other thiazide diuretics (Figure 8). Diazoxide increases cardiac output and stroke volume, and lowers peripheral vascular re-

sistance. It dilates arteries and arterioles and has little effect
on veins (Thirlwell and Zsoter, 1972). It was originally suggested
that diazoxide has a specific antagonistic effect on Ca^{2+} receptors leading to competition with Ca^{2+} for contractile proteins
(Wohl et al., 1968). More recently it was proposed that diazoxide
acts at the cell membrane inhibiting excitation–contraction
coupling (Rhodes and Sutter, 1971). This suggests a Ca^{2+} channel inhibitory action, although diazoxide has not yet been shown
to inhibit ^{45}Ca uptake by vascular tissue or to interfere with a
Ca^{2+} current in the membrane of the vascular smooth muscle
cell.

Diazoxide was reported to inhibit various vasoconstrictor
agents, including norepinephrine, Ca^{2+}, Ba^{2+}, 5-HT and K^+. Unlike most Ca^{2+} channel inhibitors, diazoxide is more effective
against norepinephrine than against K^+-induced contractions.
The effect of diazoxide on Ca^{2+}-induced contractions of rat aortic strips is non–competitive (Rhodes and Sutter, 1971). Diazoxide is thought to act at a site common to all vasoconstrictor
stimuli probably involving intracellular translocation of Ca^{2+}
(Janis and Triggle, 1973). Since diazoxide is a more potent antagonist of Ca^{2+}-induced contractions in spontaneously hypertensive than in normotensive rats, the drug may conceivably affect a mechanism involved in the development of spontaneous
hypertension in rats.

The clinical use of diazoxide is presently limited to hypertensive emergencies. The major reason for this limitation is the
hyperglycemic effect of the drug.

C. Sodium Nitroprusside

The hypotensive effect of sodium nitroprusside ($Na_2[Fe(CN)_5$
$NO]\cdot 2H_2O$) was discovered as early as 1877 (Davidsohn, 1877),
but its use in the treatment of hypertension is based primarily
on the finding of Page et al. (1955) who evaluated the drug in
animals and in hypertensive patients.

By intravenous administration, sodium nitroprusside has a
rapid hypotensive effect. Its duration of action is short, so that
continuous infusion is required. Easy reversal of the effect is
useful in surgery in "controlled hypotension," where the hypotension does not have to last longer than the surgical procedure.
Another common use of sodium nitroprusside is in hypertensive
emergencies were rapid onset of its action is particularly
important.

On vascular smooth muscle, sodium nitroprusside is active against all contractile substances including norepinephrine, vasopressin and K^+ (Kreye et al., 1975, Kreye, 1978).

The acute toxicity of sodium nitroprusside is determined by the release of free cyanide, which can lead rapidly to metabolic acidosis. To avoid acute cyanide toxicity, the dose of the drug should not exceed 0.5 mg/kg. Chronic toxicity of sodium nitroprusside is often caused by accumulation of thiocyanate. The plasma levels of thiocyanate should not exceed 5 mg/100 ml. At higher concentrations, signs of thiocyanate toxicity are observed: fatigue, headache, disorientation and muscle spasms. Some of the possible mechanism of cellular action of sodium nitroprusside were discussed above and are shown on Figure 6. Unlike Ca^{2+} antagonists, sodium nitroprusside relaxes vascular smooth muscle independently of extracellular calcium.

D. Minoxidil and RO 12-4713

Minoxidil was discovered as a metabolic product of diallyl-melamine, a hypotensive agent with a slow onset of action (Freyburger et al., 1965). The hypotensive effect of minoxidil is associated with an increase in heart rate and cardiac output. Minoxidil increases plasma norepinephrine concentration and plamsa renin activity, and it produces salt and water retention without affecting glomerular filtration rate. Total renal blood flow is not affected by minoxidil whereas outer cortical blood flow is reduced, and blood flow to the juxtamedullary region is increased (DuCharme and Zins, 1980).

In dogs, minoxidil produces right atrial degenerative lesions, the pathogenesis of which is not understood. An unique side effect of minoxidil is hypertrichosis. The hair growth on the face is particularly disturbing; it disappears with the discontinuation of the therapy. Minoxidil was introduced, in spite of its side effects, because of its unique ability to lower arterial pressure in patients resistant to other drugs.

Among the drugs with similar chemical structure (Figure 9) is Ro 12-4713 (Gerold et al., 1981). Clinical studies (Chu et al., 1981; Grimm et al., 1981) indicate that, at 300 mg/day, this drug is an effective and long-acting vasodilator. The clinical findings included relative absence of tachycardia and of salt and water retention, but an increase in plasma norepinephrine and renin levels. In spontaneously hypertensive rats or renal hypertensive

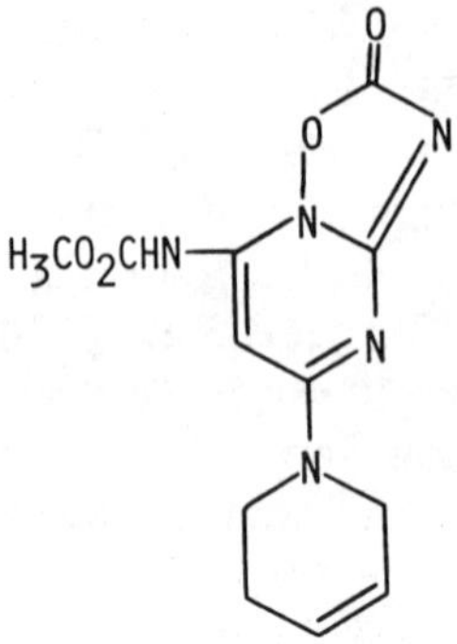

RO 12-4713 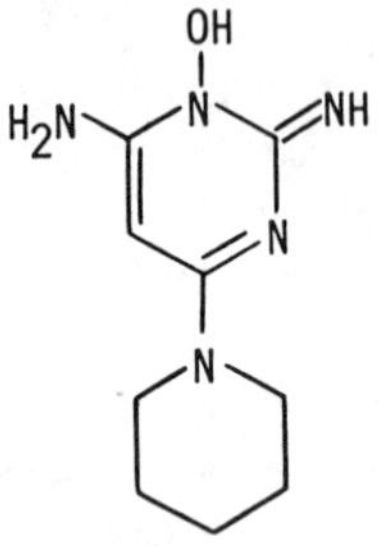   MINOXIDIL

Figure 9.   Chemical structures of Ro-12-4713 and minoxidil.

dogs, Ro 12-4713 has antihypertensive effect. In normotensive
animals no significant effect on arterial pressure was seen, although in conscious dogs, aortic blood flow was increased by the
drug. Ro 12-4713 increased coronary blood flow to a greater
extent than blood flow in femoral, renal or mesenteric vascular
beds. Unlike minoxidil, Ro 12-4713 had no antidiuretic or anti-
saluretic effect in the rat.

E. Beta-Adrenoceptor Antagonists with
Vasodilator Action

During the last few years various new antihypertensive
drugs have been developed which combine β-adrenoceptor antagonist and vasodilator properties in one molecule. The impetus
for this development was a success with combined β-antagonist
and vasodilator therapy. A single drug with these two properties
was thought to be superior to a combination of two drugs with
different mechanisms of action. It should be simpler with a single drug to find a proper dose for the majority of patients. Also,
different pharmacokinetic parameters of each of the two drugs
will be expected to complicate the optimal therapeutic regimen.

Attempts to combine structural features typical for either of the two types of drugs led to the development of MK 761 (Sweet et al., 1979a,b) and of prizidilol (Taylor et al, 1981a,b). MK 761 has a pyridine nucleus, present also in another vasodilator (MK 534, Scriabine et al., 1979), and a typical β-adrenoceptor antagonist side chain. Prizidilol combines a hydrazinopyridine moiety of hydralazine with a similar side chain (Figure 10). In pharmacological studies both drugs were shown to have β-adrenoceptor antagonist and vasodilator properties. The vasodilator activity of MK 761 was only partially antagonized by β-adrenoceptor blockade, so that the drug was thought to have two components of vasodilator action. Similarly, sulfinalol (Hernandez et al., 1979) and bucindolol (Deitchman et al., 1980) had vasodilator activity which was only partially attributable to β_2-adrenoceptor stimulation (Figure 10). Recently Sybertz et al. (1982) compared the vasodilator effects of four β-adrenoceptor antagonists and found that only prizidilol has no β_2-adrenoceptor stimulant component of action. In their experiments, the maximal obtainable vasodilator effects of pindolol or of MK 761 were considerably lower than those of sulfinalol or isoproterenol.

A successful combination of β- and α-adrenoceptor antagonist properties in one molecule was achieved with synthesis and development of labetalol (Figure 11) which blocks β_1- and β_2-adrenoceptors to a similar extent but is highly selective for α_1- as compared to α_2-adrenoceptors (Brittain and Levy, 1976; Levy and Richards, 1980). Neither heart rate nor cardiac output are significantly affected by labetalol. Clinical studies demonstrated therapeutic usefulness of labetalol (Prichard and Boakes, 1976). An isomer of labetalol, Sch 19927, was recently described (Baum et al., 1981). Another vasodilator drug with β-and α-adrenoceptor blocking activity is medroxalol (Dage et al., 1981; Figure 12).

Table 2 lists a series of compounds with β-adrenoceptor antagonist and vasodilator properties. Pindolol is used as an example of β-adrenoceptor antagonist drug with acute intrinsic sympathetic activity (ISA). With chronic administration the antagonist component plays a greater role in the overall cardiovascular action of the drug. Drugs of this group probably have no substantial advantage over β-adrenoceptor antagonists without ISA. The therapeutic utility of drugs from the other groups listed in Table 2 is likely to be dependent on the mechanism of their vasodilator action.

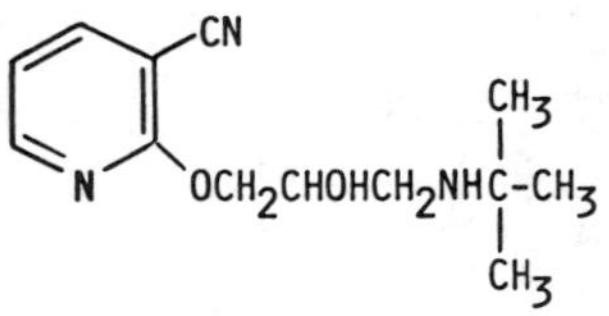

MK-761

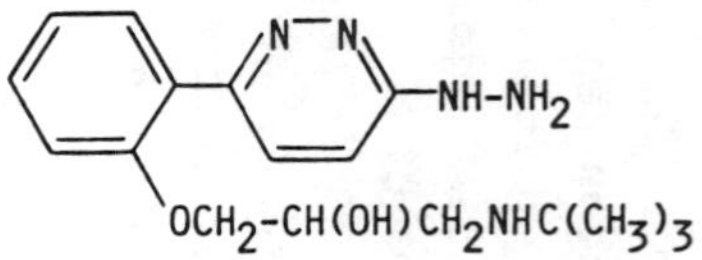

PRIZIDILOL, SKF 92657

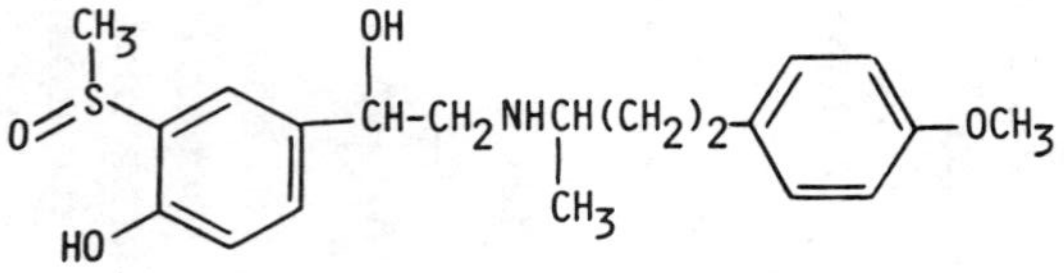

SULFINALOL

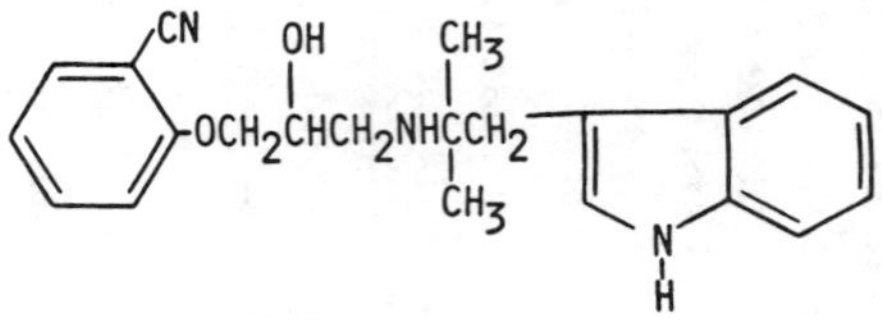

BUCINDOLOL

Figure 10. Chemical structures of β-adrenoceptor antagonists with vasodilator activity.

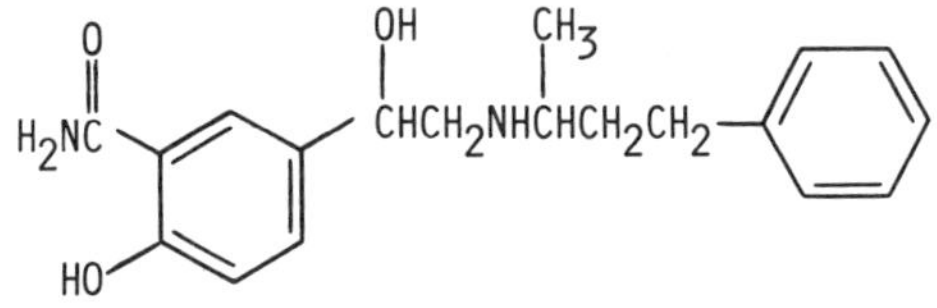

Figure 11. Chemical structure of labetalol.

F. Alpha-Adrenoceptor Antagonists with Vasodilator Activity

The first α-adrenoceptor antagonist recognized as useful in the treatment of hypertension was prazosin (Scriabine et al., 1968; Constantine et al., 1973). The major reason for its initial selection and development was a recognition that the drug differs from classical α-adrenoceptor antagonists (phentolamine and phenoxybenzamine) in producing sustained lowering of arterial pressure without reflex tachycardia. The discovery of selectivity of prazosin for α_1-adrenoceptors (Cambridge et al., 1977) has been used to explain the relative absence of tachycardia with the drug. More recent findings on the inhibition of sympathetic discharge by prazosin (Persson et al., 1981) suggested an additional central sympathetic nervous system inhibitory activity of the drug. The major side effect of prazosin is so-called "first-dose phenomenon," a collapse with loss of consciousness following the first dose prazosin. This effect was attributed to a selective blockade of visceral sympathetic nerve activity (Moulds and Jauernig, 1977). Gradual increase in prazosin dose largely eliminated the "first-dose phenomenon."

Prazosin success led to the development of many chemically related compounds which were claimed to represent improve-

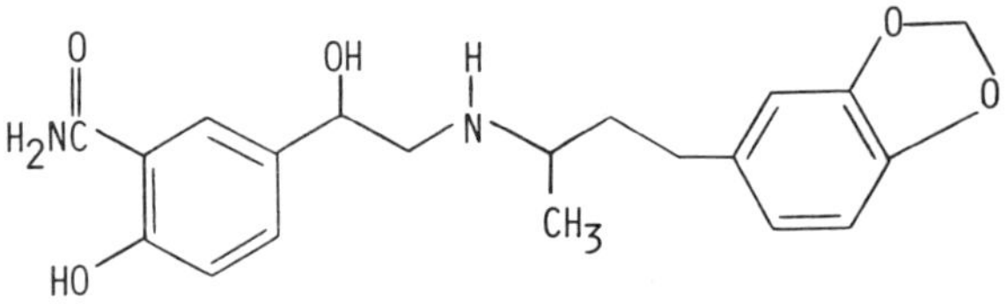

Figure 12. Chemical structure of medroxalol.

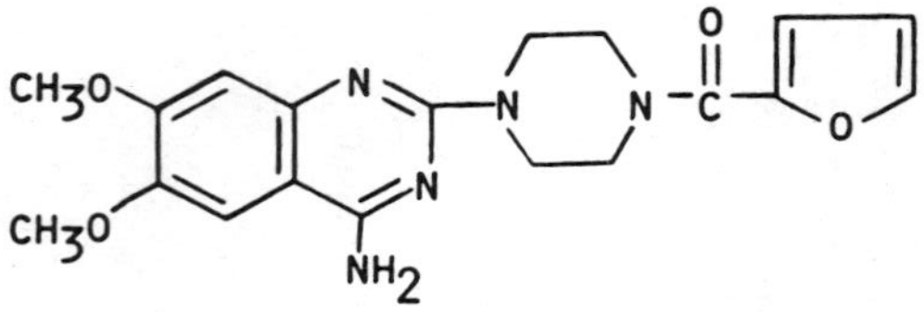

Figure 13. Chemical structures of prazosin and prazosin derivatives.

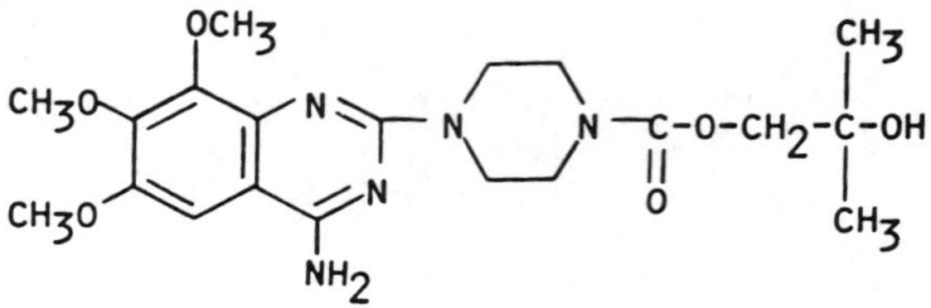

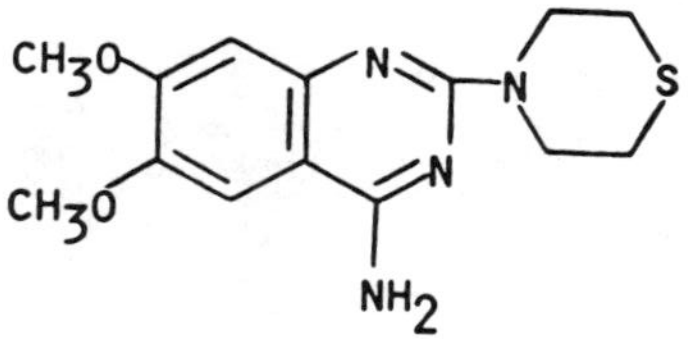

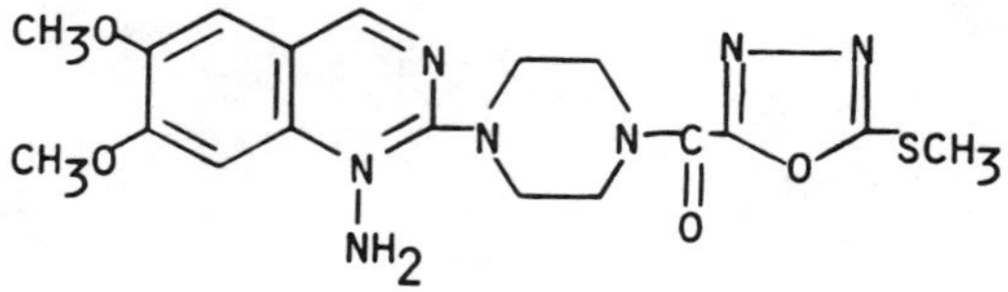

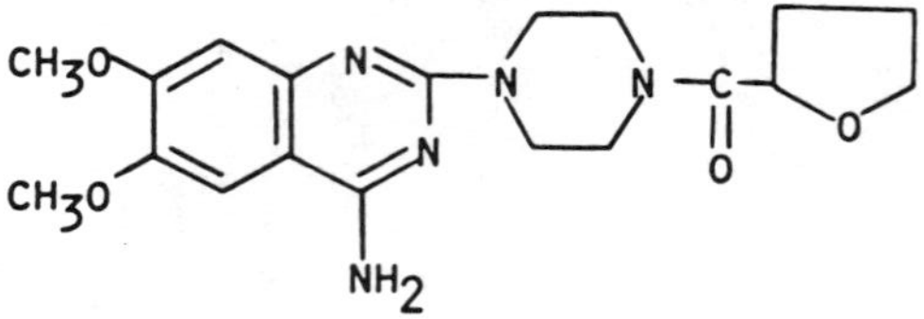

Table 2.   Beta-Adrenoceptor Antagonists with Vasodilator
           Action

Mechanism of Vasodilator Action

1.	β-Stimulation	Pindolol
2.	β-Stimulation + Direct Vascular Relaxation	MK 761 Sulfinalol Bucindolol
3.	Direct Vascular Relaxation	Prizidilol
4.	α_1-Blockade + Direct Vascular Relaxation	Labetalol Sch 19927 Medroxalol

---

ments over prazosin. The chemical structures of new prazosin
derivatives are shown in Figure 13. Trimazosin (Constantine and
Hess, 1981) is less potent than prazosin, but appears to more
suitable for the therapy of heart failure. CN 88823 (Kaplan et
al., 1980) was reported to have less tendency to tolerance development than prazosin. Tiodazosin has a longer half-life than
prazosin and appears to have a second component of vasodilator
action (Buyniski et al., 1980). The binding of terazosin to α_1-
adrenoceptors is more labile than that of prazosin (Kyncl et al.,
1982).

Indoramin is an α-adrenoceptor antagonist with a different
chemical structure (Figure 14). It is a selective α_1-adrenoceptor
antagonist with vasodilator activity. Like prazosin, indoramin
causes little or no tachycardia. Indoramin reduces sympathetic
nerve activity and has antihistaminic and antiarrhythmatic effects. Its side effects include sedation and occasional orthostatic hypotension (Alps et al., 1972a,b).

G. Other Vasodilators

The scope of this chapter does not permit review of all vasodilators discovered during the last decade. Four compounds
with different but unique mechanisms of action are reviewed

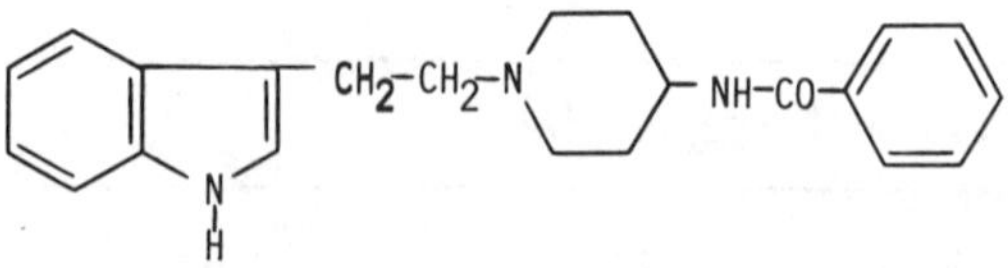

Figure 14. Chemical strucutre of indoramin.

here. They are: urapidil, nicorandil, SKF 82526 and a new prostaglandin-like compound.

Urapidil (Figure 15; Schoetensack et al., 1977) combines in
one molecule prazosin-like α_1-adrenoceptor antagonist and clon-
idine-like α_2-adrenoceptor agonist activities. The drug is a
vasodilator which does not increase heart rate or plasma renin
activity.

Nicorandil (Figure 16), an antianginal drug (Uchida et al.,
1978), improves coronary circulation by a vascular action alleg-
edly involving an interference wtih K^+ conductance in vascular
smooth muscle cell. A decrease in K^+ conductance could theo-
retically lead to a decrease in Ca^{2+} entry and nicorandil can be
expected to have pharmacological effects similar to those of
Ca^{2+} antagonists.

SKF 82526 (Figure 17) has relatively specific renal vasodilator activity which is mediated by stimulation of renovascular dopamine receptors (Ackerman et al., 1982). Another
specific renal vasodilator recently reported by Blaine et al.
(1982) is chemically related to prostaglandins. It is active orally

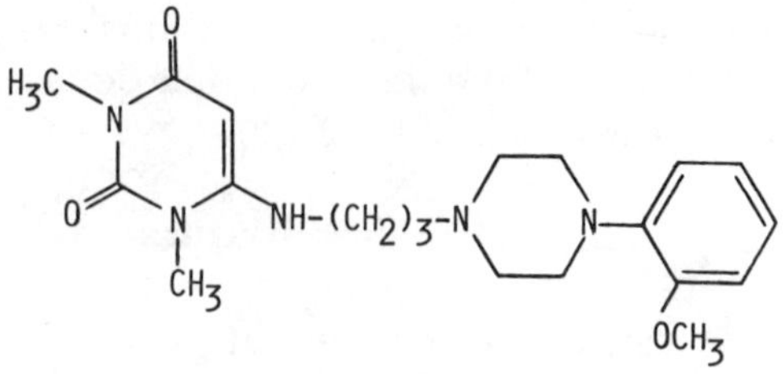

Figure 15. Chemical structure of urapidil.

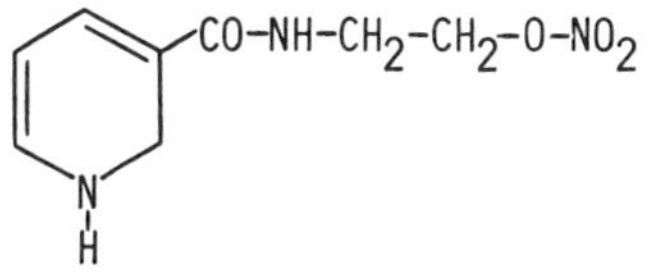

Figure 16. Chemical structure of nicorandil.

and has antihypertensive properties (Figure 18). In accordance
with the Guyton's (1974) concept, the reduction in renal vascular
resistance may provide an attractive approach to the treatment
or prevention of hypertension. The validity of this concept will
be tested with either of the two renal vasodilators.

IV. LABORATORY METHODS FOR EVALUATION OF VASODILATOR DRUGS AS ANTIHYPERTENSIVES

Demonstration of the antihypertensive activity of vasodilator drugs in the laboratory is easy: most vasodilators lower
arterial pressure in most animal models, although some of them
are more effective in hypertensive than in normotensive animals.
It is more difficult to decide whether the observed antihypertensive activity is likely to be useful clinically, whether the drug
has not only an arterial but also a venous vasodilator action, and
to establish its cellular site of action.

Before clinical usefulness of a vasodilator drug is suggested,
its duration of action, tendency to produce tolerance, and poten-

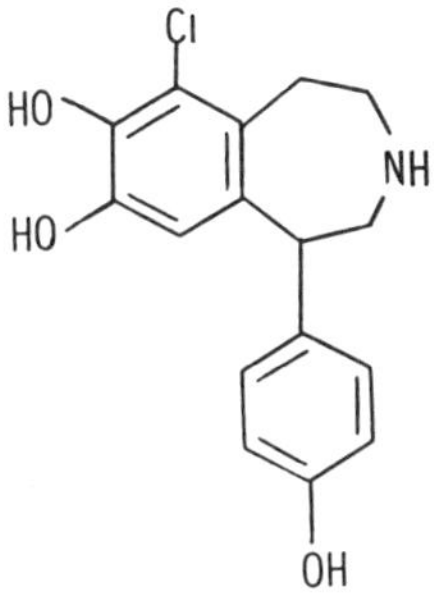

Figure 17. Chemical structure of SK & F 82526.

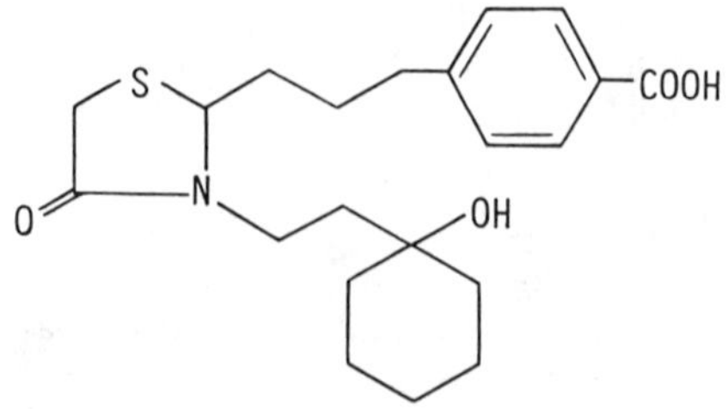

*Figure 18. Chemical structure of a new prostaglandin-like
derivative: 4-[3-[2-(1-hydroxycyclohexyl)ethyl]-4-oxo-2-
thiazolidinyl]propyl]benzoic acid.*

tial side effects should be studied. Evaluation of a potential antihypertensive drug should also include hemodynamics: effect on
cardiac output, myocardial contractility and blood flow distribution.

Since cellular sites of vasodilator action of drugs are still
highly speculative, only some biochemical determinations can be
considered obligatory. These include effects on cAMP levels,
adenyl cyclase, phosphodiesterase and ^{45}Ca uptake. The ^3H-
nitrendipine binding is now used in evaluation of Ca^{2+} channel
inhibitors. It is conceivable that specific receptors exist for other vasodilator agents and that ligand binding techniques can be
adapted to initial screening of other vasodilators as well.

In vitro pharmacological methods involving isolated vascular strip or vessel segments are routinely used in the evaluation
of vasodilators. For this purpose, we use the technique of
Steinsland et al. (1973), involving perfusion of an isolated seg-
ment of rabbit ear artery. This preparation constricts in response to electrical stimulation and to various vasoconstrictor
agents. Vasodilator effects of sodium nitroprusside can be dis-
tinguished from those of Ca^{2+} antagonists using either short or
long periods of electrical stimulation. Sodium nitroprusside or
prazosin reduce vasoconstriction caused by brief electrical
shocks, while Ca^{2+} antagonists are ineffective under the same
experimental conditions (Figure 19 and 20). With longer periods
of electrical stimulation, a biphasic response is obtained. Sodium nitroprusside or α-adrenoceptor antagonists reduce both
phases of the response (Figures 21 and 22), whereas Ca^{2+} channel
inhibitors, e.g., nifedipine or nitrendipine, selectively block only

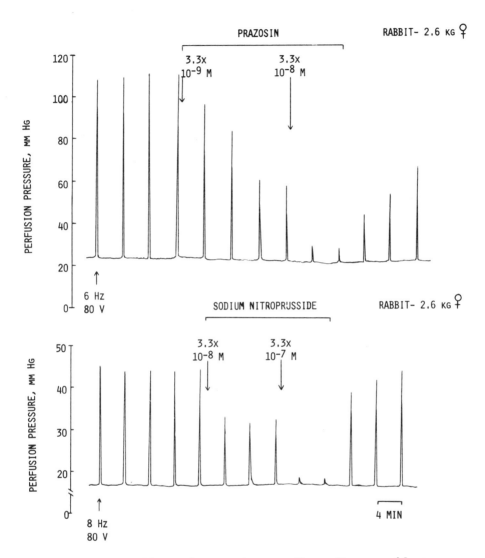

Figure 19. Effect of prazosin or sodium nitroprusside on vasoconstrictor responses of isolated perfused rabbit ear artery to short periods (3 sec) of electrical stimulation.

the second phase of the vasoconstrictor response (Figure 23). The second phase of the response to electrical stimulation is thought to depend on the entry of extracellular Ca^{2+} and is, therefore, specifically blocked by Ca^{2+} channel inhibitors. This

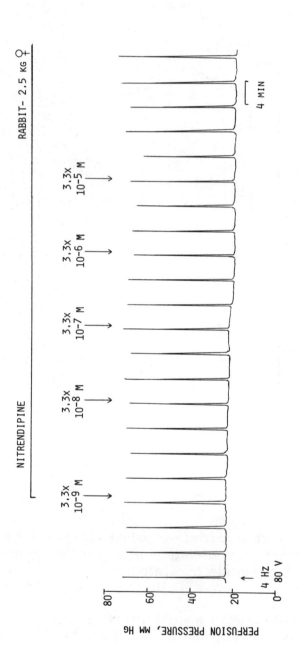

Figure 20. Lack of effect of nitrendipine on vasoconstrictor responses of isolated perfused rabbit ear artery to short periods (3 sec) of electrical stimulation.

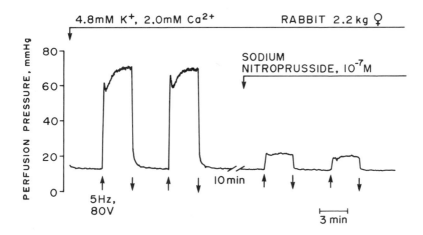

Figure 21. Effect of sodium nitroprusside on biphasic responses of isolated perfused rabbit ear artery to prolonged (3 min) electrical stimulation. Note that both phases of response are inhibited.

method allows us to distinguish between vasodilators acting on Ca^{2+} channels or associated receptors located at the cell membrane and drugs which block the intracellular release or the effect of Ca^{2+}.

V. PERSPECTIVES IN VASODILATOR
THERAPY OF HYPERTESNION

On the basis of the recent clinical experience with new vasodilators, a considerable expansion of the use of vasodilators in hypertension can be predicted. Vasodilator drugs are likely to partially replace β-adrenoceptor antagonists and diuretics, and will account for the anticipated further expansion of the anti-hypertensive market. In many instances vasodilator drugs will be used as an initial and even sole therapy of hypertension.

During the next decade attempts will be made to develop specific drugs for various types of hypertension. The basic research on the pathogenesis of hypertension can be expected to create new approaches to the development of antihypertensive drugs. Of considerable interest in this respect is the discovery of endothelial vasodilator factor (Furchgott and Zawadski, 1980;

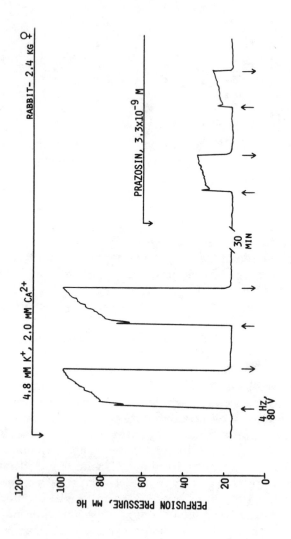

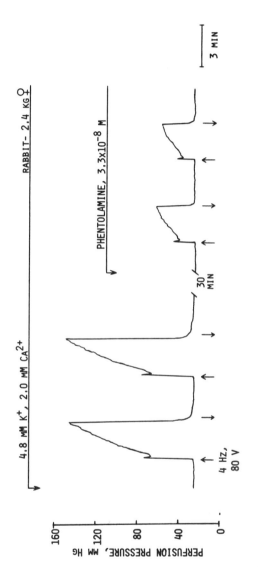

Figure 22. Effects of α-adrenoceptor antagonists on biphasic responses of isolated perfused rabbit ear artery to prolonged (3 min) electrical stimulation. Note that both phases of response are inhibited.

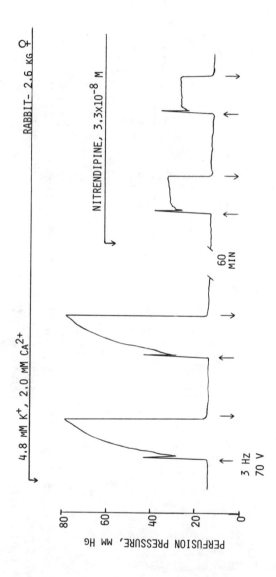

Figure 23. Selective inhibition by nitrendipine of second phase of response of isolated perfused rabbit ear artery to prolonged (3 min) electrical stimulation.

Chand and Altura, 1981) and its possible relation to acetylcholine receptors as well as to the lipoxygenase pathway. A new prostaglandin analog with long-lasting vasodilator activity has already been reported (Chan et al., 1982).

This chapter did not attempt to cover numerous new developments in the field of converting enzyme inhibitors (Gross et al., 1981, Horovitz, 1981;), although these drugs tend to reduce peripheral vascular resistance and can be viewed as indirectly acting vasodilator drugs. Many new inhibitors of converting enzyme as well as renin inhibitors will be developed during the next few years.

VI. SUMMARY

It is anticipated that the use of vasodilator drugs in the treatment of hypertension will increase considerably during the next few years. The increase will be primarily due to introduction of Ca^{2+} antagonists, but other new vasodilators will also become available. The new vasodilator drugs will have fewer side effects than those currently available.

The cellular mechanisms of action of vasodilator drugs are not precisely known, but are under active investigation. Lowering of cytosolic Ca^{2+} appears to be involved in the memechanism of cellular action of many vasodilators.

Vasodilator drugs can be effectively studied in most in vivo hypertension models. In vitro screening techniques for new vasodilator drugs include perfusion of vascular segments, ion fluxes and ligand binding techniques.

New approaches to the therapy of hypertension include development of prostaglandin-like vasodilator drugs, endothelial factor releasing agents or drugs lowing cytosolic Ca^{2+} by mechanism other than the blockade of Ca^{2+} channels.

REFERENCES

Ackerman, D. M., Weinstock, J., Wiebelhaus, V. D., and Berkowitz, B. (1982). Renal vasodilators and hypertension. Drug Dev. Res. 2, 283-297.

Adelstein, R. S. (1982). Calmodulin and the regulation of the actin-myosin interaction in smooth muscle and nonmuscle cells. Cell 30, 349-350.

Adelstein, R. S., Sellers, J. R., Conti, M. A., Pato, M. D., and de Lanerolle, P. (1982). Regulations of smooth muscle contractile proteins by calmodulin and cyclic AMP. Fed. Proc. **41**, 2873-2878.

Alps, B. J., Borrows, E. T., Johnson, E. S., Stamfortin, M. W., and Wilson, A. B. (1972a). A comparison of the cardiovascular actions of indoramin, propranolol, lignocaine and quinidine. Cardiovasc. Res. **6**, 226-234.

Alps, B. J., Hill, M., Johnson, E. S., and Wilson, A. B. (1972b). Quantitative analysis on isolated organs of the autonomic blocking properties of indoramin hydrochloride (WY 21901). Br. J. Pharmacol. **44**, 52-62.

Anderson, R. (1973). Cyclic AMP as a mediator of the relaxing action of papaverine, nitroglycerine, diazoxide and hydralazine in intestinal and vascular smooth muscle. Acta. Pharmacol. Toxicol. **32**, 321-336.

Barnett, C. A., and Whitney, J. E. (1966). The effect of diazoxide and chlorothiazide on glucose uptake in vitro. Metabolism **15**, 88-93.

Baum, T., Watkins, R. W., Sybertz, E. J., Vemulapolli, S., Pula, K. K., Eynon, E., Nelson S., Vander Vliet, G., Glennon, J., and Moran, R. M. (1981). Antihypertensive and hemodynamic actions of Sch19927, the R, R-isomer of labetalol. J. Pharmacol. Exp. Ther. **218**, 444-452.

Blaine, E. H., Russo, H. F., Schorn, T. W., and Snyder, C. (1982). An orally active prostaglandin analog with renal vasodilatory activity in the dog. J. Pharmcol. Exp. Ther. **222**, 152-158.

Brittain, R. T., and Levy, G. P. (1976). A review of the animal pharmacology of labetalol, a combined α-and β-adrenoceptor blocking drug. Br. J. Clin. Pharmacol. **3**, 681-694.

Buyniski, J. P., Pircio, A. W., Schurig, J. E., and Campbell, J. A. (1980). Effects of tiodazosin, prazosin, trimazosin and phentolamine on blood pressure, heart rate and on pre- and post synaptic α-adrenergic receptors in the rat. Clin. Exp. Hypertens. **2**, 1039-1066.

Cambridge, D., Davey, M. J., and Massingham, R. (1977). Prazosin, a selective antagonist of postsynaptic alpha-adrenoceptors. Br. J. Pharmacol. **59**, P514-P515.

Carpi, C., and Dorigotti, L. (1974). Antihypertensive activity of a new 3-hydrazinopyridazine derivative. ISF 2123. Br. J. Pharmacol. **52**, 459P.

Chan, P. S., Scully, P. A., Accomando, R. C., and Cervoni, P. (1982). Mechanisms of action of a new prostaglandin anti-hypertensive, CL 115, 347 (15-deoxy-16-hydroxy-16-vinyl-prostaglandin E_2 methyl ester). Fed. Proc. **41**, 1647.

Chand, N. and Altura, B. M. (1981). Endothelial cells and relaxation of vascular smooth muscle cells: possible relevance to lipoxygenases and their significance in vascular diseases. Microcirculation **1**, 297-317.

Chevillard, C., Mathieu, M. N., Saiag, B., and Worcel, M. (1980). Hydralazine: Effect of the outflow of noradrenaline and mechanical responses evoked by sympathetic nerve stimulation of the rat tail artery. Br. J. Pharmacol. **69**, 415-420.

Chu, D., Cocco, G., Strozzi, C., Vallini, R., Nonato, M., and Amrein, R. (1981). Antihypertensive effects of a novel peripheral vasodilator, Ro 12-4713. Eur. J. Clin. Pharmacol. **19**, 233-238.

Constantine, J. W., McShane, W. K., Scriabine, A., and Hess, H-J. (173). Analysis of the hypotensive action of prazosin. In "Hypertension: Mechanisms and Management" (G. Onesti, K. E. Kim and J. H. Moyer, eds.), pp. 429-444. Grune & Stratton, New York.

Constantine, J. W., and Hess, H-J (1981). The cardiovascular effects of trimazosin. Eur. J. Pharmacol. **74**, 227-238.

Dage, R., Cheng, H. C., and Woodward, J. K. (1981). Cardiovascular properties medroxalol, a new antihypertensive drug. J. Cardiovasc. Pharmacol. **3**, 299-315.

Davidsohn, K. (1877). Versuche uber die Wirkung des Nitroprussidnatriums. Thesis, Albertus-Universitat Koningsberg, Germany.

Deitchman, D., Perhach, J., and Snyder, R. (1980). Beta-adreno-ceptor and cardiovascular effects of MJ-13105 (bucindolol) in anesthetized dogs and rats. Eur. J. Pharmacol. **61**, 263-277.

De Mey, J., and Vanhoutte, P. M. (1981). Uneven distribution of postjunctional $alpha_1$- and $alpha_2$-like adrenoceptors in canine arterial and venous smooth muscle. Circ. Res. **48**, 875-884.

Diamond, J. (1978). Role of cylic nucleotides in control of smooth muscle contraction. Adv. Cyclic Nucleotide Res. **9**, 327-340.

Diamond, J., and Reichert, C. C. (1982). Effects of hydralazine (HYD) on tension and ATP levels in isolated vascular smooth muscle. Canadian Federation of Biological Societies **25**, 157.

DuCharme, D. W., and Zins, G. R. (1980). Minoxidil. In "Pharmacology of Antihypertensive Drugs" (A. Scriabine, ed.), pp. 415-421. Raven Press, New York.

Ebashi, S., Nonomura, Y., Nakamura, S., Nakasone, H., and Kohama, K. (1982). Regulatory mechanism in smooth muscle: actin-linked regulation. Fed. Proc. **41**, 2863-2867.

Freyburger, W. A., Weeks., J. R., and DuCharme, D. W. (1965). Cardiovascular actions of the hypotensive agent, N,N-diallylmelamine (U-7720). Naunyn-Schmiedebergs Arch. Pharmacol. **251**, 39-47.

Furchgott, R. F., and Zawadski, J. V. (1980). The obligatory role of endothelial cells in the relaxation of arterial smooth muscle by acetylcholine. Nature (London) **288**, 373-376.

Garthoff, B., Knorr, A., and Kazda, S. (1982). Nitrendipine increases sodium excretion of acutely saline-loaded rats. Biochem. Pharmacol. **31**, 3015-3016.

Gerold, M., Eigenmann, R., Hefti, F., Daum, A., and Haeusler, F. (1981). Cardiovascular effects of a novel vasoactive antihypertensive agent, Ro 12-4713. J. Pharmacol. Exp. Ther. **216**, 624-633.

Greenwald, J. E., Wong, L. K., Alexander, M., and Bianchine, J. R. (1980). In vivo inhibiton of thromboxane biosynthesis by hydralazine. In "Advances in Prostaglandin and Thromboxane Research, Vol. 6" (B. Sammuelson, P. W. Ramwell, and R. Paoletti, eds.) pp. 293-295. Raven Press. New York.

Grimm, M., Weidmann, P., Meier, A., Ziegler, W. H., and Reubi, F. C. (1981). Acute effects of a new vasodilator, Ro 12-4713 on blood pressure, plasma renin activity, aldosterone and catecholamine levels, and renal function in hypertensive and normal subjects. Eur. J. Clin. Pharmacol. **20**, 169-177.

Gross, D. M., Sweet, C. S., Ulm, E. H., Backlund, E. P., Morris, A. A. Weitz, D., Bohn, D. L., Wenger, H. C. Vassil, T. C. and Stone, C. A. (1981). Effect of N-[(S)-1-carboxy-3-phenylpropyl]-L-Ala-L-Pro and its ethyl ester (MK-421) on angiotensin converting enzyme in vitro and angiotensin I pressor responses in vivo. J. Pharmacol. Exp. Ther. **216**, 552-557.

Gross, F. (1977). Drugs acting on arteriolar smooth muscle (vasodilator drugs). In "Antihypertensive Agents" (F. Gross, ed.), pp. 397-476. Springer-Verlag, Berlin.

Gross, F., Druey, J., and Meier, R. (1950). Eine neue Gruppe blutdrucksenkender Substanzen von besonderem Wirkingscharakter. Experientia 6, 19-21.

Gruetter, D. Y., Gruetter, C. A., Barry, B. K., Baricos, W. H., Hyman, A. L., Kadowitz, P. J., and Ignarro, L. J. (1980). Activation of coronary arterial guanylate cyclase by nitric oxide, nitroprusside, and nitrosoguanidine-inhibition by calcium, lanthanum and other cations, enhancement by thiols. Biochem. Pharmacol. 29, 2943-2950.

Guyton, A. C., Colemen, T. G., Cowley, A. W., Jr., Manning, R. D., Jr., Norman, R. A., Jr., and Ferguson, J. D. (1974). A systems analysis approach to understanding long-range arterial blood pressure control and hypertension. Circ. Res. 35, 159-176.

Hardman, J. G. (1981). Cyclic nucleotides and smooth muscle contraction: some conceptual and experimental considerations. In "Smooth Muscle, And Assessment of Current Knowledge" (E. Bulbring, A. F. Brading, A. W. Jones, and T. Tomita, eds.), pp. 248-262. Universtiy of Texas Press, Austin, Texas.

Hayes, J. M., Graham, R. M., O'Connell, B. P., Speers, E., and Humphrey, T. J. (1976). Effect of prazosin on plasma-renin activity. Aust. N.Z.J. Med. 6, 90.

Hernandez, P. H., Lape, H. E., and Philion, R. E. (1979). Vasodilatory and beta-blocking activity of sulfinalol, a new antihypertensive agent. Fed. Proc. 38, 738.

Horovitz, Z. P. (Ed.) (1981). "Angiotensin converting enzyme inhibitors. Mechanism of action and clinical implications." Urban & Schwarzenberg, Baltimore.

Janis, R. A. (1981). Calcium channel blockers as probes of calcium channels. In "The Mechanism of Gated Calcium Transport across Biological Membranes" (S. T. Onishi, and M. Endo, eds.), pp. 101-110. Academic Press, New York.

Janis, R. A., and Triggle, D. J. (1973). Effect of diazoxide on aortic reactivity to calcium in spontaneously hypertensive rats. Can. J. Physiol. Pharmacol. 51, 621-626.

Janis, R. A., and Diamond, J. (1979). Relationship between cyclic nucleotide levels and drug-induced relaxation of smooth muscle. J. Pharmacol. Exp. Ther. 211, 480-484.

Kaplin, H. R., Commarato, M. A., Dugan, D. H., Essenburg, A. E., Langley, A. E., and Smith R. D. (1980). CN-88823 (6,7-Dimethoxy-2-[4-Thiormorpholinyl]-4-quinazolinamine).

Antihypertensive/autonomic profile-comparison with prazosin. Pharmacologist **23**, 155.

Karaki, H., Hester, R. K., and Weiss, G. B. (1980). Cellular basis of nitroprusside-induced relaxation of graded responses to norepinephrine and potassium in canine renal arteries. Arch. Int. Pharmacodyn. Ther. **245**, 198–210.

Kazda, A., Garthoff, B., and Thomas, G. (1982). Antihypertensive effect of a calcium antagonistic drug: regression of hypertensive cardiac hypertrophy by nifedipine. Drug Dev. Res. **2**, 313–323.

Klinner, V., Ehlers, D., Fermum, R., and Meisel, P. (1977). Versuche zum Wirkungsmechanismus von Gefäßspasmolytika, Acta Biol. Med. Ger. **36**, 1143–1148.

Kreye, V. A. W., Baron, G. D., Luth, J. B., and Schmidt-Gayk, H. (1975). Mode of action of sodium nitroprusside on vascular smooth muscle. Naunyn-Schmiedebergs Arch. Pharmakol. **288**, 381–402.

Kreye, V. A. W., Khayyal, M., and Gross, F. (1980). The response to hydralazine and its modification by ouabain and potassium ions of the rabbit renal artery. Blood Vessels **17**, 153.

Kreye, V. A. W. (1978). Organic nitrates, sodium nitroprusside, and vasodilatation. In "Mechanisms of Vasodilatation" (P. M. Vanhoutte, and I. Leusen, eds.), pp. 158–164. S. Karger, Basel.

Kreye, V. A. W. (1980). Sodium nitroprusside: approaches towards the elucidation of its mode of action. Trends Pharmacol. Sci. October, 384–388.

Kukovetz, W. R. Poech, G., and Holzmann, S. (1981). Cyclic nucleotides and relaxation of vascular smooth muscle. In "Vasodilatation" (P. M. Vanhoutte, and I. Leusen, eds.) pp. 339–353. Raven Press, N. Y.

Kyncl, J. J., Bush, E. N., and Buckner, S. A. (1982). Alpha adrenergic blocking properties of terazosin. Fed. Proc. **41**, 1648.

Levy, G. P., and Richards, D. A. (1980). Labetalol. In "Pharmacology of Antihypertensive Drugs" (A. Scriabine, ed.), pp. 325–347. Raven Press, N. Y.

Liu, T. Z., Shen, J-T., and Loken, H. F. (1974). Inhibition of dopamine-β-hydroxylase by hydralazine. Proc. Soc. Exp. Biol. Med. **145**, 294–297.

Loubatieres, A., Mariani, M. M., and Alric, R. (1968). The action of diazoxide of insulin secretion, medullo-adrenal secretion and the liberation of catecholamines. Ann. N. Y. Acad. Sci. **150**, 226–241.

McLean, A. J., Barron, K., du Souich, P., Haegele, K. D., McNay, J. L., Carrier, O., and Briggs, A. (1978). Interaction of hydralazine and hydrazone derivatives with contractile mechanisms in rabbit aortic smooth muscle. J. Pharmacol. Exp. Ther. 205, 418-425.

Meyer, V. H., Bossert, F., Wehinger, K., Stoepel. K., and Vater, W. (1981). Synthese und vergleichende pharmakologische Untersuchungen von 1,4-Dihydro-2,6-dimethyl-4-(3-nitrophenyl)pyridin-3,5-dicarbonsaureestern mit nicht-identischen Esterfunktionen. Arzneim. Forsch. 31, 407-409.

Moulds, R. F. W., and Jauernig, R. A. (1977). Mechanism of prazosin collapse. Lancet 1, 200-201.

Oates, H. F., and Stoker, L. M. (1981). Studies in the rat on endralazine, a new antihypertensive drug structurally related to hydralazine. Clin. Exp. Pharmacol. Physiol. 8, 133-139.

Packer, M. (1982). Selection of vasodilator drugs for patients with severe chronic heart failure: an approach based on a new classification. Drugs 24, 64-74.

Page, I. H., Corcoran, A. C., Dustan, H. P., and Koppanyi, T. (1955). Cardiovascular actions of sodium nitroprusside in animals and hypertensive patients. Circulation 11, 188-198.

Perry, H. M., Jr. (1953). Method of quantitating 1-hydrazino-phthalazine in body fluids. J. Lab. Clin. Med. 41, 566-573.

Persson, B., Yao, T., and Thoren, P. (1981). Correlation between decreased heart rate and central inhibition of sympathetic discharge after prazosin administration in the spontaneously hypertensive rat. Clin. Exp. Hypertens. 3, 245-255.

Prichard, B. N., and Boakes, A. J. (1976). Labetalol in long term treatment of hypertension. Br. J. Clin. Pharmacol. 3, 743-750.

Reece, P. A. (1981). Hydralazine and related compounds: chemistry, metabolism, and mode of action. Med. Res. Rev. 1, 73-96. Report of the Joint National Committee on Detection, Evaluation and Treatment of High Blood Pressure. A cooperative study (1977). J. Am. Med Assoc. 237, 255-261.

Rhodes H. J., and Sutter, M. C. (1971). The action of diazoxide on isolated vascular smooth muscle electrophysiology and contraction. Can. J. Physiol. Pharmacol. 49, 276-287.

Rubin, A. A., Roth, R. E., Winburg, M. M., Topliss, J. G., Sherlock, M. H., Sperber, N., and Black, J. (1961). New class of antihypertensive agents. Science 33, 2067.

Salzmann, V. R., Burki, H., Chu, D., Clark, B., Marbach, P., Markstein, R., Reinert, H., Siegl, H., and Waite, R. (1979). Pharmakolgische Wirkungen des Antihypertensivums (6-benzoyl-3-hydrazino-5,6,7,8-tetrahydropyrido-(4,3-c)pyridazine (BQ 22-708, Endralazin). Arzneim. Forsch. 29, 1843-1853.

Schoetensack, W., Bischler, P., Dittmann, E. C., and Steinijans, V. (1977). Tierexperimentelle Untersuchungen uber den Einflu$ des Antihypertensivums Urapidil auf den Kreislauf und die Kreislaufregulation. Arzneim. Forsch. 27, 1908-1919.

Scriabine, A., Constantine, J. W., Hess, H-J., and McShane, W. K. (1968). Pharmacological studies with some new antihypertensive aminoquinazolines. Experentia 24, 1150-1151.

Scriabine, A., Ludden, C. T., Watson. L. S., Stavorski. J. M., Morgan, G., and Baldwin. J. J. (1979). Antihypertensive and other cardiovascular effect of 2-(3-pyridyl)-and 2-(4-pyridyl)-4-trifluoromethylimidazoles. Experientia 35, 653-655.

Semeraro, C., Dorigotti, L., Banfi, S. and Carpi, C. (1981). Pharmacological studies on cadralazine: a new antihypertensive vasodilator drug. J. Cardiovasc. Pharmacol. 3, 455-567.

Spokas, E. G. Quilley, J., Rossoni, G., McGiff. J. C., and Folco. G. C. (1982). The endothelium as a determinant of the vascular actions of antihypertensive drugs. Abstracts of 36th Annual Fall Conference of the Council for High Blood Pressure Research. American Heart Asociation, Abstract 31.

Steinsland, O. S., Furchgott, R. F., and Kirpekar, S. M. (1973). Biphasic vasoconstriction of the rabbit ear artery. Circ. Res. 32, 49-58.

Stoepel. K., Heise, A., and Kazda, S. (1981). Pharmacological studies of the antihypertensive effect nitrendipine. Arzneim. Forsch. 31, 2056-2061.

Sweet, C. S., Hall, R. A., Columbo, J. M., Wenger, H. C., Backlund, E., Morgan, G., Gaul, S. L., and Scriabine, A. (1979a). Beta adrenoceptor blocking properties of MK-761. J. Pharmacol. Exp. Ther. 211, 195-199.

Sweet, C. S., Scriabine, A., Weitz, D., Ludden, C. T., Minsker, D. H., and Stone, C. a. (1978b). Antihypertensive and hemodyanamic properties of 2-(3-ter-butylamino-2-hydroxy-propoxy)-3-cyanopyridine HCl (MK761). J. Pharmacolo. Exp. Ther. 211. 201-206.

Sybertz, E. J., Baum, T., Pula, K. K., Nelson, S., Eynon, E., and

Sabin, C. (1982). Studies on the mechanism of the acute antihypertensive and vasodilator actions of several β-adrenoceptor antagonists. J. Cardiovasc. Pharmacol. 4, 749-758.

Taylor, D. G. Jr. (1980). Hydralazine. In "Pharmacology of Antihypertensive Drugs" (A. Scriabine, ed.), pp. 407-414. Raven Press, New York.

Taylor, E. M., Cameron, D., Eden, R. J., Fielden, R., and Owen, D. A. A. (1981a). Hemodynamic profile of a new antihypertensive agent, D,L-3-[2-(3-t-butylamino-2-hydroxypropoxy)phenyl]-6-hydrazinopyridazine (SK&F 92657). J. Cardiovasc. Pharmacol. 3, 337-354.

Taylor, E. M., Eden, R. J., Fielden, R., and Owen, D. A. A. (1981b). Studies on the autonomic nervous system with SK β F 92657, a new antihypertensive agent causing direct arterial vasodilatation and β-adrenoceptor blockade. J. Cardiovasc. Pharmacol. 3, 355-368.

Thirlwell, M. P., and Zsoter, T. T. (1972). The effect of diazoxide on the veins. Am. Heart J. 83, 512-517.

Uchida, Y., Yoshimoto, N., and Murao, S. (1978). Effects of 2-nicotinamidoethyl nitrate (SG-75) on coronary circulation. Jpn. Heart J. 19, 112-124.

Van Nueten, J. M. (1978). Vasodilatation or inhibition of peripheral vasoconstriction. In "Mechanism of Vasodilatation" (P. M. Vanhoutte, and I. Leusen, eds.), pp. 137-143. Karger, Basel.

Van Zwieten, P. A., Van Meel, J. C. A., and Timmermans, P. B. M. W. M. (1981). Vascular aspects of calcium antagonists. Pharm. Weekbl. 3, 237-247.

Webb, R. C., Lockette, W. E., Vanhoutte, P. M., and Bohr, D. F. (1981). Sodium potassium-adenosine triphosphatase and vasodilation. In "Vasodilatation" (P. M. Vanhouttte, and I. Leusen, eds.), pp. 319-330. Raven Press, New York.

Wohl, A. J., Hausler, L. M., and Roth, R. E. (1968). Mechansim of antihypertensive effect of diazoxide: in vitro vascular studies in the hypertensive rat. J. Pharmacol. Exp. Ther. 162, 109-114.

Worcel, M. (1978). Relationship between the direct inhibitory effects of hydralazine and propildazine on arterial smooth muscle contractility and sympathetic innervation. J. Pharmacol. Exp. Ther. 207, 320-33.

Some Aspects of the Chemical Pharmacology of Calcium Channel Antagonists

David J. Triggle

Department of Biochemical Pharmacology
School of Pharmacy
State University of New York at Buffalo
Buffalo, New York

I. INTRODUCTION

Although the group of drugs known as calcium (Ca^{2+}) channel antagonists have been available for some twenty years, their recent introduction into clinical medicine in the United States has served to direct new attention to the cellular roles of calcium.

The Ca^{2+} channel antagonists, also referred to as Ca^{2+} antagonists, slow channel blockers or Ca^{2+} entry blockers (Henry, 1979; Stone et al., 1980; Cano and Henry, 1982; Flaim and Zelis, 1982), are a chemically heterogeneous group of compounds that includes verapamil, D 600, diltiazem and nifedipine (Figure 1). They are of considerable interest because of their clinical use and indications for a number of cardiovascular disorders (Table 1). It is likely that new Ca^{2+} antagonists, representing second and third generations of drugs, may have a wider range of application and may also exhibit greater tissue selectivity, including cardioselectivity, selectivity for defined vascular beds or nonvascular smooth muscles.

Since Ca^{2+} is clearly recognized to play fundamental roles in the maintenance and control of cellular function and excitability, Ca^{2+} antagonists have often been considered as a rather nonspecific and non-selective class of drugs. That this is not

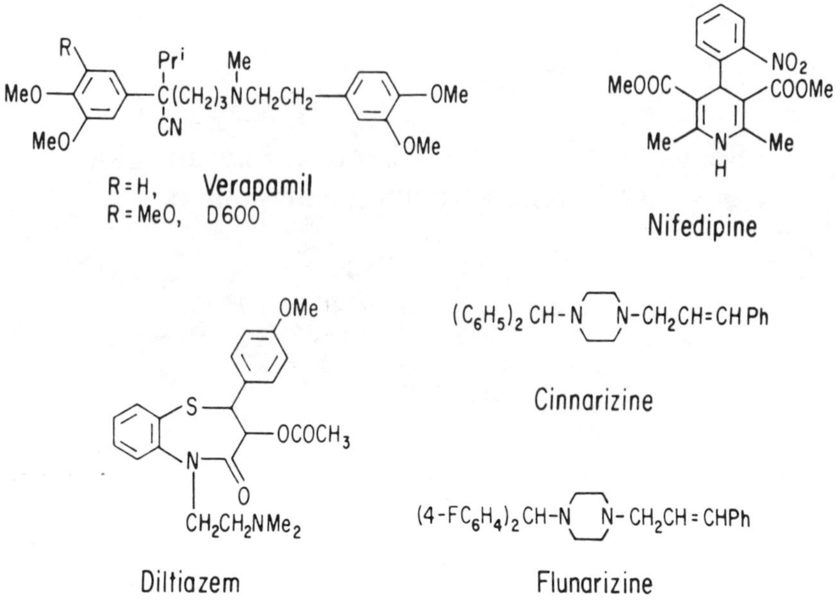

Figure 1. Structural formulae of calcium channel antagonists.

automatically true is documented by the existence of drugs with considerable specificity for certain Ca^{2+}-mediated processes (Figure 1), and may be more clearly realized by brief consideration of the factors controlling cellular Ca^{2+} concentrations and movements.

II. CELLULAR CALCIUM REGULATION

There are three key features to the understanding of cellular Ca^{2+} regulation (Kretsinger, 1977; Rosenberger and Triggle, 1977; Cheung, 1980a,b):

(1) The resting intracellular concentration of free (ionized) Ca^{2+} is normally low, $\leq 10^{-7}$ M, and during excitation it rises to $10^{-7} - 10^{-5}$ M.

(2) There exist within the cell some specific, Ca^{2+}-regulated, target proteins whose binding affinities for Ca^{2+} are in the range of $10^{-7} - 10^{-5}$ M.

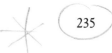

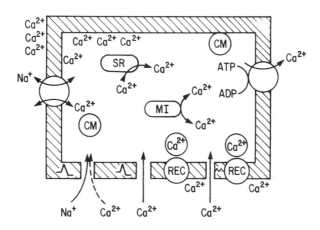

Figure 2. Schematic representation of cellular Ca^{2+} regulation. Depicted are Ca^{2+} entry processes through the Na^+ channel and through voltage-dependent and receptor-operated Ca^{2+} channels. Ca^{2+} efflux mechanisms depicted include Na^+-Ca^{2+} counter transport and a Ca^{2+}-ATPase. Intracellular Ca^{2+} sequestration (and release) can occur in mitochondria (MI) and sarcoplasmic reticulum (SR). Some intracellular Ca^{2+} binding may also occur at internal plasmalemmal surfaces. The calcium binding protein calmodulin (CM) is shown in both cytosolic and membrane-bound localization.

(3) There are a number of Ca^{2+}-specific entry, exit and sequestration processes that are critical to both the maintenance and restoration of low resting intracellular Ca^{2+} levels, and to the increased levels of ionized Ca^{2+} during excitation.

These three features make possible the messenger role of intracellular Ca^{2+} and permit translation of membrane events into cellular responses.

A generalized view of cellular Ca^{2+} regulation is depicted in Figure 2. Cellular Ca^{2+} is sequestered in intracellular organelles including mitochondria (MI) and sarcoplasmic reticulum (SR) for which specific energy-dependent Ca^{2+} uptake processes exist. These stores, notably SR, also serve as a source of intracellular activator Ca^{2+}. Although mitochondria, sarcoplasmic reticulum and other intracellular sites do serve to sequester

Table 1. *Clinical Uses and Indications for Calcium Channel Antagonists*[a]

	Verapamil	Diltiazem	Nifedipine
Cardiac arrhythmias:			
Supraventricular tachycardia	Yes	Likely	No
Atrial flutter, fibrillation	Likely[b]	—	—
Myocardial Ischemia:			
Variant (Prinzmetal's) angina	Yes	Yes	Yes
Exertional (classic) angina	Likely	Likely	Likely
Hypertension:			
Arterial hypertension	—	Likely	Likely
Pulmonary hypertension	?	?	?
Hypertrophic Cardiomyopathy	Likely	—	—
Cardiac Failure	No	Likely	No
Cardiac Preservation	Likely	Likely	Likely

a. Compiled from Henry, 1979; Stone et al., 1980; Flaim and Zelis, 1982.
b. Probably not as efficacious as in supraventricular tachycardia.

Ca^{2+}, ultimately the cell must, in order to maintain total Ca^{2+} sensibly constant, remove Ca^{2+} to the extracellular medium. There are at least two mechanisms involved, a plasma membrane Ca^{2+}-ATPase and a Na^{+}-Ca^{2+} exchange process.

Within the cell the target for free cytoplasmic Ca^{2+} is a group of Ca^{2+} binding proteins including troponin C, parvalbumin, and calmodulin. These proteins, which enjoy a considerable degree of structural homology, serve as the intracellular Ca^{2+} receptors to confer Ca^{2+}-dependent regulation on mechanical, secretory and enzyme activation pathways (Kretsinger and Nelson, 1976; Cheung, 1980; Means and Dedman, 1980). Calmodulin is of particular interest in this regard for it is ubiquitously distributed, shows extreme conservation of structure, and enjoys multiple roles including involvement in mechanical, motility and secretory processes (Cheung, 1980a,b, 1981; Means and Dedman, 1980; Means et al., 1982; Triggle and Swamy, 1983; Table 2).

Finally, there must exist specific Ca^{2+} entry and mobilization pathways which serve to transmit those membrane signals that lead to changes in intracellular Ca^{2+} levels (Rosenberger and Triggle, 1978; Triggle and Swamy, 1983). A summary view of these mobilization processes is shown in Figure 3. Quite generally, Ca^{2+} may be mobilized from both intracellular and extracellular sources and the relative importance of these sources can be both tissue- and stimulus-dependent. Thus, there is considerable interest (and difficulty) in distinguishing the several sources of Ca^{2+} involved in stimulus-function coupling systems.

Membrane channels mediating Ca^{2+} entry have been designated as two major types. Potential-dependent Ca^{2+} channels (PDC) are activated by membrane depolarization whilst receptor-operated Ca^{2+} channels (ROC) are activated by membrane ligand-receptor interactions (Rosenberger and Triggle, 1978; Bolton, 1979; van Breemen et al., 1980; Meisheri et al., 1981; Triggle and Swamy, 1983). Thus a solely depolarizing stimulus (elevated K^{+}_{EXT}) will activate PDC whilst a hormone- or transmitter-receptor stimulus will activate ROC and, depending upon the extent of membrane depolarization, may also activate PDC or mobilize intracellular Ca^{2+} (Figure 3). The relative contributions of the several Ca^{2+} mobilization pathways shown in Figure 3 will thus be both stimulus- and tissue-dependent.

Much remains to be learned about the properties of plasma membrane Ca^{2+} channels. It is unlikely that either channel type is absolutely specific for Ca^{2+} and it is probable that their dis-

Table 2. Partial Listing of Calmodulin-Dependent Processes[a]

A. Enzyme activation

Cyclic nucleotide phosphodiesterase
Adenylate cyclase
Myosin light chain kinase
Ca^{2+}, Mg^{2+}-ATPase
Phosphorylase-B kinase
Glycogen synthetase kinase
Phospholipase A_2
Tryptophan 5'-monooxygenase
Phosphoprotein phosphatase

B. Cellular Events

Muscle (smooth) contraction
Hormone and neurotransmitter secretion
Cellular architecture
Ca^{2+} transport
Cellular motility
Axonal transport
Phospholipid breakdown
Cl^- transport

---

a. From Means et al., 1982.

tribution within the membrane is quite distinct. Receptor-operated channels may well be components of specific receptors whilst potential-dependent channels are probably independent entities, responding to a change in membrane potential which may be initiated by a number of stimulants. Thus, while there may be a single major class of potential-dependent Ca^{2+} channels, receptor-operated channels may be of many distinct types, each unique to the specific receptor of which the channel may be a component. Nonetheless, both ROC and PDC must have a common ability to translocate Ca^{2+}. The linkage(s) between membrane stimulus and channel activation remains to be established, and biochemical events could be involved. In cardiac tissue potential-dependent Ca^{2+} channel activation evoked by beta-adrenergic receptor stimulation may involve a cAMP mediated

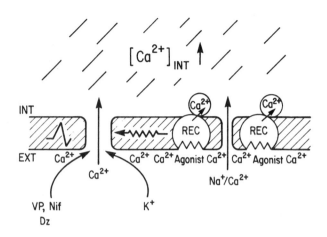

Figure 3. Representation of Ca^{2+} mobilization in excitable tissue. Ca^{2+} entry (extracellular Ca^{2+} mobilization) may occur through voltage-dependent (–∿) channels which are activated by K^+ depolarization and also by agonist-receptor interactions (–∿∿∿→). These channels are blocked by the calcium channel antagonists verapamil (VP), nifedipine (Nif) and diltiazem (DZ). The latter interactions may also mobilize extracellular Ca^{2+} through receptor-operated (potential-independent) channels. Ca^{2+}-mobilization from receptor-associated Ca^{2+} may also be a consequence of specific agonist-receptor interactions.

phosphorylation step (Reuter and Scholz, 1977; Vogel and Sperelakis, 1981). In a number of smooth muscle and secretory systems a role for stimulus-evoked phosphatidylinositol breakdown in the direct control of Ca^{2+} channel gating has been proposed (Michell et al., 1981; Putney, 1981).

Differentiation between the several Ca^{2+} sources and mobilization pathways is obviously of importance. In this regard, much remains to be achieved, but valuable information is being obtained through the use of Ca^{2+} antagonists, compounds which have pharmacologic selectivity for defined Ca^{2+}-mediated events.

III. CALCIUM ANTAGONISTS

Given the various sites of cellular Ca^{2+} control the possible existence of site-selective Ca^{2+} antagonists may be considered. This possibility is far from full realization, although there is no shortage of chemical structures possessing to varying degrees the ability to inhibit some Ca^{2+}-dependent processes. These structures range from inorganic di- and tri-valent cations, to local anesthetics, to antipsychotics, to complex antibiotics including neomycin C. Their Ca^{2+}-antagonistic properties are, however, often secondary to other and better defined pharmacologic activites. In recent years considerable attention has been paid to two major groups of compounds exerting Ca^{2+} antagonistic effects — the calmodulin antagonists (Figure 4) and the Ca^{2+} channel blockers (Figure 1). Both groups of compounds are diverse in chemical structure, this diversity being their major common attribute (Figure 4).

Although some of the calmodulin antagonists, notably trifluoperazine, have been widely employed in the attempted definition of calmodulin-dependent pathways (Roufogalis, 1983), there is considerable uncertainty about their specificity of action, particularly in cellular systems. The ability of these compounds to bind to calmodulin and to inhibit Ca^{2+}-calmodulin dependent processes is nonstereoselective and appears to be largely determined by the hydrophobicity of the molecule (Levin and Weiss, 1979; Norman et al., 1979; Raess and Vincenzi, 1980; Roufogalis, 1983), a finding quite consistent with observations that Ca^{2+} binding to calmodulin exposes hydrophobic sites (LaPorte et al., 1980). Thus considerable caution should be exercised in assigning the pharmacologic effects to calmodulin antagonism since such nonspecific hydrophobic associations are likely to perturb many cellular functions. Even though it is well recognized that the calmodulin-antagonistic effect of the phenothiazine and related antagonists is secondary to their far more potent effects on dopamine receptors (Norman et al., 1979; Raess and Vincenzi, 1980; Roufogalis, 1983), it is also clear that these agents inhibit other receptor events including alpha-adrenergic, muscarinic and serotonergic mediated events at concentrations less than or equal to those at which they interfere with calmodulin function (Roufogalis, 1983). Whether these cautionary comments should apply to all calmodulin antagonists including the highly potent R 24571 (Figure 4) is not yet certain. It is, however, quite certain that further research into the development of more specific calmodulin antagonists is urgently needed.

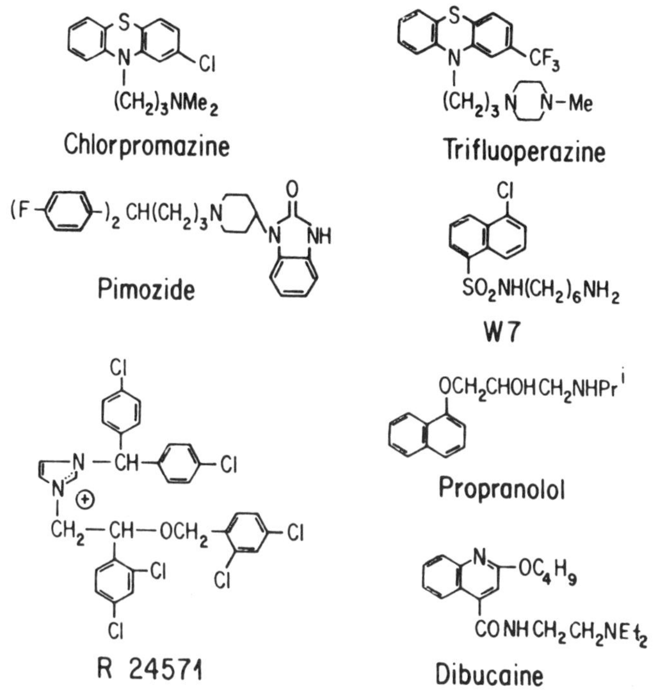

Figure 4. *Structural formulae of some calmodulin antagonists.*

Although the group of compounds known as the Ca^{2+} channel antagonists is also structurally heterogeneous, evidence for their specificity of major action at a defined site, i.e., the potential dependent Ca^{2+} channel, is quite convincing. The remainder of this chapter will therefore focus on this group of compounds.

IV. CALCIUM CHANNEL ANTAGONISTS

The description of the activity of the Ca^{2+} channel antagonists owes much to the pioneering work of Fleckenstein who recognized the ability of a number of compounds, including verapamil/D 600, prenylamine and subsequently nifedipine and diltiazem, to mimic the effects of Ca^{2+} withdrawal in cardiac

tissue (Fleckenstein, 1964, 1971). These effects extended to
vascular smooth muscle, including coronary arteries (Fleckenstein, 1977), and later work showed that these agents inhibited
quite specifically the slow Ca^{2+} current of cardiac tissue
(Tritthart et al., 1973; Bayer et al., 1977; Bayer and Ehara, 1978;
Fleckenstein, 1981). Several reviews by Fleckenstein detail
the development of this area (Fleckenstein, 1971, 1977, 1981).

To define more precisely the actions of this group of compounds several important aspects of their actions must be discussed. These include:
  (1) Specificity of action
  (2) Structure-activity correlations
  (3) Selectivity of action
  (4) Differences in action
  (5) Sites and mechanisms of action

Table 3. Calcium Channel Antagonist Activites in Smooth Muscle

System		Antagonist	ID_{50}, M
Rabbit aorta[a]	NE	Verapamil	1.2×10^{-4}
	K^+	Verapamil	2.7×10^{-8}
Rabbit saphenous artery[b]	5-HT	Nimodipine	2×10^{-5}
	K^+	Nimodipne	2.5×10^{-10}
Rabbit basilar artery[b]	5-HT	Nimodipine	7.3×10^{-10}
	K^+	Nimodipine	1.7×10^{-10}
Guinea pig ileum[c]	ACh	Nifedipine	5.1×10^{-9}
	K^+	Nifedipine	3.4×10^{-9}
Canine coronary[d]	NE	D 600	5×10^{-7}
	K^+	D 600	2×10^{-7}
Rabbit ear artery[e]	NE	Diltiazem	1×10^{-6}
	5-HT	Diltiazem	8×10^{-7}
	K^+	Diltiazem	2×10^{-6}

a. From Schumann et al., 1975.
b. From Towart, 1981.
c. From Rosenberger et al., 1979.
d. From Van Breemen and Siegel, 1980.
e. From Bevan, 1982.

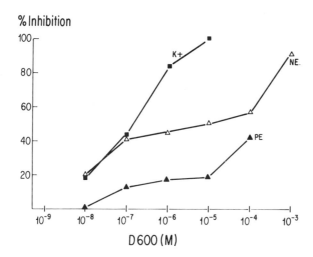

Figure 5. *Inhibition of responses of rat aorta by D 600 to maximally effective concentrations of phenylephrine (PE), norepinephrine (NE) and K^+.*

A. Specificity of Action and Structure–Activity Correlations

Although the activities of the Ca^{2+} channel antagonists were originally described for cardiac tissue, it was soon realized that they had potent inhibitory effects on both vascular and nonvascular smooth muscle (Fleckenstein, 1977; Rosenberger and Triggle, 1978; Triggle and Swamy, 1980). Quite generally the antagonists are effective against K^+-induced responses (a depolarizing stimulus) but have varying degrees of effectiveness against agonist-induced responses. This is illustrated by the representative data shown in Table 3.

These data suggest that the relative sensitivities of the agonist-induced responses depend, at least in part, upon the relative mobilization of Ca^{2+} through PDC, ROC and intracellular stores (Figure 3). This is further illustrated in Figure 5 which compares Ca^{2+}_{EXT} dependence and D 600 sensitivity of response in aortic tissue to K^+-depolarization, norepinephrine and phenylephrine.

Additional support is provided by a number of studies which have demonstrated that the Ca^{2+} channel antagonists inhibit stimulus-evoked $^{45}Ca^{2+}$ uptake in smooth muscle (Rosenberger

Table 4. *Comparison of Calcium Antagonist Activities against mechanical responses and $^{45}Ca^{2+}$ Uptake in Smooth Muscle.*

System		Antagonist	ID_{50}, M	
			$^{45}Ca^{+2} \uparrow$	Contraction
Rabbit pulmonary artery[a]	K^+	Verapamil	3.0×10^{-7}	4.0×10^{-7}
Rabbit aorta[b]	K^+	Nicardipine	1.0×10^{-9}	1.9×10^{-9}
		Verapamil	6.8×10^{-8}	1.7×10^{-7}
		D 600	1.5×10^{-7}	2.0×10^{-7}
Rat aorta[c]	NE	Flunarizine	7.0×10^{-7}	5.0×10^{-7}
	K^+	Flunarizine	1.8×10^{-7}	2.2×10^{-7}
Rat superior mesenteric[d]	NE	Flunarizine	5.0×10^{-8}	2.4×10^{-8}

a. From Thorens and Haeusler, 1979.
b. From Terai et al., 1981.
c. From Meisheri et al., 1981.
d. From Godfraind and Dieu, 1981.

et al., 1979; Thorens and Haeusler, 1979; Meisheri et al., 1981; Terai et al., 1981; Godfraind and Dieu, 1981). Moreover, there is good agreement between the concentrations at which inhibition of $^{45}Ca^{2+}$ uptake and inhibition of mechanical response occur (Table 4).

The apparent specificity of action revealed in the preceding data finds support from structure-activity studies of the Ca^{2+} channel antagonists (Loev et al., 1974; Rosenberger and Triggle, 1978; Mannhold et al., 1978; Rodenkirchen et al., 1979; Fossheim et al., 1982). These studies do not yield a single all-encompassing structure-activity relationship for Ca^{2+} channel antagonists, but such a relationship would not have been anticipated from the structural heterogeneity of this class of agents. However, the structure-activity data do indicate, for each chemical category, the existence of discrete structure-activity relationships. This is particularly true for the 1,4-dihydropyridine (nifedipine) series of compounds, due in part to the relative ease of chemical synthesis

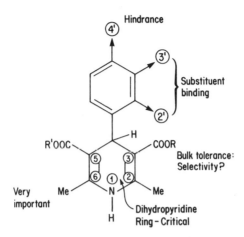

Figure 6. Structural requirements for activity in the 1,4-dihydropyridines (see test for further discussion).

of these agents (Bossert et al., 1981). For this series (Figure 6) the structural requirements may be summarized as follows (Loev et al., 1974; Rosenberger and Triggle, 1978; Bossert et al., 1981; Fossheim et al., 1982):

(1) N-1 of the 1,4-dihydropyridine ring should be unsubstituted.

(2) The 2,6-substituents of the 1,4-dihydropyridine ring should be lower alkyl (Me), although one NH_2 group can substitute for an alkyl group.

(3) Ester functions are optimal for the 3- and 5-positions of the dihydropyridine ring. The most frequent substitution has been carbomethoxy, but higher ester functions maintain or increase activity and may even confer a degree of tissue selectivity.

(4) An aryl substituent, usually substituted phenyl, in the 4-position of the 1,4-dihydropyridine ring is required for maximal activity. Placement of the substituent in the phenyl ring is critical; C_2'- and C_3'-substituents increase or maintain activity whereas substitution at C_4' is invariably detrimental.

(5) The 1,4-dihydropyridine ring is essential: oxidation or reduction (to pyridines or piperidines) abolishes the Ca^{2+} antagonist activity.

Qualitatively the same structural features appear necessary regardless of whether vasodilatation (antihypertensive activity), negative inotropic activity or in vitro inhibition of smooth muscle (vascular or nonvascular) is measured. This suggests a considerable degree of similarity between the sites of 1,4-dihydropyridine interaction.

The existence of structure-activity correlations is obviously consistent with the concept of specific, rather than with nonspecific, sites of action. This conclusion is supported by the stereoselectivity of action exhibited by diltiazem, verapamil/D 600 and compounds of the nifedipine series. Thus, for diltiazem with two asymmetric centers, the activity of the (+)-cis-isomer is greater than the (-)-cis-isomer (Nagao et al., 1972). Similarly, the (-)-isomers of both verapamil and D 600 are the more potent than their enantiomers in both cardiac and smooth muscle preparations (Satoh et al., 1980; Raschack and Engelmann, 1980; Nawrath et al., 1981; Jim et al., 1981). Several dihydropyridines bearing different ester functions at the 3- and 5-positions of the dihydropyridine ring have been examined. Stereoselectivity of antagonism is also exhibited by this series of compounds (Table 5, 6). In marked contrast, however, neither verapamil nor D 600 exhibit stereoselectivity as competitive antagonists of adrenergic α_1 and muscarinic receptor binding in smooth and cardiac muscle membranes (Shibanuma et al., 1980; Nayler et al., 1982).

B. Selectivity of Action

The apparent tissue selectivity of the Ca^{2+} channel antagonists is clearly one of the most exciting concepts that are developing in this field. Indeed the Ca^{2+}-channel blockers appear heterogeneous both with respect to chemical structure and pharmacologic activity. This pharmacologic heterogeneity is expressed in differences in cardiodepressant and vasodilatory properties, onset times and durations of action, use dependence, discrimination between different vascular beds, inhibition of excitation-contraction and stimulus-secretion coupling processes, as well as the extent to which antagonism of non-Ca^{2+} dependent events occur.

Apparent selectivity of action may arise from the disproportionate use of the Ca^{2+}-channel antagonist sensitive pathways utilized by a common stimulant acting in different tissues, or by different stimulants acting in the same tissue. Two exam-

Table 5. Stereoselective Actions of Verapamil and D 600

Antagonist		Isomer Ratio[a]			
		Canine Heart (inotropic) ↓	Cat papillary (inotropic) ↓	G.P. ileum (K⁺)	Rat vas deferens (K⁺)
Verapamil	(−) : (+)	15	10	—	—
D600	(−) : (+)	—	100	10	40

a. Compiled from Satoh et al., 1980; Raschak and Engelmann, 1980: Newrath et al., 1981; Jim et al, 1981.

Table 6. Stereoselective Actions of 1,4-Dihydropyridines

| Antagonist | | | Isomer Ratio[a] | | | | |
R	R¹		Rabbit aorta (K+)	Rabbit basilar (K+)	Rabbit saphenous (K+)	G.P. bladder (K+)	G.P. ileum (K+)
Me₂CH	(CH₂)₂OMe	(−) : (+)	5	7.5	4.5	—	—
Me	CHMe₂	(−) : (+)	10	—	—	8	10
Et	CHMe₂	(−) : (+)	—	—	—	—	2.5
Me	(CH₂)₂NMe CH₂Ph	(+) : (−)	4	—	—	—	—

a. Compiled from Shibanuma et al., 1980; Towart et al., 1981, 1982; Triggle, unpublished results.

ples may make this situation clearer. Nimodipine is quite ineffective against 5-HT-induced responses in rabbit saphenous artery yet is highly effective against 5-HT-induced mechanical responses in the basilar artery (Towart, 1981; Table 3). Since the responses to K^+ in either artery are equisensitive to nimodipine, it is likely that the apparent selectivity arises from the inability of 5-HT to activate the antagonist-sensitive PDC in the saphenous artery. In the rat aorta responses to K^+ are very sensitive to D 600, responses to phenylephrine (an α_1-agonist) are insensitive and those to norepinephrine (α_1,α_2-agonist) show a range of mixed sensitivity (Figure 5). This can be interpreted by assuming that, in this tissue, α_2-responses are linked to the pathways sensitive to channel antagonists, whereas α_1-responses are not.

Selectivity can also arise from apparently more fundamental causes. Thus, differences in relative cardiodepressant and vasodilatory actions between different classes of antagonists have long been recognized (Fleckenstein, 1977; Rosenberger and Triggle, 1978; Henry, 1979, 1980; Stone et al., 1980). Nifedipine has a higher vasodilator: cardiodepressant ratio than verapamil or diltiazem (Hashimoto et al., 1979; Henry, 1980; Kawai et al., 1981; Lindner et al., 1982) being some 10-20 fold more potent as a vasodilator. Even higher ratios of vasodilator:cardiodepressant have been found amongst analogs of nifedipine. For example, nisoldipine is some 10 times more potent than nifedipine as a vasodilator but has the same cardiac activity as nifedipine (Kazda et al., 1980). Flordipine is reported to have even greater selectivity with only 0.001 times the activity of nifedipine as a cardiac depressant (Smith et al., 1982). Thus, separation of pharmacologic effects in cardiac and vascular tissue appears to be well established.

Of further interest are recent conclusions that it is possible to separate the negative inotropic and negative chronotropic effects of the Ca^{2+} channel antagonists. In guinea-pig atria the order of activity for negative chronotropy was diltiazem >D 600 >verapamil > nifedipine whilst the potency order for negative inotropy was nifedipine >D 600 >verapamil >diltiazem (Perez et al., 1982). These are potentially very important findings and have implications for the design of ino- and chrono-selective antagonists. However, it remains to be determined to what extent the "other effects" (local anesthesia, receptor blockade) of the Ca^{2+} antagonists, which are markedly more prominent for D 600, verapamil and diltiazem than for nifedipine, contribute to

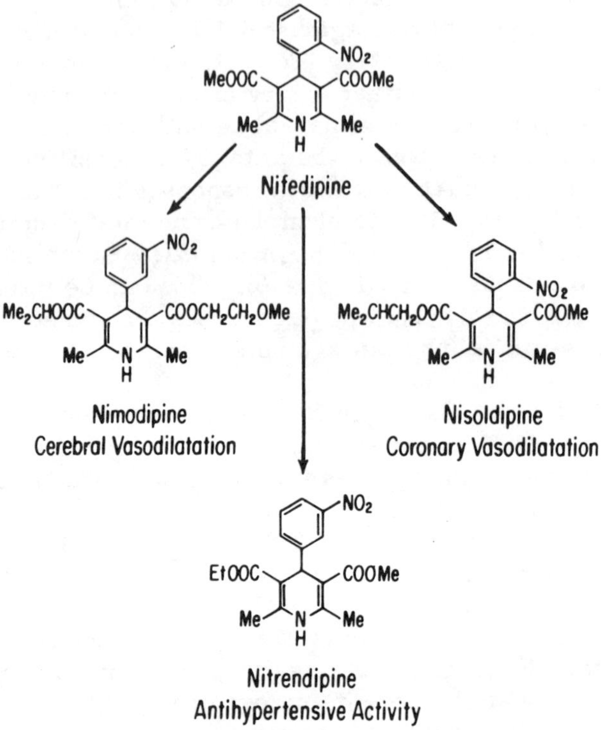

Figure 7. Potential tissue-selective analogs of nifedipine.

this apparent discrimination.

Of comparable importance is the potential ability of the calcium channel antagonists to selectively antagonize responses in specific vascular beds. Several reports have appeared indicating such selectivity. Thus, nisoldipine is reported to be selective for the coronary vascular bed (Kazda et al., 1980), nimodipine to be selective for the cerebral vasculature (Kazda et al., 1982) and nitrendipine to be selective for blood vessels of the skeletal musculature (Stoepel et al., 1981). This suggests that nisoldipine, nimodipine and nitrendipine may, respectively, have therapeutic utility for angina, cerebral ischemia and hypertension (Figure 7).

However, selectivity reported for in vivo systems may arise from distribution and other pharmacokinetic effects as well as from specific differences at the site of interaction of the Ca^{2+}-channel antagonists. It is therefore of particular interest that selectivity differences have been reported for in vitro preparations of smooth muscles. Thus, nisoldipine is some 100 times more potent than nifedipine against Ca^{2+}-induced contractions in rabbit portal vein, but only 10 times more effective in the rabbit aortic strip preparation (Kazda et al., 1980). Such selectivity is not confined to antagonists of the 1,4-dihydropyridine series; in a comparison of diltiazem activity in rabbit basilar, ear and mesenteric artery, the basilar artery was the most sensitive regardless of the nature of stimulant (Bevan, 1982). Van Nueten and Vanhoutte (1981) have shown a 200-fold sensitivity difference for flunarizine inhibition of Ca^{2+} responses in K^+-depolarized canine veins and arteries.

Both the heterogeneity of chemical structure and the evidence for selectivity of action of the Ca^{2+} channel blockers are consistent with the view that these agents probably act by different mechanisms to impair Ca^{2+} channel function. This view is further strengthened by a number of clear-cut differences in the pharmacologic actions of these agents. Thus, flunarizine and cinnarizine differ markedly from verapamil, diltiazem and nifedipine in their slowness of onset and offset of action (Van Nueten and Janssen, 1973; Spedding, 1982). This, together with the marked vascular selectivity of these agents, suggests that flunarizine and cinnarizine fall into a separate category of Ca^{2+} antagonist.

An additional difference between Ca^{2+} channel antagonists is to be found in the marked rate- or use-dependence exhibited by some agents. As may be anticipated this has been best described for cardiac tissue where both frequency- and voltage-dependence, activity increasing with frequency of stimulation and decreasing membrane potential, has been described for verapamil and D 600 but not for nifedipine (Bayer et al., 1975; McDonald et al., 1980; Kohlhardt, 1981). Both verapamil and D 600 impede the voltage-dependent recovery of the Ca^{2+} channel from inactivation (McDonald et al., 1980; Kohlhardt, 1981). Thus, the activities of verapamil and D 600 are state-dependent and they may exhibit preferential interaction with the Ca^{2+} channel in its non-resting configuration(s). Because of the paucity of electrophysiologic data in smooth muscle, it remains to be established whether use-dependence equivalent to that seen in cardiac muscle also occurs. However, Godfraind (Godfraind and Dieu, 1981) has reported that the inhibitory action of flunarizine increases with the duration of stimulation.

Despite the apparent differences in actions among the various types of Ca^{2+} channel antagonist, it is likely that they exert their primary actions at the level of the plasma membrane. This is strongly indicated by the inactivity of these agents as inhibitors of Ca^{2+} movements in intracellular organelles (Entman et al., 1972; Godfraind and Miller, 1982) and by their inactivity as inhibitors of Ca^{2+}-dependent tension responses in skinned cardiac and smooth muscle (Fleckenstein, 1971; Frey and Janke, 1975; Itoh et al., 1981). This indication of a plasma membrane site of interaction has received strong support from several very recent investigations documenting direct binding of Ca^{2+} channel antagonists to membrane fractions derived from smooth and cardiac muscle.

C. Sites and Mechanisms of Action

The accumulated evidence that the Ca^{2+} channel antagonists interact at a specific site to inhibit Ca^{2+} channel function is confirmed by several demonstrations of specific binding of [^{3}H]-nitrendipine and [^{3}H]-nimodipine to crude membrane preparations (Bellemann et al., 1981, 1982; Murphy and Snyder, 1982; Ehlert et al., 1982a,b; Bolger et al., 1982, 1983; Gould et al., 1982; Janis et al., 1982; Triggle et al., 1982). Subsequent to the original report by Belleman et al. (1981) which described the binding of [^{3}H]-nitrendipine to cardiac membranes, binding has been reported also for smooth muscle and brain membranes, and the effects of different structural classes of Ca^{2+} antagonists on [^{3}H]-nitrendipine and [^{3}H]-nimodipine binding have been examined.

The characteristics derived from such radioligand binding studies are consistent with the concept that an interaction occurs at a site (or sites) at which the pharmacologic actions of these compounds are exerted. Thus, binding of [^{3}H]-nitrendipine or [^{3}H]-nimodipine is saturable, reversible, of high affinity and pharmacologically appropriate; competition for the specific binding by 1,4-dihydropyridines reveals a broad parallel with the pharmacologic potencies of these compounds. A representative selection of equilibrium binding data is shown in Table 7. Consistently found is a high affinity binding component, $K_D \sim 0.1$-0.2 nM, but Bellemann et al. (1981) have also reported a low affinity binding component for [^{3}H]-nitren-

Table 7. Binding Characteristics of [^{3}H]-Nitrendipine and [^{3}H]-Nimodipine

System	[^{3}H]-Nitrendipine		[^{3}H]-Nimodipine	
	K_D,nM	B_{MAX}[a]	K_D,nM	B_{MAX}[a]
Guinea-pig heart[b]	0.1	300		
	67	35000		
Guinea-pig brain[c]			0.3	340
Rat heart[d]	0.24	120		
Rat cerebral cortex[d]	0.11-0.16	102		
Rat ileum[d]	0.26	25		
Rat ventricle[e,f]	0.18	400	0.21	350
Guinea-pig ileum[f,g]	0.16	1100	0.12	750

a. Maximum number of binding sites is expressed as f mol/mg protein.
b. From Bellemann et al., 1981.
c. From Bellemann et al., 1982.
d. From Ehlert et al., 1982a,b.
e. From Bolger et al., 1982.
f. From Janis et al., 1982.
g. From Bolger et al., 1983.

dipine in heart membranes. Specific binding is unaffected by a variety of receptor active ligands (muscarinic, adrenergic, nicotinic etc.) and appears sensitive only to those agents which have pharmacologically defined activities at the Ca^{2+} channel (organic and inorganic Ca^{2+} channel antagonists).

A good correlation has been found between the abilities of a series of 1,4-dihydropyridines to inhibit [^{3}H]-nitrendipine binding and to inhibit K^+-induced responses in guinea-pig ileal longitudinal smooth muscle (Figure 8; Bolger et al., 1982, 1983). Binding is sensitive to both di- and trivalent metal cations; La^{3+}, Co^{2+}, Ni^{2+}, Mn^{2+} and Cd^{2+}, which block Ca^{2+} channel function,

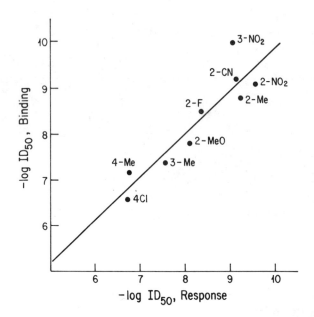

Figure 8. Correlation between ID_{50} values for inhibition of K^+-induced mechanical response (tonic phase) of guinea-pig ileal longitudinal muscle and inhibition of $[^3H]$-nitrendipine binding to microsomal fractions of the same tissue for a series of 2,6-dimethyl-3,5-dicarbomethoxy-4-substituted-phenyl-1,4-dihydropyridines. The position and nature of the substituent in the phenyl ring is shown in the figure.

also block $[^3H]$-nitrendipine binding (Ehlert et al., 1982b; Gould et al., 1982; Bolger et al., 1983). It is of particular interest that $[^3H]$-nitrendipine binding is Ca^{2+}-dependent and removal of Ca^{2+} produces a reversible reduction in binding affinity, an effect which is particularly marked in brain tissue. The ability of Ca^{2+} to stimulate $[^3H]$-nitrendipine binding is shared by some other divalent cations, including Sr^{2+} and Ba^{2+}, which can serve as current carrying species (Gould et al., 1982). These provocative findings suggest that the interaction of cations with the Ca^{2+} channel may generate two conformational states, "active" and "blocked", which differentially modulate the binding of Ca^{2+}-channel antagonists.

The structural heterogeneity of the Ca^{2+} channel blockers suggests, as discussed previously that the various structural classes may interact with the Ca^{2+} channel by different mechanisms. The inhibition of [^{3}H]-nitrendipine binding by verapamil and D 600 confirms this suggestion. Verapamil and D 600 produce only partial inhibition (~50%) of [^{3}H]-nitrendipine binding in rat heart, rat brain and guinea-pig ileum (Ehlert et al., 1982a,b; Bolger et al., 1983) and this is achieved by a concentration-limited decrease in the affinity of [^{3}H]-nitrendipine. This effect of D 600 has also been shown to be stereoselective, consistent with the degree of stereoselectivity determined pharmacologically (Bolger et al., 1983). The actions of verapamil and D 600 are consistent with an allosteric mode of antagonism and suggest that there are probably several distinct components to the Ca^{2+} channel at which binding of antagonists can modulate function.

Although the collective data for [^{3}H]-nitrendipine and [^{3}H]-nimodipine binding are highly suggestive of a pharmacologically appropriate interaction, some inconsistencies remain to be addressed (Triggle, 1982). Cardiac tissue (mechanical responses or Ca^{2+} currents) is known to be less sensitive to the dihydropyridine series of antagonists than smooth muscle, although the same basic structural requirements hold for both tissues. The comparably high affinity binding found in both cardiac and smooth muscle represents, therefore, a discrepancy that needs further investigation. Similarly, the high affinity binding found in brain tissue does not appear to manifest itself in any major profile of pharmacologic effects associated with the central nervous system.

V. CA^{2+} AND SMOOTH MUSCLE DEFECTS

There is considerable evidence that changes in contractile function of vascular smooth muscle occur during the development of hypertension (Daniel, 1981; Daniel and Kwan, 1981). These changes include an increase in nonspecific reactivity of some intact arterial beds (McGregor and Smirk, 1970; Folkow et al., 1970; Finch and Haeusler, 1974), selective increases of sensitivity in isolated vascular smooth muscles (Clineschmidt et al., 1970; Field et al., 1972; Hallback et al., 1971; Swamy and Triggle, 1980; Harris et al., 1980), decreased maximum tension responses in tissues from hypertensive animals (Hallback et al.,

1971; Field et al.,, 1972; Shibata et al., 1973) and decreased rates of poststimulus relaxation (Field et al., 1972; Cohen and Berkowitz, 1976). Several proposals have been advanced which attempt to provide a unifying account of these changes of contractile function of arteries from hypertensive animals. These proposals include structural changes (hypertrophy and hyperplasia) of the vascular smooth muscle (Folkow et al., 1970; Mulvany et al., 1978; Daniel, 1981) and altered Na^+ pump activity (Jones, 1973; Hermsmeyer, 1976; Friedman and Friedman, 1976; Pammani et al., 1981). Critical comments on the merits of these and other related hypotheses are available (Daniel, 1981; Daniel and Kwan, 1981).

Of particular interest is the possibility that the vascular smooth muscle changes seen in hypertension are linked to a defect or defects in smooth muscle Ca^{2+} metabolism. Interest in this proposal is heightened because of recent reports that dietary Ca^{2+} intake and serum concentrations of ionized Ca^{2+} are both significantly reduced in human hypertension (McCarron, 1982; McCarron et al., 1982). Decreased relaxation rates following stimuli suggest that Ca^{2+} transport, either by sequestration into intracellular organelles or by extrusion across the plasma membrane, is reduced. A defect in Ca^{2+} handling by the hypertensive vascular smooth muscle cell could also underlie an increased basal active tension and the observed altered reactivities as well as maximum tension responses. Consistent with this possibility, decreased ATP-dependent Ca^{2+} accumulation is found not only in crude microsomal fractions from hypertensive aortae (Bhalla et al., 1970; Moore et al., 1975), but also in highly enriched plasma membrane fractions of rat mesenteric arteries from spontaneously hypertensive, renal hypertensive and DOC-hypertensive rats (Kwan et al., 1979, 1980a,b). This suggests that the defect in Ca^{2+} metabolism in hypertension is located at the plasma membrane and could represent a decrease in Ca^{2+}-ATPase activity or an increase in permeability of the membrane to Ca^{2+}. The latter possibility would be consistent with reports of altered sensitivity to Ca^{2+} of stimulant-evoked responses in hypertensive smooth muscle (Sutter and Ljung, 1977; Pedersen et al., 1978; Mulvany and Nyborg, 1980; Mulvany et al., 1981; Pang and Sutter, 1981).

Because of their vasodilatory properties the Ca^{2+} channel antagonists have been shown in several clinical trials to have antihypertensive activity. As anticipated, this activity is most prominent with nifedipine, the antihypertensive action of which is achieved primarily through peripheral arteriolar vasodilatation (Toggart and Zelis, 1982). Of particular interest in connection with the proposed Ca^{2+} defect in hypertension are several observations that the effects of the Ca^{2+} channel blockers on vascular smooth muscle are enhanced in the hypertensive animal and human (Pedersen et al., 1978; Pang and Sutter, 1981; Pedersen, 1981; Robinson et al., 1982). Thus, both D 600 (methoxyverapamil) and nifedipine are more potent in SHR than in WKY in mediating relaxation and inhibiting contractions in the aorta (Pedersen et al., 1978; Pang and Sutter, 1981; Pedersen, 1981). In human primary hypertension the dilator response of forearm resistance vessels to verapamil was more pronounced than in a control group (Robinson et al., 1982). These intriguing observations suggest that one component of the defect in Ca^{2+} regulation in hypertensive tissues may be at the level of the Ca^{2+} channel or in the process which couples receptors to the Ca^{2+} channels.

Alterations in Ca^{2+} regulation may also underlie other pathologic states in which changes in smooth muscle function are apparent. A characteristic feature of asthma is the associated bronchial hyperreactivity, characterized by an increased responsiveness to a wide variety of stimuli (Boushey et al., 1980). As with the altered reactivity of smooth muscle associated with hypertension, a variety of explanations have been advanced to accommodate this defect including changes in airway caliber, smooth muscle hypertrophy and changes at the receptor level. However, any postulated mechanism(s) of hyperreactivity must accommodate the fundamental observation that reactivity to a wide variety of discrete stimuli is increased. This suggests that a defect in the pathway which couples the stimuli with the response may exist. Thus, the hypothesis of altered Ca^{2+} mobilization is an attractive candidate for this type of defect (Triggle, 1983).

ACKNOWLEDGMENTS

Preparation of this review was assisted by a grant from the National Institutes of Health (HL 16003). Additional assistance from the Miles Institute for Preclinical Pharmacology is gratefully acknowledged.

REFERENCES

Bayer, R., and Ehara, T. (1978). Comparative studies on cal-
    cium antagonists. Prog. Pharmacol. 2, 31-37.
Bayer, R., Henneckes, R., Kaufmann, R., and Mannhold, R.
    (1975). Inotropic and electrophysiological actions of vera-
    pamil and D 600 action in mammalian myocardium. I.
    Pattern of inotropic effects of the racemic compounds.
    Naunyn-Schmiedeberg's Arch. Pharmacol. 290, 49-68.
Bayer, R., Rodenkirchen, R., Kaufmann, R., Lee, J. H., and
    Hennekes, R. (1977). The effects of nifedipine on con-
    traction and monophasic action potentials of isolated cat
    myocardium. Naunyn-Schmiedeberg's Arch. Pharmacol.
    30, 29-37.
Bellemann, P., Ferry, D., Lubbecke, F., and Glossmann, H.
    (1981). [^{3}H]-Nitrendipine, a potent calcium antagonist,
    binds with high affinity to cardiac membranes. Arzneim.
    Forsch. 31, 2064-2067.
Bellemann, P., Ferry, D., Lubbecke, F., and Glossmann, H.
    (1982). [^{3}H]-Nimodipine and [^{3}H]-nitrendipine as tools
    to directly identify the sites of action of 1,4-dihydropy-
    ridine calcium antagonists in guinea-pig tissues. Arzneim.
    Forsch. 32, 361-363.
Bevan, J. A. (1982). Selective action of diltiazem on cerebral
    vascular smooth muscle in rabbit: antagonism of extrinsic
    but not intrinsic maintained tone. Am. J. Cardiol. 49,
    519-524.
Bhalla, R. C., Webb, R. C., Singh, D., Ashley, T., and Brack, T.
    (1978). Calcium fluxes, calcium binding and adenosine
    cyclic 3'5'-monophosphate-dependent protein kinase ac-
    tivity in the aorta of spontaneously hypertensive and Kyoto
    Kyoto Wistar normotensive rats. Mol. Pharmacol. 14, 468-
    477.
Bolger, G. T., Gengo, P. J., Luchowski, E. M., Siegel, H., Triggle,
    D. J., and Janis, R. A. (1982). High affinity bind-
    ing of a calcium channel antagonist to smooth and cardiac
    muscle. Biochem. Biophys. Res. Commun. 104, 1604-1609.

Bolger, G. T., Gengo, P., Klockowski, R., Luchowski, E., Siegel, H., Janis, R. A., Triggle, A. M., and Triggle, D. J. (1983). Characterization of the binding of the Ca^{2+}-channel antagonist [^3H]-nitrendipine to guinea-pig ileal smooth muscle. J. Pharmacol. Exp. Ther., 225, 291-309.

Bolton, T.B. (1979). Mechanisms of action of transmitters and other substances on smooth muscle. Physiol. Rev. 59, 606-718.

Bossert, F., Meyer, H., and Wehinger, E. (1981). 4-Aryldihydropyridines, a new class of highly active calcium antagonists. Angew. Chem. 20, 762-769.

Boushey, H. A., Holtzman, M. J., Sheller, J. R., and Nadel, J. A. (1980). State of the art. Bronchial hyperreactivity. Am. Rev. Respir. Dis. 121, 389-413.

van Breemen, C., and Siegel, B. (1980). The mechanism of α-adrenergic activation of the dog coronary artery. Circ. Res. 46, 426-429.

van Breemen, C., Aaronson, P., Loutzenhiser, R., and Meisheri, K. (1980). Ca^{2+} movements in smooth muscle. Chest (Suppl.) 78, 157-165.

Cano, S. B., and Henry, D. W. (1982). Calcium channel blockers: pharmacology and therepeutic uses of a new class of drugs. Hospital Formulary 17, 376-384.

Cheung, W. Y. (ed.) (1980a). "Calcium and Cell Function, Vol. I. Calmodulin." Academic Press, London and New York.

Cheung, W. Y. (1980b). Calmodulin plays a pivotal role in cellular regulation. Science 207, 19-24.

Cheung, W. Y. (ed.) (1981). "Calcium and Cell Function, Vol. III." Academic Press, London and New York.

Clineschmidt, B. V., Gella, R. G., Govier, W. C., and Sjoerdsma, A. (1970). Reactivity to norepinephrine and nature of the alpha adrenergic receptor in vascular smooth muscle of a genetically hypertensive rat. Eur. J. Pharmacol. 10, 45-50.

Cohen, M. L., and Berkowitz, B. (1976). Decreased vascular relaxation in hypertension. J. Pharmacol. Exp. Ther. 196, 396-406.

Daniel, E. E. (1981). Role of altered vascular smooth muscle function in hypertension. In "Vasodilation" (P. M. Vanhoutte and I. Leusen, eds.), Raven Press, New York.

Daniel, E. E., and Kwan, C. Y. (1981). Control of contraction of vascular muscle: relation to hypertension. Trends in Pharmacol. Sci. 3, 220-223.

Ehlert, F. J., Itoga, E., Roeske, W. R., and Yamamura, H. I. (1982a). The interaction of [^{3}H]-nitrendipine with receptors for calcium antagonists in the cerebral cortex and heart of rats. Biochem. Biophys. Res. Commun. **104**, 937-943.

Ehlert, F. J., Roeske, W. R., Itoga, E., and Yamamura, H. J. (1982b). The binding of [^{3}H]-nitrendipine to receptors for calcium channel antagonists in the heart, cerebral cortex, and ileum of rats. Life Sci. **30**, 2191-2202.

Entman, M. L., Allen, J. C., Bornet, E. P., Gillette, P. C., Wallick, E. T., and Schwartz, A. (1972). Mechanisms of calcium accumulation and transport in cardiac relaxing system (sarcoplasmic reticulum membrane): effects of verapamil, D 600, X-537A and A 23187. J. Mol. Cell. Cardiol. **4**, 681-687.

Field, F. P., Janis, R. A., and Triggle, D. J. (1972). Aortic reactivity of rats with genetic and experimental renal hypertension. Can. J. Physiol. Pharmacol. **50**, 1072-1079.

Finch, L., and Haeusler, G. (1974). Vascular resistance and reactivity in hypertension. Blood Vessels **11**, 145-158.

Flaim, S. F., and Zelis, R. (eds.) (1982). "Calcium Blockers: Mechanisms of Action and Clinical Applications." Urban and Schwarzenberg, Baltimore.

Fleckenstein, A. (1964). Die bedeutung der energiereichen phosphate fur kontraktiltaet und tonus der myokards. Verh. Dtsch. Ges. Inn. Med. **70**, 81-99.

Fleckenstein, A. (1971). Specific inhibitors and promoters of calcium action in the excitation-contraction coupling of heart muscle and their role in the prevention or production of myocardial lesions. In "Calcium and The Heart" (P. Harris and L. Opie, eds.), pp. 135-188. Academic Press, London.

Fleckenstein, A. (1977). Specific pharmacology of calcium in myocardium, cardiac pacemakers and vascular smooth muscle. Annu. Rev. Pharmacol. Toxicol. **17**, 149-166.

Fleckenstein, A. (1981). Fundamental actions of calcium antagonists on pacemaker cell membranes. In "New Perspectives on Calcium Antagonists" (G. B. Weiss, ed.), pp. 59-81, American Physiological Society, Bethesda.

Folkow, B., Hallback, M., Lundgren, Y., and Weiss, L. (1970). Structurally based increase of flow resistance in spontaneously hypertensive rat. Acta Phys. Scand. **79**, 373-378.

Fossheim, R., Svarteng, K., Mostad, A., Rømming, C., Shefter, E., and Triggle, D. J. (1982). Crystal structures and pharmacological activity of calcium channel antagonists: 2,6-dimethyl-3,5-dicarbomethoxy-4-(unsubstituted, 3-methyl,4-methyl,3-nitro,4-nitro, and 2,4-dinitrophenyl)-1,4-dihydropyridine. J. Med. Chem. 25, 126-131.

Frey, M., and Kanke, J. (1975). The effect of organic Ca-antagonists (verapamil, prenylamine) on the calcium transport system in isolated mitochondria of rat cardiac muscle. Pfluegers Arch. 356, R26.

Friedman, S. M., and Friedman, C. L. (1976). Cell permeability, sodium transport and the hypertensive process in the rat. Circ. Res. 39, 433-441.

Godfraind, T., and Dieu, D. (1981). The inhibition by flunarizine of the norepinephrine-evoked contraction and calcium influx in rat aorta and mesenteric arteries. J. Pharmacol. Exp. Ther. 217, 510-515.

Godfraind, T., and Miller, R. C. (1982). Actions of prostaglandin $F_2\alpha$ and noradrenaline on calcium exchange and contraction in rat mesenteric arteries and their sensitivity to calcium entry blockers. Br. J. Pharmacol. 75, 229-236.

Gould, R. J., Murphy, K. M. M., and Snyder, S. H. (1982). [^{3}H]-Nitrendipine-labeled calcium channels discriminate inorganic calcium agonists and antagonists. Proc. Nat. Acad. Sci. U.S.A. 79, 3656-3660.

Hallback, M., Lundgren, Y. and Weiss, L. (1971). Reactivity to noradrenaline of aortic strips and portal veins from spontaneously hypertensive and normotensive rats. Acta. Phys. Scand. 81, 176-181.

Harris, A., Swamy, V. C., Triggle, D. J., and Waters, D. H. (1980). Responses to noradrenaline of portal vein strips from normotensive and spontaneously hypertensive rats. J. Auton. Pharmacol. 1, 617-623.

Hashimoto, K., Takeda, K., Katano, Y., Nakagawa, Y., Tsukada, T., Hashimoto, T., Shimamoto, N., Sakai, K., Otorrii, T., and Imai, S. (1979). Effects of niludipine (Bay a 7168) on the cardiovascular system. With a note on its calcium-antagonistic effects. Arzneim. Forsch. 29, 1368-1373.

Henry, P. D. (1979). Calcium ion (Ca^{++}) antagonists: mechanisms of action and clinical applications. Prac. Cardiol. 5, 145-156.

Henry, P.D. (1980). Comparative pharmacology of calcium antagonists: nifedipine, verapamil and diltiazem. Am. J. Cardiol. 46, 1047-1058.

Hermsmeyer, K. (1976). Cellular basis for increased sensitivity of vascular smooth muscle in spontaneously hypertensive rat. Circ. Res. (Suppl. II), **38**, II53–II57.

Holtje, H. D. (1982). Theoretische untersuchung zu struktur-wirkungsbeziehungen von ringsubstituierten verapamil-derivaten. Arch. Pharm. **315**, 317–323.

Itoh, T., Kijiwara, M., Kitamura, K., and Kuriyama, H. (1981). Effect of vasodilator agents on smooth muscle cells of the coronary artery of the pig. Br. J. Pharmacol. **74**, 455–468.

Janis, R. A., Maurer, S. C., Sarmiento, J. G., Bolger, G. T., and Triggle, D. J. (1982). Binding of [^{3}H]-nimodipine to cardiac and smooth muscle membranes. Eur. J. Pharmacol., **182**, 191–194.

Jim, K., Harris, A., Rosenberger, L. B., and Triggle, D. J. (1981). Stereoselective and nonstereoselective effects of D 600 (methoxyverapamil) in smooth muscle preparations. Eur. J. Pharmacol. **76**, 67–72.

Jones, A. W. (1973). Altered ion transport in vascular smooth muscle from spontaneously hypertensive rats. Circ. Res. **33**, 563–572.

Kawai, C., Konishi, T., Matsuyama, E., and Okazaki, H. (1981). Comparative effects of three calcium antagonists, diltiazem, verapamil and nifedipine on the sinoatrial and atrioventricular nodes. Circulation **63**, 1035–1042.

Kazda, S., Garthoff, B., Meyer, H., Schlossmann, K., Stoepel, K., Towart, R., Vater, W., and Wehinger, E. (1980). Pharmacology of a new calcium antagonist compound, isobutylmethyl-1,4-dihydro-2,6-dimethyl-4-(2-nitrophenyl)-3,5-pyridinedicarboxylate (Nisoldipine, Bay k 5552). Arzneim. Forsch. **30**, 2144–2162.

Kazda, S., Garthoff, B., Krause, H., and Schlossmann, K. (1982). Cerebrovascular effects of the calcium antagonistic dihydropyridine derivative nimodipine in animal experiments. Arzneim. Forsch. **32**, 331–338.

Kohlhardt, M. (1981). Slow channel kinetics in heart muscle. Basic Res. Cardiol. **76**, 589–601.

Kretsinger, R. H., and Nelson, D. J. (1976). Calcium in biological systems. Coord. Chem. Rev. **18**, 29–124.

Kretsinger, R. H. (1977). Evaluation of the informational role of calcium in eukaryotes. In "Calcium Binding Proteins and Calcium Function" (R. H. Wassermann, ed.), pp. 63–72. Elsevier, Amsterdam.

Kwan, C. Y., Belbeck, L., and Daniel, E. E. (1979). Abnormal biochemistry of vascular smooth muscle plasma membrane as an important factor in the initiation and maintenance of hypertension in rats. Blood Vessels 16, 259-268.

Kwan, C. Y., Belbeck, L., and Daniel E. E. (1980a). Abnormal biochemistry of vascular smooth muscle plasma membrane isolated from hypertensive rats. Mol. Pharmacol. 17, 137-140.

Kwan, C. Y., Belbeck, L., and Daniel, E. E. (1980b). Characteristics of arterial plasma membrane in renovascular hypertension in rats. Blood Vessels 17, 131-140.

La Porte, D. E., Wierman, B. M., and Storm, D. R. (1980). Calcium-induced exposure of a hydrophobic surface on calmodulin. Biochemistry 19, 3814-3819.

Levin, R. M., and Weiss, B. (1979). Selective binding of antipsychotics and other psychoactive agents to the calcium-dependent activator of cyclic nucleotide phosphodiesterase. J. Pharmacol. Exp. Ther. 208, 454-459.

Lindner, E., and Ruppert, D. (1982). Effects of calcium antagonists on coronary spasm and pulmonary artery contraction in comparison to their antagonistic action against K-stropanthin in isolated guinea-pig artria. Pharmacology 24, 294-302.

Loev, B., Goodman, M. M., Snader, K. M., Tedeschi, R., and Macko, E. (1974). "Hantzsch-type" dihydropyridine hypotensive agents. J. Med. Chem. 17, 956-965.

Mannhold, R., Steiner, R., Haas, W., and Kaufmann, R. (1978). Investigations on the structure-activity relationship of verapamil. Naunyn-Schmiedeberg's Arch. Pharmacol. 302, 217-226.

McCarron, D. A. (1982). Low serum concentrations of ionized calcium in patients with hypertension. New Engl. J. Med. 307, 226-228.

McCarron, D. A., Morris, C. D., and Cole, C. (1982). Dietary calcium in human hypertension. Science 217, 267-269.

McDonald, T. F., Pelzer, D., and Trautwein, W. (1980). On the mechanism of slow calcium channel block in heart. Pfluegers Arch. 385, 175-179.

McGregor, D. D., and Smirk, F. H. (1970). Vascular responses to 5-hydroxytryptamine in genetic and renal hypertensive rats. Am. J. Physiol. 219, 687-690.

Means, A. R., and Dedman, J. R. (1980). Calmodulin - an intracellular calcium receptor. Nature 285, 73-77.

Means, A. R., Tash, J. S., and Chafouleas, J. G. (1982). Physiological implications of the presence, distribution and regulation of calmodulin in eukaryotic cells. Physiol. Rev. 62, 1-39.

Meisheri, K., Hwang, O., and van Breeman, C. (1981). Evidence for two separate Ca^{2+} pathways in smooth muscle plasmalemma. J. Membr. Biol. **59**, 19-25.

Michell, R. H., Kirk, C. J., Jones, L. M., Downes, C. P., and Creba, J. A. (1981). The stimulation of inositol lipid metabolism that accompanies calcium mobilization in stimulated cells: defined characteristics and unanswered questions. Philos. Trans. R. Soc. London B. **296**, 123-137.

Moore, L., Hurwitz, L., Davenport, G. R., and Landon, E. J. (1975). Energy dependent calcium uptake activity of microsomes from the aorta of normal and hypertensive rats. Biochim. Biophys. Acta. **413**, 432-443.

Mulvany, M. J., and Nyborg, N. (1980). An increased calcium sensitivity of mesenteric resistance vessels in young and adult spontaneously hypertensive rats. Br. J. Pharmacol. **17**, 585-596.

Mulvany, M. J., Hansen, P. K., and Aalkjaer, C. (1978). Direct evidence that the greater contractility of resistance vessels in spontaneously hypertensive rats is associated with a narrowed lumen, a thickened media and an increased number of smooth muscle cell layers. Circ. Res. **43**, 854-864.

Mulvany, M. J., Korsgaard, N., and Nyborg, N. (1981). Evidence that the increased calcium sensitivity of resistance vessels in spontaneously hypertensive rats is an intrinsic defect of their vascular smooth muscle. Clin. Exp. Hypertension **3**, 749-761.

Murphy, K. M. M., and Snyder, S. H. (1982). Calcium antagonist receptor binding sites labeled with [^{3}H]-nitrendipine. Eur. J. Pharmacol. **77**, 201-202.

Nagao, T., Sato, M., Iwasawa, Y., Takada, T., Ishida, R., Nakajima, H., and Kiyomoto, A. (1972). Studies on a new 1,5-benzothiazepine derivative (CRD-401). III. Effects of optical isomers of CRD-401 on smooth muscle and other pharmacological properties. Jpn. J. Pharmacol. **22**, 467-478.

Nawrath, H., Blei, I., Gegnor, R., Ludwig, C., and Zang, X. G. (1981). Stereospecific effects of the optical isomers of verapamil and D 600 on the heart. In "Calcium Antagonists in Cardiovascular Therapy" (A. Zanchetti and D. M. Krikler, eds.), pp. 523-63. Excerpta Med., Amsterdam.

Nayler, W. G., Thompson, J. E., and Jarrott, B. (1982). The interactions of calcium antagonists (slow channel blockers) with myocardial alpha adrenoceptors. J. Mol. Cell. Cardiol. **14**, 185-188.

Norman, J. A., Drummond, A. H., and Moser, P. (1979). Inhibition of calcium-dependent regulator-stimulated phosphodiesterase activity by neuroleptic drugs is unrelated to their clinical efficacy. Mol. Pharmacol. 16, 1089-1094.

Pammani, M. B., Clough, D. L., Huot, S. J., and Haddy, F. J. (1981). Sodium-potassium pump activity in experimental hypertension. In "Vasodilatation" (P. M. Vanhoutte and I. Leusen, eds.), pp. 391-403. Raven Press, New York.

Pang, C. Y. C., and Sutter, M. C. (1981). Differential effects of D 600 on contractile response of aorta and portal vein from spontaneously hypertensive rats. Blood Vessels 18, 120-127.

Pedersen, O. L. (1981). Calcium blockade as a therapeutic principle in arterial hypertension. Acta Pharmacol. Toxicol. 49, Suppl. II, 1-31.

Pedersen, O. L., Mikkelsen, E., and Andersson, K. E. (1978). Effects of extracellular calcium on potassium and noradrenaline induced contractions in the aorta of spontaneously hypertensive rats - increased sensitivity to nifedipine. Acta Pharmacol. Toxicol. 43, 137-144.

Perez, J. E., Borda, L., Schuchleib, R., and Henry, P. D. (1982). Inotropic and chronotropic effects of vasodilators. J. Pharmacol. Exp. Ther. 221, 609-613.

Putney, J. W. (1981). Recent hypotheses regarding the phosphatidylinositol effect. Life Sci. 29, 1183-1194.

Raess, B. U., and Vincenzi, F. F. (1980). Calmodulin activation of red blood cell $(Ca^{2+} + Mg^{2+})$-ATPase and its antagonism by phenothiazines. Mol. Pharmacol. 18, 253-258.

Raschack, M., and Engelmann, K. (1980). Calcium-antagonistic activity and myocardial ischemia protection by both stereoisomers of verapamil. J. Mol. Cell Cardiol. 12, Suppl. I, 132-138.

Reuter, H., and Scholz, H. (1977). Regulation of the calcium conductance of cardiac muscle by adrenaline. J. Physiol. 264, 49-62.

Robinson, B. F., Dobbs, R. J., and Bayley, S. (1982). Response of forearm resistance vessels to verapamil and sodium nitroprusside in normotensive and hypertensive men. Evidence for a functional abnormality of vascular smooth muscle in primary hypertension. Clin. Sci. 63, 33-42.

Rodenkirchen, R., Bayer, R., Steiner, R., Bossert, F., Meyer, H., and Moller, E. (1979). Structure-activity studies on nifedipine in isolated cardiac muscle. Naunyn-Schmiedeberg's Arch. Pharmacol. 310, 69-78.

Rosenberger, L., and Triggle, D. J. (1978). Calcium, calcium translocation and specific calcium antagonists. In "Calcium and Drug Action" (G. B. Weiss, ed.), pp. 3-31. Plenum Press, New York.

Rosenberger, L. B., Ticku, M. K. and Triggle, D. J. (1979). The effects of Ca^{2+} antagonists on Ca^{2+} movements and mechanical responses in guinea-pig ileal longitudinal smooth muscle. Can. J. Physiol. Pharmacol. 57, 333-347.

Roufogalis, B. D. (1983). Specificity of trifluoperazine and related phenothiazines for Ca^{2+} binding proteins. In "Calcium and Cell Function", Vol. 3 (W. Y. Cheung, ed.), Academic Press, London and New York.

Satoh, K., Yanagisawa, T., and Taira, N. (1980). Coronary vasodilator and cardiac effects of optical isomers of verapamil in the dog. J. Cardiovas. Pharmacol. 2, 309-318.

Schumann, H. J., Gorlitz, B. D., and Wagner, J. (1975). Influence of papaverine, D 600 and nifedipine on the effects of noradrenaline and calcium on the isolated aorta and mesenteric artery of the rabbit. Naunyn-Schmiedeberg's Arch. Pharmacol. 289, 409-417.

Shibanuma, T., Iwanani, M., Okuda, K., Takenaka, K. T., and Murakami, M. (1980). Synthesis of optically active 2-(N-benzyl-N-methylamino)ethyl methyl 2,6-dimethyl-4-(m-nitrophenyl)-1,4-dihydropyridine-3,5-dicarboxylate (Nicardipine). Chem. Pharm. Bull. 28, 2809-2812.

Shibata, S., Kurahashi, K., and Kuchii, M. (1973). A possible etiology of contractile impairment of vascular smooth muscles from spontaneously hypertensive rats. J. Pharmacol. Exp. Ther. 185, 406-417.

Smith, R. D., Romano, D. V., Loev, B., Pruss, T. P., and Wolf, P. S. (1982). Comparison of the calcium antagonism and negative inotropic effects of flordipine (F) and nifedipine (N) in isolated canine vascular tissue and cat papillary muscle preparations. The Pharmacologist 24, 241 (abstract).

Spedding, M. (1982a). Assessment of "Ca^{2+}-antagonist" effects of drugs in K^+-dependent smooth muscle. Differentiation of antagonist subgroups. Naunyn-Schmiedeberg's Arch. Pharmacol. 318, 234-240.

Spedding, M. (1982b). Comparison of "Ca^{2+}-antagonists" and trifluoperazine in skinned smooth muscle fibres. Br. J. Pharmacol. 75, 25P.

Stone, P. H., Antman, E. M., Muller, J. E., and Braunwald, E. (1980). Calcium channel blocking agents in the treatment of cardiovascular disorders part II.: hemodynamic effects and clinical applications. Ann. Intern. Med. **93**, 886-904.

Stoepel, K., Heise, A., and Kazda, S. (1981). Pharmacological studies of the antihypertensive effect of nitrendipine. Arzneim. Forsch. **31**, 2056-2060.

Sutter, M. C., and Ljung, B. (1977). Contractility, muscle mass and agonist sensitivity of isolated portal veins from normo- and hypertensive rats. Acta Physiol. Scand. **99**, 484-495.

Swamy, V. C., and Triggle, D. J. (1980). The reactivity of iliac vascular strips from spontaneously hypertensive and normo-tensive rats. Blood Vessels **17**, 246-256.

Terai, M., Takenaka, T., and Maeno, H. (1981). Inhibition of calcium influx in rabbit aorta by nicardipine hydrochloride. Biochem. Pharmacol. **30**, 375-378.

Thorens, S., and Haeusler, G. (1979). Effects of some vasodila-tors on calcium translocation in intact and fractionated vascular smooth muscle. Eur. J. Pharmacol. **54**, 79-91.

Toggart, E. J., and Zelis, R. (1982). The role of calcium block-ers in the treatment of other cardiovascular disorders. In "Calcium Blockers. Mechanisms of Action and Clinical Applications" (S. F. Flaim and R. Zelis, eds.), pp. 265-283. Urban and Schwarzenberg, Baltimore.

Towart, R. (1981). The selective inhibition of serotonin-induced contractions of rabbit cerebral vascular smooth muscle by calcium-antagonistic dihydropyridines. Circ. Res. **48**, 650-657.

Towart, R., Wehinger, E., and Meyer, H. (1981). Effects of unsymmetrical ester substituted 1,4-dihydropyridine derivatives and their optical isomers on contraction of smooth muscle. Naunyn-Schmiedeberg's Arch. Pharmacol. **317**, 183-185.

Towart, R., Wehinger, E., Meyer, H., and Kazda, S. (1982). The effects of nimodipine, its optical isomers and metabolites on isolated vascular smooth muscle. Arzneim. Forsch. **32**, 338-346.

Triggle, D. J. (1982). Counting Calcium Channels? Trends Pharmacol. Sci., **3**, 465.

Triggle, D. J. (1983). Calcium, the control of smooth muscle function and bronchial hyperreactivity. Allergy **38**, 1-9.

Triggle, D. J., and Swamy, V. C. (1980). Pharmacology of agents that affect calcium. Chest **78**, Suppl. 174-180.

Triggle, D. J., and Swamy, V. C. (1983). Calcium antagonists: some chemical pharmacologic aspects. Circ. Res., **52** (suppl I), I-17-I-28.

Tritthart, H., Volkmann, R., Weiss, R., and Fleckenstein, A.
    (1973). Calcium-mediated action potentials in mammal-
    ian myocardium. Naunyn-Schmiedeberg's Arch. Pharma-
    col. **280**, 239-252.
Van Nueten, J. M., and Janssen, P. A. J. (1973). Comparative
    study of the effects of flunarizine and cinnarizine on
    smooth muscles and cardiac tissues. Arch. Int. Pharma-
    codyn. **204**, 37-55.
Van Nueten, J. M., and Vanhoutte, P. M. (1981). Selectivity of
    calcium antagonism and serotonin antagonism with re-
    spect to venous and arterial tissues. Angiology **32**, 476-
    484.
Vogel, S., and Sperelakis, N. (1981). Induction of slow action
    potentials by microiontophoresis of cyclic AMP into heart
    cells. J. Mol. Cell. Cardiol. **13**, 51-64.

Calcium Channel Blockers as a New Therapeutic Concept: Cardiovascular Physiology and Clinical Applications

Stephen F. Flaim

Department of Biological Research
McNeil Pharmaceutical
Spring House, Pennsylvania

Paul H. Ratz and Rudyard J. Ress

Division of Cardiology
M. S. Hershey Medical Center
The Pennsylvania State University
Hershey, Pennsylvania

I. INTRODUCTION

The therapeutic impact of the calcium blockers at present is with relation to their effectiveness as coronary vasodilators and, consequently, their usefulness in the treatment and prevention of coronary spasm leading to Printzmetal's as well as possibly other forms of angina. The vasodilatory capacity of these agents may also be useful in the treatment of other disease states associated with hyperactivity of the peripheral vessels such as hypertension, Raynaud's syndrome, and cerebral vasospasm. Since calcium blocking activity is also associated with alterations in the cardiac muscle cell electrical potential, another major proven area of therapeutic efficacy for these compounds is as antiarrhythmic agents. There are numerous calcium dependent processes in the body, thus it is not surprising to find that some of the calcium blocking agents have significant negative effects. The effects can be associated not only with the inhibition of noncardiovascular vital calcium–dependent processes but also with inappropriate vasodilator activity leading to deleterious cardiovascular effects. To maximize the beneficial aspects and minimize the deleterious effects of the calcium blockers, it becomes vital to understand as precisely as possible the mechanisms of action of these agents both at the cellular and at the systemic level.

HYPERTENSION: PHYSIOLOGICAL
BASIS AND TREATMENT

Since much of our own experience with calcium blockers has been derived from studies of the agent, diltiazem (Cardizem, Marion Laboratories, Kansas City, Missouri), a major portion of this chapter will be based upon these data. However, it must be emphasized that one cannot fully comprehend this group of drugs from studies on a single member. This is the case since not only are the calcium blockers highly heterogenous in structure but also since they have varying spectra of effects throughout the cardiovascular system over a wide dosage range. Furthermore, although there are ample data showing that numerous members of this group have inhibitory effects on calcium influx across the cell membrane, it is clear that a number of other cellular effects may be involved and in no single case is the precise mechanism of action completely understood.

II. THE PHYSIOLOGY OF ANGINA PECTORIS

Although calcium blocking agents have been extensively studied and used clinically in western Europe for more than a decade, these agents have appeared on the American clinical scene only within the past five years. The primary reason for this recent clinical interest in calcium blockers coincides with the recent recognition of coronary artery spasm as a definite disease entity, as well as the finding that calcium blockers such as nifedipine are highly effective for the treatment and reversal of this inappropriate coronary artery constrictor activity. Before proceeding, a brief review of our present understanding of the mechanism of coronary spasm and how it fits under the general heading of angina pectoris is in order.

It is now thought that angina pectoris results from an imbalance between myocardial oxygen requirements and oxygen supply levels available within the coronary arterial circulation. Figure 1 schematically summarizes this concept. The major factors governing myocardial oxygen consumption are heart rate, myocardial contractility which is an index of the strength and velocity of the myocardial contraction, and the magnitude of tension within the wall of the ventricle. On the other side of the balance is oxygen supply which is primarily determined by coronary blood flow. Because of the high level of wall tension which occurs during cardiac systole, coronary flow to the muscle of the left ventricle occurs primarily during diastole. For this reason, an increase in the rate of cardiac contraction (heart rate) will reduce the duration of diastole and will, therefore, result in a lowering

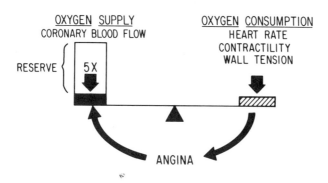

DYNAMICS OF ANGINA PECTORIS

Figure 1. The classical approach to the description of the pathophysiology of angina pectoris. Under normal conditions at rest, a balance exists between the rate of oxygen consumption by the heart and the supply of oxygen to the muscle of the myocardium. Any event which increases heart rate, myocardial contractility and/or myocardial wall tension will also increase oxygen requirements of the heart. In this situation, if oxygen supply to the myocardium is compromised for any reason reducing the oxygen reserve (i.e., coronary atherosclerosis), an imbalance results producing the symptoms of angina pectoris. In cases of variant or Printzmetal's angina, coronary spasm appears to have an important role in reducing oxygen supply. Thus, in classical angina pectoris, angina results from a change in the right side of the balance whereas in variant angina, the symptom results from changes in the left side of the balance shown. Reproduced from "Cardiovascular Drug Therapy", Cardiovascular Clinics Series, Vol. 6, No. 2, Melmon, K.L. (ed.), Philadelphia, F.A. Davis Company, 1974, with permission.

of blood flow and oxygen supply to the left ventricle. A reduction in blood pressure during diastole will have essentially the same effect to lower oxygen supply to the myocardium. Under normal conditions, coronary blood flow is determined primarily by the local production of vasodilator metabolites. Because of the large portion of time spent by the cardiac muscle in the state of systole, the heart is constantly in a state of hyperemia, and the rate of oxygen extraction by the cardiac muscle is near maximum even under resting conditions. Unlike skeletal muscle,

the heart is almost exclusively aerobic being unable to derive a
significant amount of energy from anaerobic metabolic processes.
Therefore, the heart requires a fully functional coronary arterial
supply for the normal basal level of activity. The heart can
accomodate to the increased oxygen consumption which occurs
during such activity as exercise since the coronary circulation
has a tremendous reserve capacity as indicated in Figure 1. The
normal coronary circulation can increase its rate of delivery of
oxygenated blood to the myocardium by as much as five times.
This reserve, however, is compromised not only by elevated heart
rate and reduced blood pressure as indicated earlier, but also
by several phenomena which physically limit the ability of the
coronary arteries to dilate. When the supply cannot meet the
oxygen consumption demand, the result is ischemia within the
myocardium and chest pain or angina. One major cause of
angina is atherosclerotic coronary artery disease which results
in the build up of plaques within the lumen of the coronary
arteries. These plaques constitute fixed areas of narrowing of
the artery. In this situation, angina is a predictable occurrence
and is associated with, and can be precipitated by, a variety of
activities which raise the myocardial oxygen demand: e.g.,
exercise, exposure to cold which increases cardiac work secondary to increases in peripheral vascular resistance primarily in
the cutaneous circulation, smoking which results in similar circulatory phenomena, eating which increases the need for blood
flow to the gastrointestinal circulation thus competing with
the coronary supply, or a combination of these activities.
Angina under these conditions can be relieved simply by termination of the activity. Standard therapy for this typical type
of angina is directed toward the reduction of myocardial oxygen
requirements. For example, nitrate therapy causes both veno-
and arteriolar dilatation which result in lowered peripheral
vascular resistance and ventricular wall tension thus lowering
myocardial oxygen demand. Beta blocker therapy on the other
hand reduces myocardial oxygen demand simply via an inhibitory
effect on the heart rate and inotropic response to exercise
however strenuous.

Associated with the recent recognition of the importance
of the calcium blockers has been the definition of a subset of
angina termed variant or Printzmetal's angina. This type of
angina results from what appears to be a focal narrowing of a
major coronary artery secondary to a spastic contractile event
in the vascular smooth muscle of the wall of the artery. Variant
angina cannot be associated with a specific type of activity which

would be expected to create increased myocardial oxygen demand. On the contrary, variant angina can spontaneously develop at rest, even during sleep. Although the precise mechanism of variant angina or coronary vasospasm has not been defined, it can be artificially precipitated during cardiac catheterization by the local injection of certain vasoactive agents into the lumen of the coronary circulation. Although ergonovine is the standard agent used to test for vasospasm under these conditions, it is known that any number of agents such as norepinephrine, histamine, serotonin and similar vasoconstrictors can precipitate vasospasm in the susceptible coronary circulation. Thus, variant angina appears to be associated with a supersensitivity within the vascular smooth muscle of the coronary arteries. Although large intracoronary injections of nitroglycerin will reverse ergonovine-induced coronary spasm in the cardiac catherization laboratory, the calcium blockers primarily represented by nifedipine (Procardia - Pfizer), verapamil (Isoptin - Knoll; Calan - Searle), and diltiazem are now known to effectively prevent or reduce the frequency of variant angina as well as exertional angina in the normal population.

From the proceeding discussion, it is fairly clear that the subset of angina pectoris which is termed Printzmetal's or variant angina and which is clearly treatable with calcium blocking agents is a disease event associated with vascular smooth muscle. Therefore, in order to understand the mechanism of the antianginal effects of calcium blockers, it is necessary to understand not only the mechanism of contraction of vascular smooth muscle in the normal blood vessel, but also how this process is altered to allow the inappropriate vasoconstrictor event which is associated with coronary vasospasm.

III. HETEROGENOUS NATURE OF VASCULAR SMOOTH MUSCLE

There are several major problems which must be addressed before one can properly understand the "normal" mechanism of contraction in vascular smooth muscle. One major difficulty lies in the fact that there appears to be a great deal of heterogeneity with respect to vascular smooth muscle, not only between species but also within regions of the circulation.

Catecholamines such as norepinephrine cause contractions in vascular smooth muscle primarily by way of activation of alpha-adrenergic receptors. The exact molecular mechanism of this event is not completely understood. Norepinephrine causes a biphasic contractile event in isolated segments of rabbit aorta (Bohr, 1963; Deth and Van Breeman, 1974), rabbit (Godfraind and Kaba, 1972) and dog (Sitrin and Bohr, 1971) mesenteric arteries, rat aorta (Godfraind and Kaba, 1972; Godfraind, 1976), and rabbit ear artery (Bevan et al., 1973; Steinsland et al., 1973). This biphasic contractile pattern may not be uniform as is the case with the rabbit ear artery and the rabbit aorta (Bevan et al., 1973; Steinsland et al., 1973). The contractile phases are more apparent in the rabbit ear artery simply because it appears that the rapid phase develops more quickly in this artery type. Contractions due to norepinephrine during beta-blockade with propranolol in large coronary artery of the dog are monophasic (Van Breemen and Siegel, 1980; Van Nueten and Vanhoutte, 1980). However, bovine ventricular marginal and diagonal coronary arteries respond poorly (Ratz et al., 1980) and bovine large circumflex, left anterior descending, and right coronary arteries (Altura, 1966) as well as large ventral interventricular coronary arteries of the dog (Muller–Schweinitzer, 1980) show no response to norepinephrine during beta-blockade with pro-pranolol. Basilar arteries of the bovine (Yamashita et al., 1977) and dog (Muller–Schweinitzer, 1980) exhibit no response to 10^{-7}M norepinephrine and only a minimal response to higher norepinephrine concentrations. Pial arteries from rabbit show no response to either exogenous or endogenous norepinephrine released from periarterial nerves during electrical stimulation, despite the observation that pial arteries show histofluorescence suggesting extensive adrenergic innervation (Duckles and Bevan, 1979). Isolated rabbit vertebral, internal carotid, and basilar arteries respond to norepinephrine at 10^{-7}M with a rapid tran-sient contraction; at higher norepinephrine concentrations, a biphasic contractile response occurs (Bevan, 1979). Norepi-nephrine elicits a strong but transient contractile response in isolated human coronary arteries (Ross et al., 1980) and in cat mesenteric arteries (Fara, 1971). It is possible to obtain rhyth-mic contractions in response to norepinephrine in some vascula-tures such as the rabbit femoral (Flaim et al., 1980b) and gracilis (Suzuki and Casteels, 1979) arteries, the cat mesen-teric artery (Ross, 1975), and the isolated human coronary artery (Ginsburg et al., 1980). Spike potentials associated with rhythmic contractile activity have been reported in small arteries (Steedman, 1966) and veins (Somlyo and Somlyo, 1968; Hermsmeyer, 1971; Haeusler, 1978; Takata, 1980), and the frequency of this activity can be increased with norepinephrine.

Thus, it is clear that the norepinephrine-induced contractile response in vascular smooth muscle is nonhomogenous. Figure 2 schematically summarizes and compares the basic types of re-

α-Receptor Mediated Tension Profiles

Schematized Tension Profile	Blood Vessel	Reference
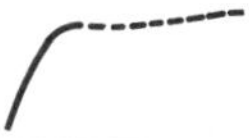	Rabbit aorta	Deth and van Breemen, 1974; Deth and van Breemen, 1977
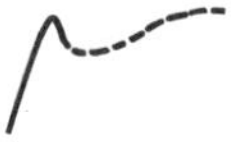	Rabbit ear artery	Bevan et al., 1973; Steinsland et al., 1973
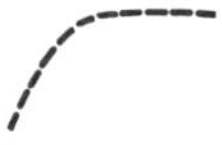	Dog large coronary arteries	van Breemen and Siegel, 1980
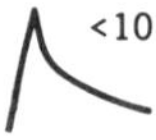 $<10^{-7}$ M $>10^{-7}$ M 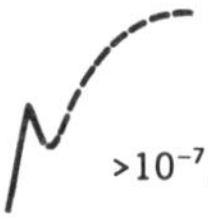	Rabbit basilar artery	McCalden and Bevan, 1980; McCalden and Bevan, 1981; Bevan, 1979
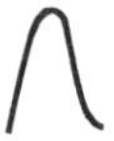 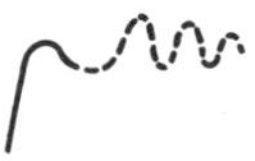	Human large coronary arteries	Ross et al., 1980; Ginsberg et al., 1980

Figure 2. Schematic of a series of selected vascular tension responses to norepinephrine demonstrating the heterogeneous contractile response patterns observed when vascular smooth muscle from different areas of the circulation and from different species is subjected to identical receptor stimulation. Diagrams are not drawn to scale and cannot be compared in a quantitative fashion. Solid and dotted lines represent the component of the tension profile that may be primarily dependent on, respectively, intracellular calcium and extracellular calcium mobilization mechanisms. A transient contraction is elicited in rabbit basilar artery at low norepinephrine (NE) concentrations (no greater than 10^{-7} M) whereas a biphasic contraction is induced by higher NE concentrations (greater than 10^{-7} M) in this vessel. (From Ratz and Flaim, 1982, with permission.)

sponses to norepinephrine in various blood vessels. Those parts of the tension response thought to be secondary to the release of intracellularly stored calcium are shown by solid lines and portions which may be due to the influx of extracellular calcium across the cell membrane are depicted as dashed lines. At this time, it is unclear if these apparent differences are the result of heterogenous alpha-receptor structure or function, design of the actual transduction event associated with the activation of the receptor, inherent differences in the mechanism of operation of the calcium channel, or differences in the degree of intracellularly stored calcium. These and other aspects of the heterogenous nature of the vascular smooth muscle response to agonists have been reviewed recently in considerable detail (Ratz and Flaim, 1982).

The tension response in vascular smooth muscle to other vasoactive agents can be equally variable. A primary example is acetylcholine which induces contraction in most veins (Shepherd and Vanhoutte, 1975) and many arteries (Altura, 1966; Ito et al., 1979; Kitamura and Kuriyama, 1979) in vitro. However, when

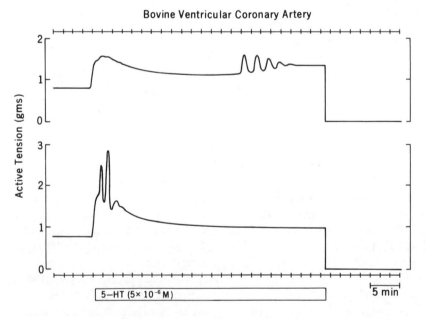

Figure 3. Tracings of two tension profiles obtained from isolated rings of bovine coronary artery during stimulation with 5-hydroxytryptamine exhibiting rhythmic contractile activity. (From Ratz and Flaim, 1982, with permission.)

added in vivo, acetylcholine causes potent vasodilatation in both the periphery (Mellander and Johansson, 1968; Brody, 1978) as well as the coronary circulation (Hackett et al., 1971; Gross et al., 1981). Acetylcholine also causes vasodilatation in cerebral arteries in vitro (Lee et al., 1978; Duckles, 1979; 1980). Similarly, histamine can be either an agonist or a relaxant depending on the experimental conditions as well as the specific vasculature studied (Owen, 1977; Ohhashi and Azuma, 1980; Sakai, 1980). In large arteries, serotonin is generally a contractile agent while, in arterioles, it appears to be a relaxant (Burrows and Vanhoutte, 1981). The source of calcium which supports serotonin-induced contraction in different vessel types appears to vary. In bovine basilar (Yamashita et al., 1977) and both marginal and diagonal ventricular coronary (Ratz and Flaim, 1981a) arteries, influx of calcium from the extracellular space appears to have a minimal input whereas this calcium source contributes substantially to serotonin-induced contraction in rabbit basilar (Towart, 1981) and dog large circumflex and right coronary (Van Nueten et al., 1980; Van Nueten and Vanhoutte, 1980). Although no clear explanation for these phenomena is available, they can conceivably be explained in several ways. Major possibilities are differences in the architectural relationships within the walls of the vessels and differences in the environment within which the vessel must function.

Given this large degree of heterogeneity in the performance characteristics of vascular smooth muscle, it is not surprising that there have been no successful experimental models of the human coronary smooth muscle. This tissue type is of obvious interest due to its probable association with angina, but is not readily available for experimental evaluation. As mentioned previously, one unusual characteristic of this tissue observed by Ginsburg and coworkers (Ginsburg et al., 1980) was the presence of rhythmic contractile activity elicited by various agonists. In recent attempts in our laboratory to identify an experimental model for the human coronary artery, we utilized this characteristic to guide our search. Another factor which was involved in the selection of a model was the ability of the vessel to respond to serotonin. Serotonin receptors have been shown to be activated during stimulation of vascular smooth muscle with ergonovine, an agonist which is used chemically to identify patients subject to coronary artery spasm (Mueller-Schweinitzer, 1980). We observed in the bovine coronary artery some rhythmic contractile activity induced by serotonin (Ratz and Flaim, 1982), and two examples of such responses are shown in Figure 3. The bovine coronary artery is somewhat unique since it responds with active tension generation to stimulation with serotonin, but is relatively insensitive to both histamine and norepinephrine during beta-blockade with propranolol (Figure 4). In the absence of propranolol, norepinephrine induces a vasodilatation as shown in Figure 5.

IV. CALCIUM HANDLING MECHANISMS IN VASCULAR SMOOTH MUSCLE

There are considerable differences between the mechanisms involved in the contraction of smooth muscle and those involved

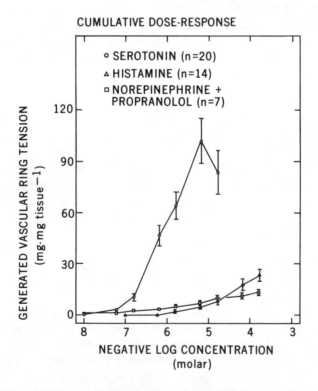

Figure 4. Cumulative dose-response relationships for several agonists in isolated rings of bovine ventricular coronary arteries. Rings were preset at 1 g of resting preload tension prior to stimulation. Vertical axis represents actively generated tension in response to stimulation by addition of the respective agonist to the bathing media.

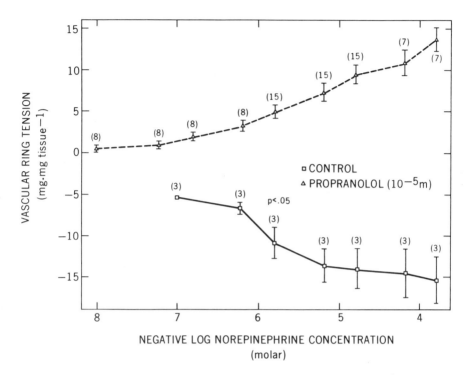

*Figure 5. Cumulative dose-response relationships for norepi-
nephrine in isolated rings of bovine ventricular coronary arteries.
Rings were preset at 1 g of resting preload tension prior to stimulation. Vertical axis represents actively generated tension levels
in response to stimulation by addition of norepinephrine alone
(control) or norepinephrine plus beta-blockade with propranolol
to the bathing media.*

in the contraction of either cardiac or skeletal muscle. In the
latter two cases, transmembrane influx of calcium ions contribute
either to a small extent (cardiac) or not at all (skeletal) to the
stimulus-induced rise in free cytoplasmic calcium ion which
supports the contractile process. In these muscles, the elevated
cytoplasmic calcium ion concentration allows the initiation of
the contractile event by binding to the regulator protein, troponin.
This event allows the binding of action to myosin, followed by
hydrolysis of ATP and the resultant muscle-shortening. In cardiac
and skeletal muscle, relaxation occurs when the free intracellular

calcium is reduced by uptake into the sarcoplasmic reticulum where calcium is actively sequestered. Much less is known about the calcium handling processes in vascular smooth muscle. However, it is possible to construct a hypothetical picture of how an analogous process may operate in the vascular smooth muscle by piecing together information obtained with tissue from different parts of the circulation as well as from the nonvascular gastrointestinal and uterine smooth muscle. Such a hypothetical model is schematically depicted in Figure 6.

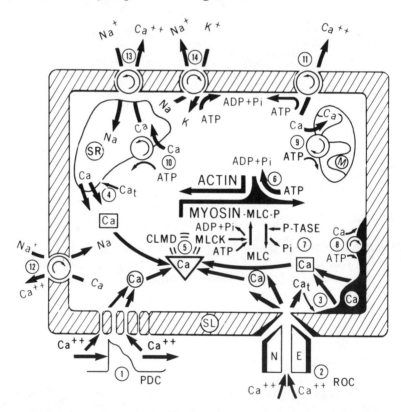

Figure 6. Schematic representation of the mechanisms involved in vascular smooth muscle contraction and relaxation. Vacular smooth muscle contraction can be initiated by the activation of potential-dependent calcium channels (PDC) ① or by the activation of receptor-operated channels (ROC) ② e.g., norepinephrine (NE). Calcium ion (Ca^{++} or Ca) entering through ROC can release Ca (Ca_t) from storage sites in the sarcolemmal (SL) ③ or sarcoplasmic reticulum (SR) ④. When intracellular Ca in-

Contraction of vascular smooth muscle appears to be strikingly different by comparison to cardiac and skeletal muscle. Excitation–contraction coupling can be achieved by two distinctly different processes: electromechanical coupling and pharmacomechanical coupling. Electromechanical coupling appears to involve the opening of potential-dependent calcium channels across the cell membrane (PDC, #1), a process which may be analogous to the "slow channel" of cardiac muscle and is probably more common to smooth muscle outside of the vasculature. However, it appears that almost all vascular smooth muscle possess the PDC and can be stimulated to contract via this mechanism by either increasing extracellular potassium concentration or by strong electrical field stimulation such as the 30 volt stimulus using platinum field electrodes described below in studies on the bovine coronary artery. Pharmacomechanical coupling involves the

Figure 6 (cont.) creases, it combines with calmodulin (CLMD, the calcium modulating protein) to activate myosin light-chain kinase (MLCK)⑤. With phosphorylation of the myosin light-chain (MLC-P) actin and myosin interact, consume energy, and result in contraction⑥. The initial rapid phasic contraction of vascular smooth muscle appears to depend upon release of intracellular Ca from its storage sites via some type of trigger mechanism. The tonic phase of the contraction response of vascular smooth muscle appears to depend more on the movement of Ca from the extracellular to the intracellular space across the SL. Relaxation occurs when a phophatase-mediated (P-TASE) dephosphorylation of myosin light-chain-P ⑦ predominates over the MLCK phosphorylation reaction ⑤. MLCK activity decreases with the uptake of Ca into intracellular storage sites in the SL ⑧, SR ⑩, and possibly mitochondria (M) ⑨, although the latter is probably unimportant in healthy cells. Calcium can also be extruded from the cell via a calcium-activated pump ⑪ which utilizes energy or possibly via a sodium-calcium interaction ⑫ and ⑬ which may occur at the SL. Beta-receptor stimulation induces relaxation by activating a cyclic AMP-mediated protein kinase that phosphorylates MLCK, reducing its affinity for Ca and CLMD. The sodium-potassium pump ⑭ may also play an important role in the regulation of intracellular Ca levels by its effect upon the SL sodium-calcium interaction secondary to its direct effect in intracellular sodium levels. (From Zelis and Flaim, 1981, with permission.)

receptor-operated calcium channel (ROC, #2) which apparently
can be activated by binding of pharmacologically agonistic agents
such as norepinephrine to specific membrane receptors (for norepinephrine, the receptor is the alpha-adrenergic receptor). It is
probably true that the primary excitation-contraction coupling
process under physiological conditions is the ROC. In Figure 6,
the ROC which is depicted is the alpha-receptor being activated
by a molecule of norepinephrine (NE). When this process is started,
there appears to be some influx of calcium from the extracellular space across the cell membrane and into the cytoplasm where
some contraction is initiated. This initial puff of calcium appears
to trigger (Ca_t) further release of intracellularly stored calcium
from sites of sequestration within the cell such as sarcoplasmic
reticulum (SR, #4) and also some not so well defined storage
sites near the inner surface of the cell membrane or sarcolemma
(SL, #3). Intracellular calcium release into the cytoplasm has
been associated with the rapid initial increase in isometric tension
in vitro (sometimes called the phasic tension component). At a
slightly later point in time, tension continues to increase but at
a much slower rate. This slower phase (sometimes called the
tonic tension component) has been associated with an increasing
yet more slowly developing contribution of calcium ion moving
into the cell from the extracellular space. It appears that calcium causes contraction in vascular smooth muscle by combining
with calmodulin (CLMD) and activating the enzyme myosin light
chain kinase (MLCK, #5). After phosphorylation of the myosin
light chain has occurred, an interaction between actin and myosin
is allowed, ATP is then hydrolyzed (#6) and the shortening occurs.

In general, for relaxation to occur in muscle, cytoplasmic
free calcium must be reduced below some critical concentration
level. In skeletal muscle, removal of calcium is effected by the
active sequestration of calcium into intracellular sites of storage
such as the sarcoplasmic reticulum. In cardiac muscle, this process appears to be achieved by pumping calcium out of the cell
using a sodium-calcium exchange mechanism. In vascular smooth
muscle, this process is much more complicated since relaxation
can be achieved by a number of different mechanisms. First, a
relatively specific phosphatase enzyme (P-TASE, #7) causes
dephosphorylation of the myosin light chain which can result in
calcium-independent relaxation. Calcium-dependent relaxation
can occur secondarily to the lowering of cytoplasmic calcium
concentration which can be achieved by several different processes. Calcium ions can be actively sequestered by the sarcolemma (#8), by the mitochondria (#9) - although it is now gener-

ally thought that this process is not important in healthy vascular smooth muscle cells - and by the sarcoplasmic reticulum (#10) secondary to ATP-dependent enzyme processes
which have been shown to exist in these areas of the cell. Of
these various processes, #10 appears to be the most important.
Calcium ions can also be actively pumped out of the cell by
similar ATP-dependent enzymatic processes (#11). It has also
been proposed that intracellular calcium levels are dependent
to some extent upon a not so well defined sodium-calcium
interaction at the cell membrane (#12, #13). This process is
energized by the transmembrane sodium gradient which itself is
governed by the level of activity of the sodium-potassium pump
present on the cell membrane (#14). Thus, the regulation of
contractile activity in vascular smooth muscle is extremely
complex, especially considering the heterogenous nature of this
tissue described previously.

Many attempts have been made to describe the precise cellular mechanisms of various agents which we naively call "calcium
channel blockers" at the present time. In fact, considering the
previous discussion, it is conceivable that these agents may cause
a lowering of intracellular calcium not only by blocking calcium
influx but also, or instead, by stimulating the intracellar calcium
efflux or sequestration. In addition, several agents have been
shown to interact with the calcium-calmodulin complex, rendering
this step inactive and resulting in an inhibition of contractile
activity. Worthy evidence has been put forth which demonstrates
that some calcium blockers such as verapamil, nifedipine, and
diltiazem can inhibit calcium influx via the potential-dependent
calcium channel. The ability of these agents to have a similar
effect on the receptor-operated calcium channel is less firmly
established and appears to be somewhat tissue specific (Flaim,
1982).

V. STUDIES IN THE BOVINE CORONARY ARTERY

In order to characterize the bovine coronary artery more
carefully, we used electrical field stimulation via platinum field
electrodes (Ratz et al., 1980). Isolated vessels were stimulated
using either 9 or 30 volts to differentiate between contractions
due to norepinephrine release from sympathetic nerve terminals,
resulting in alpha-adrenergic receptor stimulation and the subsequent activation of receptor-operated calcium channels (9 volts),
and contractions due to electrical depolarization of the vascular

smooth muscle cell membrane and the subsequent opening of
potential-dependent calcium channels (30 volts). The entire
voltage-response relationship of this preparation is illustrated in
Figure 7. Norepinephrine release from sympathetic nerve terminals which is effected during low voltage stimulation (9 volts) resulted in approximately 20 mg/mg tissue of active tension, a
value approximately equal to the maximal tension level generated
by addition of exogenous norepinephrine to the bathing medium
(Figure 5). However, a 30 volt electrical stimulation, which
clearly causes cellular depolarization, resulted in approximately
75-100 mg/mg tissue of active tension, indicating a significantly
greater degree of vessel activation. These data suggest that there
are relatively few norepinephrine receptor-operated calcium
channels in the bovine coronary artery and that the majority of
these are located near the sympathetic nerve terminals. In order
to further substantiate the fact that the 9 volt but not the 30 volt

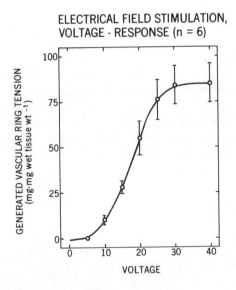

*Figure 7. Cumulative voltage-response relationship for
isolated rings of bovine coronary artery. Rings were preset at
1 g of resting preload tension prior to electrical stimulation
using parallel platinum field electrodes.*

response is dependent on activation of norepinephrine receptors, the study was repeated in the presence of the alpha-blocker, phentolamine. Figure 8 shows the results of this study. Phentolamine at 10^{-4}M significantly reduced the 9 volt response but had no significant effect on the 30 volt response. These data indicate that the 30 volt response is not dependent on the receptor-operated calcium channel. A further study was conducted to determine the effect of 10^{-5}M phentolamine on responses induced by two subsequent 9 and 30 volt stimulations in the same vessel (Figure 9). It can be seen that phentolamine's ability to reduce the 9 volt response improved during the subsequent stimulation, but no such effect occurred in the 30 volt response.

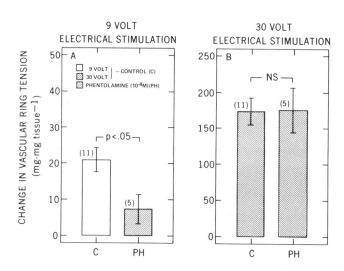

Figure 8. Change in active tension response of isolated rings of bovine ventricular coronary arteries to electrical stimulation at 9 volts (inducing release of norepinephrine from sympathetic nerve terminals) and at 30 volts (inducing depolarization of the vascular smooth muscle cells) before (control, C) and after alpha-receptor blockade secondary to pretreatment with phentolamine (PH).

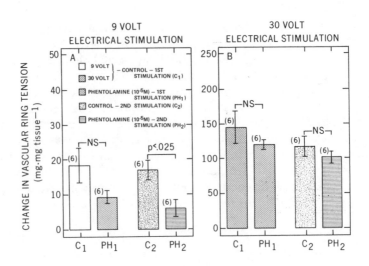

Figure 9. *Change in active tension response of isolated rings of bovine ventricular coronary arteries to electrical stimulation, at 9 and 30 volts, before (C) and after alpha-receptor blockade secondary to pretreatment with phentolamine (PH). In each ring, the first and second stimulus challenge is presented demonstrating that prolonged PH treatment did not alter the response characteristics.*

We proceeded to determine the degree of dependency of these responses to electrical stimulation on extracellular calcium. Hypothetically, if these contractile responses are due to the influx of extracellular calcium, they should be eliminated simply by removal of the available extracellular calcium. We used 2 mM EGTA added to a HEPES buffer containing zero extracellular calcium as a bathing medium and the experiments were repeated.

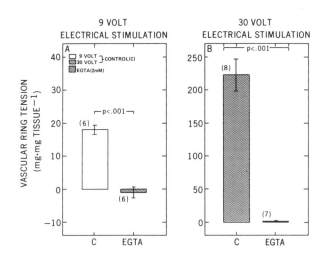

Figure 10. Bovine ventricular coronary artery ring tension generated in response to 9 and 30 electrical stimulation before (C) and after treatment with the extracellular chelator, EGTA.

As shown in Figure 10, EGTA completely eliminated both the 9 and the 30 volt responses. These results support the conclusion that few norepinephrine receptor-operated calcium channels exist in the bovine coronary artery and those which do exist are completely dependent upon extracellular calcium for the generation of contractile activity. Similarily, and not surprisingly, the entire 30 volt response could also be completely eliminated by using zero extracellular calcium plus 2 mM EGTA-HEPES buffer as the bathing media. This indicates that the potential-dependent calcium channels in this tissue are also entirely dependent upon extracellular calcium for the generation of contractile activity. We next tested the effect of the calcium blocker diltiazem on the 9 and 30 volt responses. Diltiazem significantly reduced both responses suggesting that, in this preparation, it acts as a

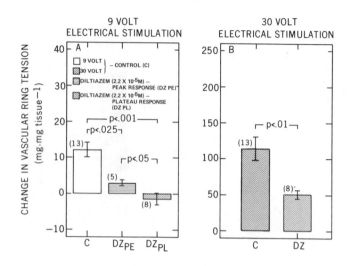

Figure 11. Change in active tension response of isolated rings of bovine ventricular coronary arteries to electrical stimulation at 9 and 30 volts, before (C) and after treatment with the calcium blocker, diltiazem (DZ). For the 9 volt stimulation, both the peak (PE) and the plateau (PL) response data are presented.

calcium influx blocker (Figure 11). In order to determine if diltiazem has any beta-adrenergic mediated effects in this tissue, we repeated the same study in the presence of propranolol, a nonselective beta-blocking agent. The change in contractile tension induced by both 9 and 30 volt electrical simulation plus diltiazem, and plus diltiazem and propanolol, are shown in Figure 12. The lack of statistically significant differences between data obtained with diltiazem alone and those generated in the presence of beta-blockade suggests that diltiazem is not a beta-receptor stimulator in the bovine coronary artery. This confirms previous data from our laboratory demonstrating that diltizem exerts no effect on the beta-adrenergic receptors in cardiac muscle (Flaim et al., 1980a).

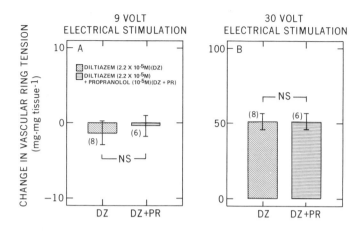

Figure 12. Change in active tension induced by 9 and 30 volt electrical stimulation during treatment with diltiazem alone (DZ) and diltiazem plus beta-blockade with propranolol (PR). NS = not significantly different.

In more recent studies on the bovine coronary artery, we have evaluated the serotonin-induced tension response (Ratz and Flaim, 1981a). Stimulation of isolated rings of bovine coronary artery using serotonin at $5 \times 10^{-6}M$ caused a biphasic constrictor response, with a peak contraction of approximately 126 mg/mg tissue at 2.3 min after stimulation. The tension response subsequently fell to a plateau of approximately 23 mg/mg tissue at 40 min post stimulation. When the serotonin response was repeated in rings previously incubated in zero calcium buffer, a biphasic response to serotonin remained, but the peak response was reduced to 80 mg/mg tissue occurring at 1 min post stimulation. The plateau response, which was relatively unaffected, was approximately 32 mg/mg tissue occurring at 23 min post stimulation. Thus, although the serotonin response was changed in the presence of zero extracellular calcium, the basic biphasic configuration as well as the peak response remained unaffected. These data indicate that a significant part of the serotonin-induced tension response in vascular smooth muscle of the bovine coronary artery is independent of extracellular calcium. This component must, therefore, be regulated by a serotonin-stimulated release of intracellular calcium. The fact that the tension profile in zero calcium was to some degree altered, primarily in the

early phase, indicates that the activation of the serotonin
receptor-operated calcium channels does involve some influx of
extracellular calcium. However, the observation that the
plateau response, achieved at 30–40 min after serotonin stimulation, was unaffected by the zero calcium buffer suggests that
this plateau is entirely dependent upon some intracellular
calcium release processes.

This model was subsequently used to test the effects of the
calcium blockers, diltiazem and verapamil. Hypothetically, an
agent which is a pure calcium influx blocker should produce an
effect on the serotonin tension profile identical to the effect
caused by the removal of extracellular calcium from the bathing
media. That is, it should change the profile and shift the peak
response to a slightly lower level at a slightly earlier time point
without changing the magnitude of the plateau response. The
effects of diltiazem and verapamil were compared to lanthanum
chloride, a known inorganic calcium influx blocker (Ratz and
Flaim, 1981b). The results of this study demonstrated that
lanthanum's effects were similar to those obtained by removing
extracellular calcium using zero calcium HEPES buffer, whereas
the effects of diltiazem and verapamil were associated with
significant supression of both the peak response and the plateau
response. Therefore, these data suggest that, unlike lanthanum
and zero extracellular calcium, both diltiazem and verapamil act
to block the calcium influx as well as to inhibit the release of
intracellularly stored calcium in bovine coronary artery. These
results represent the first findings which suggest that verapamil
and diltiazem cannot be simply classified as calcium influx
blockers.

VI. STUDIES IN RABBIT AORTA

It is imperative that one does not rely entirely on data from
tension studies as a basis to determine the mechanisms of action
of calcium blockers in vascular smooth muscle. It is well known
that changes in tension are not necessarily linked directly to
changes in calcium flux in this tissue. For this reason, we have
devoted considerable effort to perfecting the technique of measuring ^{45}Ca flux in isolated rings of vascular smooth muscle as a
means to determine the effects of calcium blockers on the transmembrane movement of calcium in this tissue (Flaim, 1982).

The results from some of this work have been recently presented (Ress and Flaim, 1982). The basic protocols used in these
studies are summarized in Figure 13. In each protocol, a three-

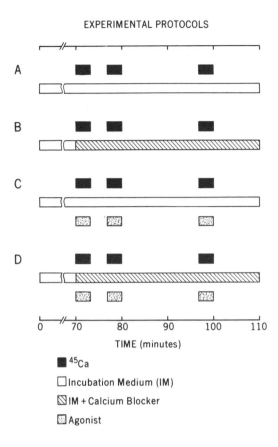

EXPERIMENTAL PROTOCOLS

■ ⁴⁵Ca — ^{45}Ca
□ Incubation Medium (IM)
▨ IM + Calcium Blocker
▨ Agonist

Figure 13. Schematic representation of the experimental protocols used to test calcium influx using radioactive calcium marker (^{45}Ca) via the leak channel, in the presence of incubation medium (IM) alone, via the receptor-operated and potential-dependent calcium channels, in the presence of an agonist (norepinephrine and high potassium respectively), and via these three channels in the presence of various calcium blockers (lanthanum chloride, diltiazem, verapamil, and nifedipine). Data resulting from these protocols are summarized in Figure 14.

minute pulse of ^{45}Ca was exposed to different groups of tissue at three different time points within the protocol, corresponding to the 3, 10 and 30-minute time points after initiation of the protocol. Protocol A represented the control study where the tissue was exposed only to the ^{45}Ca pulse. Protocol B added calcium blockers only to Protocol A. Protocol C added a vaso-active agonist (norepinephrine, 10^{-6} M; potassium chloride, 80 mM; or saline). Protocol D added both calcium blocker and agonist. After each ^{45}Ca pulse, rings were removed from the labelled solution, washed, and analyzed for the amount of ^{45}Ca taken up into the cell, thus providing an index of calcium influx. We compared the effects of the inorganic calcium blocker, lanthanum (5 mM), the organic blockers diltiazem (10^{-6} M), nifedipine (10^{-6} M), and verapamil (10^{-6} M) on calcium influx via the receptor-operated calcium channel (using norepinephrine), via the potential-dependent calcium channel (using potassium chloride), and via the leak channel for calcium influx (in the presence of saline addition alone without agonists). The results, expressed as percent inhibition of control influx (no calcium blocker), are summarized in Figure 14. In Figure 14a, it can be seen that lanthanum alone was able to significantly inhibit calcium influx via the leak channels, and this effect appeared to be attenuated over time. In Figure 14b, both lanthanum and nifedipine significantly inhibited norepinephrine-stimulated calcium influx via the receptor-operated calcium channels, the effect of lanthanum appeared to be augmented with time whereas that of nifedipine was not. Verapamil and diltiazem, on the other hand, had no significant effect on calcium influx via the potential-dependent calcium channels (Figure 14c). All but verapamil's effect appeared to be augmented with time. The observation that organic calcium blockers were capable of inhibiting calcium influx via the receptor-operated and poten-tial-dependent calcium channels, but not via the leak channels, suggests that the latter may represent a discrete class of calcium channels in the vascular smooth muscle. However, it remains possible that the leak channels are synonymous with one or both of the other channels operating at an unstimulated level. From these data we conclude that at the concentrations tested, the organic calcium blockers are not equally potent as blockers of the potential-dependent calcium channels and the receptor-operated calcium channels, nor are they equipotent with each other on these channels. Furthermore, the effects of these agents appear to be attenuated, in different fashions, with time of exposure to the tissue.

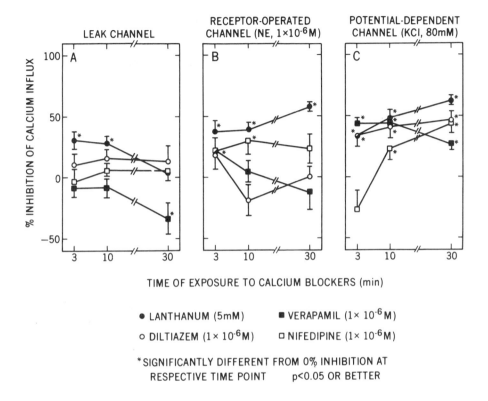

Figure 14. Data presented as percent of inhibition of calcium influx via the leak channel (Panel A), via the receptor-operated calcium channel stimulated by norepinephrine (NE) (Panel B), and via the potential-dependent calcium channel stimulated by high potassium (KCl) (Panel C) obtained at 3, 10, and 30 minutes of exposure to four different blocking agents.

VII. EFFECTS OF CALCIUM BLOCKERS
ON THE DISTRIBUTION OF CARDIAC OUTPUT

While studies at the tissue and cellular level are important for the determination of the mechanism of action of agents such as the calcium blockers, it is also important to determine their effects in the whole animal. To achieve this goal we have employed a conscious rat model utilizing hemodynamic measurements as well as the radioactive microsphere technique for the determination of cardiac output distribution (Flaim and Kanda, 1982).

Data summarizing the effects of diltiazem on cardiovascular hemodynamics are presented in Figure 15. Compared to

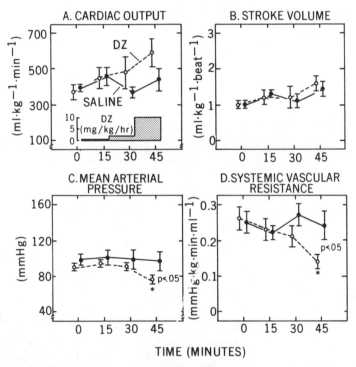

Figure 15. Effects of intravenous diltiazem (DZ) at increasing dose levels on cardiovascular hemodynamics in the normal, conscious rat. P values indicate level of statistical significance for comparison of parallel data for DZ and saline control. *Statistically significant difference between indicated data and respective control pre-infusion data. (From Flaim and Zelis, 1982, with permission.)

saline control, diltiazem at sequentially increasing dosages appeared to increase sequentially the cardiac output while saline alone had no consistent effect. Neither diltiazem nor saline control showed consistent effects upon stroke volume. Diltiazem at the highest dose level significantly reduced the mean arterial pressure in comparison with the pre-diltiazem control and the respective saline control data. The highest dose of diltiazem also significantly reduced systemic vascular resistance compared to both the pre-diltiazem control and the respective saline control data. Furthermore, diltiazem reduced peak systolic pressure at the highest dose as well as the left ventricular end diastolic pressure. While saline control infusion had no significant effect upon systolic arterial pressure or diastolic arterial pressure, diltiazem at the highest infusion level resulted in significantly reduced values for both pressures when compared to the saline control data. The effect of diltiazem on diastolic arterial pressure was also substantial and statistically significant with respect to pre-diltiazem control data; neither diltiazem nor control saline infusion had a significant effect on heart rate or central venous pressure.

The effects of diltiazem infusion on the total coronary flow and vascular resistance are presented in Figure 16. Increasing diltiazem infusion sequentially increased the total coronary blood flow; this effect was statistically significant compared to pre-diltiazem control data only at the highest diltiazem infusion level. Saline control infusion, on the other hand, caused a slight but nonsignificant increase in the total coronary blood flow. At all three infusion levels diltiazem caused a significant decrease in total coronary vascular resistance compared to pre-diltiazem control data, whereas saline infusion at all three levels caused a nonsignificant reduction in the total coronary vascular resistance. At the highest dose of diltiazem, the total coronary vascular resistance was significantly lower compared to the respective saline control infusion data.

Saline control infusion apparently had no statistically significant effect on regional blood flow or vascular resistance, although there was a tendency for blood flow to increase and vascular resistance to decrease during saline loading. Compared to the control pre-diltiazem data, diltiazem at 2 mg/kg/hr both significantly increased blood flow and decreased vascular resistance in vessels supplying the atria and right ventricle, as well as vessels supplying the left ventricle. At 10 mg/kg/hr, diltiazem increased blood flow and decreased resistance in all regions of the heart compared to the pre-diltiazem control levels. Compared to the

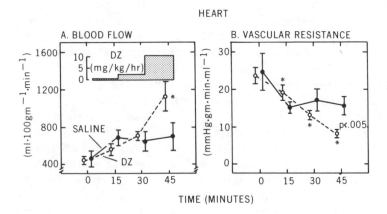

Figure 16. Effects of intravenous diltiazem (DZ) at increasing dose levels on total coronary blood flow (Panel A) and total coronary vascular resistance (Panel B) in the normal, conscious rat. P values indicate level of statistical significance for comparison of parallel data for DZ and saline control. *Statistically significant difference between indicated data and respective control pre-infusion data. (From Flaim and Zelis, 1982, with permission.)

respective control saline infusion data, diltiazem at 10 mg/kg/hr increased right ventricular blood flow and decreased atrial, right ventricular, and left ventricular resistance. At 2 mg/kg/hr, diltiazem also decreased right ventricular resistance compared to the saline control group. Thus, diltiazem significantly increased coronary blood flow and reduced coronary vascular resistance in all three regions studied, although coronary circulation in the right ventricular region appeared to be slightly more sensitive to the effects of diltiazem than in the other regions.

In order to determine if diltiazem exerts differential effects on the skeletal muscle blood flow in different regions, eight different beds were studied: psoas, gastrocnemius, quadriceps, tibialis, triceps, latissimus dorsi, soleus, and biceps. It is clear from these data that diltiazem had no substantial effect upon the skeletal muscle circulatory bed in the resting animal. Neither saline control nor diltiazem infusion caused significant changes in either blood flow or vascular resistance in the various skeletal muscle regions studied. In the latissimus dorsi muscle, blood flow at control level in the diltiazem group was higher than the respective control value in the saline group. This difference, also noted in the vascular resistance studies and not readily explained, suggests the existence of some intergroup variation.

In all other circulatory regions studied, the saline control infusion had no significant effect on either blood flow or vascular resistance. On the other hand, when comparing the diltiazem data to their respective pre-infusion control data, several statistically significant changes were noted; e.g., the hepatic arterial blood flow increased and vascular resistance significantly decreased during diltiazem infusion at 10 mg/kg/hr. Diltiazem also markedly reduced vascular resistance in the ileum and jejunum. At the highest dose studied, diltiazem significantly increased blood flow and reduced vascular resistance in the testes; it also tended to increase blood flow and reduce vascular resistance in the cerebral circulation. These effects were statistically significant at the highest dose of diltiazem for cerebellar blood flow, cerebellar vascular resistance, and vascular resistance in the midbrain regions.

Comparing animal data using diltiazem to saline control data, several significant differences were found. Blood flow to the cerebral hemispheres and the midbrain regions in the diltiazem group at both 0.4 and 2 mg/kg/hr was reduced compared to the control values. It should be noted that blood flow to these regions generally tended to increase during both infusions. Compared to pre-infusion control, the increase, although not statistically significant, was greater in the saline group than in the diltiazem group. It is, therefore, unclear whether diltiazem tended to suppress an infusion-related cerebral vasodilatation at the lower doses of the drug or if the response of the control saline group was artifactually high. It is clear, however, that at the highest infusion level, the values in the saline control group returned to the pre-infusion level while those in the diltiazem group diverged significantly from the control data in favor of vasodilatation.

Saline control infusion had no significant effects on the total distribution of cardiac output to the various regions. During diltiazem infusion, however, the percentage of total cardiac output distributed to the coronary circulation was significantly increased relative not only to the diltiazem control, but also to the respective saline control data. While a number of other circulatory systems seemed to be affected in a similar manner by diltiazem, as opposed to saline (muscle, brain, liver, gastrointestinal tract), the observed differences were not statistically

significant. Thus, diltiazem infusion significantly altered the
distribution of cardiac output in favor of the coronary arterial
circulation.

These results strongly suggest that intravenous diltiazem
preferentially reduces coronary vascular resistance in the conscious rat and that this vasodilator effect is rather specific for
the coronary circulation. Because of technical problems, it was
not possible to obtain a direct and reliable index of cardiac function. Nevertheless, it was feasible to evaluate other major determinants of cardiac function, both before and during diltiazem
infusion. These data, as summarized in Figure 17, are presented
as percent change from control during the highest dose of drug
infusion. As shown, diltiazem substantially reduced systemic
vascular resistance while control saline infusion had little or no
effect. Diltiazem also reduced coronary vascular resistance as
previously noted. However, the saline control infusion also reduced
coronary resistance in this circulation although this effect was

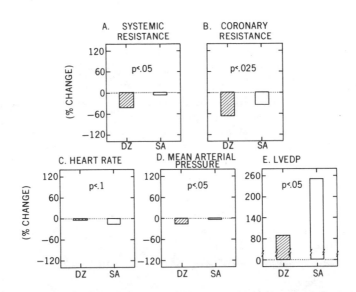

*Figure 17. Effects presented as average percent change
from control pre-infusion data of intravenous diltiazem (DZ) and
saline control (SA) at the highest dose levels (10 mg/kg/hr) on
the determinants of cardiac function. P values indicate level of
statistical significance between indicated DZ and SA data.
LVEDP = left ventricular end-diastolic pressure. (From Flaim
and Zelis, 1982, with permission.)*

significantly less than that caused by diltiazem. Heart rate was
not substantially affected by either treatment, although a decrease in rate occurred during diltiazem infusion. Mean arterial
pressure was reduced during diltiazem infusion while essentially
no change occurred with saline. Left ventricular end-diastolic
pressure increased during both diltiazem and saline infusion; however, the volume loading effect of saline was substantially greater
than that of diltiazem despite the fact that the volumes infused
were identical. From these results, therefore, the effects of both
saline and diltiazem on cardiac function can be indirectly assessed. During saline, the substantial increase in preload, coupled
with essentially no change in afterload and only a slight decrease
in heart rate, resulted in increased cardiac work which was reflected in a substantial decrease in coronary vascular resistance.
During diltiazem infusion under identical volume loading conditions, preload increased only slightly while afterload dropped
more extensively with diltiazem than with saline. These changes
caused by diltiazem would be expected to reduce cardiac work.
Despite this effect to unload the heart, coronary vascular resistance was lowered even more during diltiazem infusion, due
apparently to the direct coronary vasodilator effect of this agent.
Since cardiac ouput actually increased during diltiazem, it can
be concluded that diltiazem even at the highest dosage did not
have a significant negative inotropic effect in the resting conscious rat (Flaim and Zelis, 1982).

Similar studies have been completed using verapamil and
nifedipine. For the sake of brevity, only data obtained with the
highest dose of each of these drugs (verapamil, 6 mg/kg/hr;
nifedipine, 1.5 mg/kg/hr) will be discussed and compared to those
previously described from diltiazem (10 mg/kg/hr). It should be
noted that these dosage levels were selected since they had comparable effects in reducing mean arterial pressure by approximately 20% in the conscious resting rat.

Figure 18 summarizes the effects of these three calcium
blockers on cardiovascular hemodynamics. As noted above, all
three agents lowered mean arterial pressure by approximately
20% although none had a significant effect on heart rate. One
would normally expect the hypotensive effect of calcium blockers to cause a reflex increase in the sympathetic tone which
would result in a variety of cardiovascular changes, and a
prominent effect would be reflex tachycardia. It has been shown
that these three agents exert different effects on heart rate,
diltiazem having a greater negative chronotropic effect and a

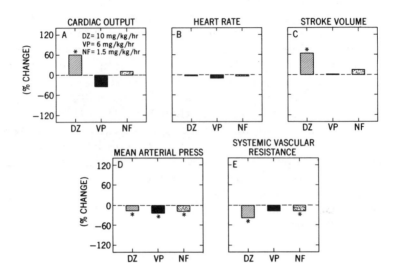

*Figure 18. Comparative effects of the three calcium block-
ers diltiazem (DZ), verapamil (VP), and nifedipine (NF) on cardiovascular hemodynamics in the conscious resting rat model. The
dose of agents used were selected based on their ability to reduce
mean arterial pressure by approximately 20%. Values plotted
are the average percent change from control levels at the indicated dose (i.v.). *Statistically significant change from control.
PRESS = pressure.*

lesser negative inotropic effect than either verapamil or
nifedipine (Henry, 1980). From Figure 18, it can be suggested
that the lack of a change in heart rate during diltiazem administration in the face of 20 mmHg drop in mean arterial pressure
may be due to its negative chronotropic effect, negating a
positive chronotropic contribution from reflex sympathetic
stimulation. This interpretation apparently cannot be applied to
verapamil and nifedipine. Diltiazem caused a 60% increase in
cardiac output whereas both verapamil and nifedipine caused
cardiac ouptut reductions. Diltiazem also increased stroke
volume whereas verapamil and nifedipine had little effect.
Finally, all three agents induced decreases in systemic vascular
resistance but diltiazem was the most potent in this respect.

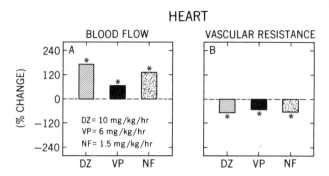

*Figure 19. Comparative effects of the three calcium blockers diltiazem (DZ), nifedipine (NF), and verapamil (VP) on coronary blood flow and vascular resistance in the conscious resting rat model. Values plotted are the average percent change from control levels at the indicated dosages of each drug (i.v.). *Statistically significant change from control.*

In our studies, all three calcium blockers were potent coronary vasodilators as shown in Figure 19. Nifedipine and diltiazem were approximately equipotent and verapamil was less effective in this regard. All three agents had approximately equal effects in reducing coronary vascular resistance, and all three agents were also potent vasodilators of the skeletal muscle bed at the highest dose administered (Figure 20); however, diltiazem and verapamil appeared to be of slightly higher potency than nifedipine. These effects are also reflected in the corresponding data for skeletal muscle vascular resistance. Diltiazem had little effect in the cutaneous circulation whereas both verapamil and nifedipine were potent vasoconstrictors; furthermore, diltiazem increased renal blood flow by approximately 30% whereas verapamil reduced flow and nifedipine had little or no effect. Similar diverse effects were noted in the cerebral, hepatic arterial, and gastrointestinal circulations (Figure 21). Thus, diltiazem and nifedipine appear to be vasodilators in the cerebral and hepatic arterial circulations, whereas verapamil is a mild vasoconstrictor in these regions. In the gastrointestinal circulation, diltiazem is a potent vasodilator, verapamil a vasoconstrictor, and nifedipine has minimal effects.

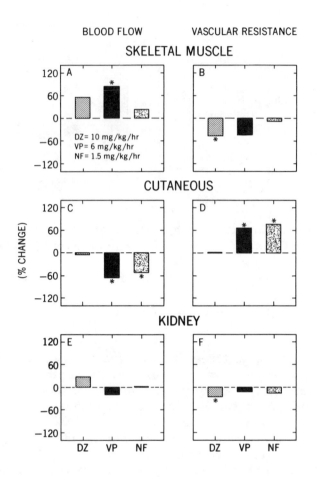

*Figure 20. Comparative effects of the three calcium block-ers diltiazem (DZ), verapamil (VP), and nifedipine (NF) on blood flow and vascular resistance in the skeletal muscle, cutaneous, and renal circulations. Values are the average percent change from control levels at the indicated dosages of each drug (i.v.). *Statistically significant change from control.*

It is highly probable that the results summarized here repre-sent an interaction of the direct vasodilator effects of the calci-um blockers in the different regions with the sympathetic reflex-induced vasoconstrictor effects that would occur secondary to the central hypotensive effects of these agents. Therefore, it might be expected that the regions of peripheral circulation,

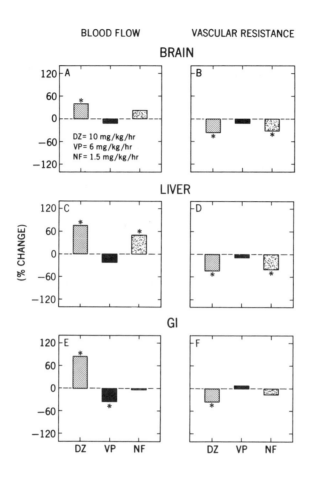

*Figure 21. Comparative effects of diltiazem (DZ), nifedipine (NF), and verapamil (VP) on blood flow and vascular resistance in the brain, hepatic arterial (liver), and gastrointestinal (GI) circulations. Values are plotted as the percent change from control levels. *Statistically significant change from control.*

which are most heavily innervated by sympathetic nerves, would show a lesser net vasodilator response as a direct effect of the calcium blocker. The most heavily innervated circulations of the body are those in the cutaneous regions. In these regions, it appeared that the direct vasodilating effects of verapamil and nifedipine were completely overridden by an increase in sympathetic tone secondary to the central hypotensive effects of these two agents, and this resulted in a dramatic vasoconstrictor effect. The fact that such effect was obtained secondary to treatment with diltiazem may indicate a capability of diltiazem to override, or possibly, to inhibit the sympathetic tone. This conclusion is supported by results obtained from the three agents on blood flow and vascular resistance in the gastrointestinal circulation, which is another region densely innervated with sympathetic nerves. In this region, verapamil and nifedipine showed little or no effect while diltiazem caused potent vasodilatation. These results tend to support the hypothesis that diltiazem and, possibly to a lesser extent, nifedipine, are capable of overriding the sympathetic reflex vasoconstrictor effects induced by the hypotensive effects of these drugs. Since it has been shown that calcium is an important component in the release process for the sympathetic neurotransmitter (Katz and Miledi, 1967), it is not surprising to find that the calcium blockers may interact with this process to result in an inhibition of sympathetic nervous function.

More recently, we investigated the effects of diltiazem (2 mg/kg/hr), compared to saline control at equal infusion rate, on cardiocirculatory dynamics and cardiac output distribution in the conscious rat, both at rest and during treadmill excercise at a rate equal to approximately 30% of maximum exercise capacity for this preparation. It was found that, while exercise significantly increased heart rate (Figure 22) in both groups, the left ventricular end diastolic pressure in the diltiazem treated group was reduced. Central venous pressure increased significantly in the saline control group and decreased significantly in the diltiazem group during exercise. Diltiazem significantly reduced systemic vascular resistance compared to saline control both at rest and during exercise, and a significant elevation of central venous pressure was observed only at rest.

Regional blood flow and vascular resistance data were obtained in eight skeletal muscle regions. Exercise induced significant increases in blood flow to all muscle regions studied (with the exception of the latissimus dorsi) during both saline and diltiazem treatment (Figure 23), while decreases in vascular resistance in seven of the eight muscles during saline and six of the eight muscles during diltiazem treatment were also noted. Diltiazem treatment had no significant effect on muscle blood flow or vascular resistance at rest compared to saline control, with the exception of the soleus muscle where a significant reduction of rest vascular resistance induced by diltiazem was noted. During exercise, however, diltiazem treatment resulted in

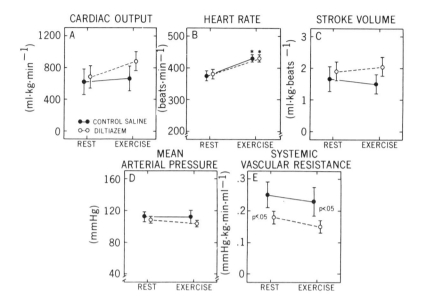

*Figure 22.   Effects of intravenous diltiazem (0.5 mg/kg) compared to saline control on various cardiovascular hemodynamic parameters in the conscious rat model at rest and during submaximal treadmill excercise. *Significant exercise-induced change; presence of P value indicates significant drug-induced change.*

significantly higher blood flow levels in four muscles compared to saline control. The average effects of exercise and diltiazem on skeletal muscle blood flow and vascular resistance are plotted in Figure 24. During saline infusion, exercise significantly increased skeletal muscle flow by 141% and significantly decreased resistance by 68%, whereas the comparable values for the diltiazem treated group were a 267% increase in flow and a 69% decrease in resistance. Thus, compared to saline control, diltiazem significantly increased exercise-induced muscle hyperemia by over 120%, and reduced resistance by 31%.

Diltiazem, compared to saline control, signifcantly increased blood flow in all three regions of the coronary circulation, both at rest and during exercise, and reduced vascular resistance in three coronary regions at rest and in two regions during exercise. The

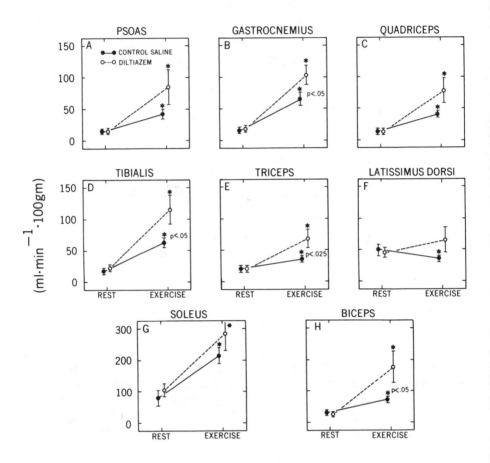

Figure 23. *Effects of intravenous diltiazem (0.5 mg/kg) compared to saline control on blood flow in eight different skeletal muscle beds in the conscious rat model at rest and during submaximal treadmill excercise. *Significant exercise-induced change; presence of P value indicates significant drug-induced change.*

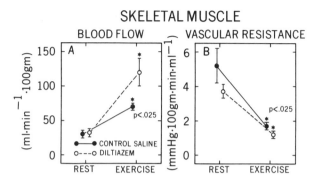

*Figure 24. Average skeletal muscle blood flow and vascular resistance at rest and during exercise in saline control and dil- tiazem-treated animals. *Significant exercise-induced change; presence of P value indicates significant drug-induced change. (From Flaim et al., 1982, with permission.)*

effects of diltiazem and exercise on the average coronary flow and resistance are summarized in Figure 25. Thus, compared to saline treatment, diltiazem significantly increased flow and reduced resistance both at rest and during exercise.

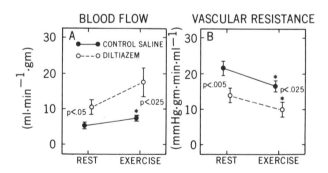

*Figure 25. Average coronary blood flow and vascular resis- tance at rest and during exercise in saline control and diltiazem- treated animals. *Significant exercise-induced change; presence of P value indicates significant drug-induced change. (From Flaim et al., 1982, with permission.)*

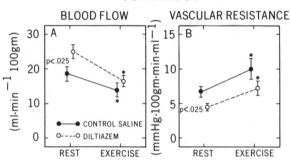

Figure 26. Average cutaneous blood flow and vascular resistance at rest and during exercise in saline control and diltiazem-treated animals. *Significant exercise-induced change; presence of P value indicates significant drug-induced change. (From Flaim et al., 1982, with permission.)

In the dorsal cutaneous region, diltiazem significantly increased blood flow and reduced vascular resistance at rest but had no significant effect during exercise. No such effect was noted in the lateral hindlimb region. The effects of exercise and diltiazem on the average cutaneous blood flow and vascular resistance are illustrated in Figure 26.

Exercise had no significant effect on renal blood flow or vascular resistance in either the saline control or the diltiazem treated groups (Figure 27). Diltiazem treatment significantly increased renal blood flow and reduced renal vascular resistance, both at rest and during exercise, compared to the respective saline control data. In the gastrointestinal bed, diltiazem treatment significantly increased blood flow compared to saline control both at rest and during exercise in the jejunum, and significantly lowered vascular resistance in both the jejunum and the stomach. Exercise appeared to have no significant effect on gastrointestinal blood flow or vascular resistance during saline treatment. However, during diltiazem treatment, exercise significantly reduced blood flow in the ileum, jejunum, colon, as well as the stomach; it also significantly elevated vascular

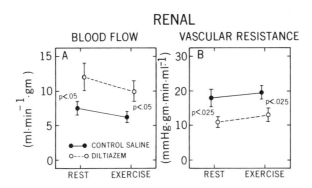

*Figure 27. Average renal blood flow and vascular resistance at rest and during exercise in saline control and diltiazem-treated animals. *Significant exercise-induced change; presence of P value indicates significant drug-induced change. (From Flaim et al., 1982, with permission.)*

resistance in the latter. The average effects of exercise and diltiazem treatment on gastrointestinal blood flow and vascular resistance are plotted in Figure 28. Thus, diltiazem treatment

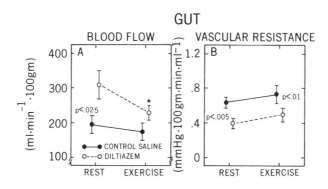

*Figure 28. Average gastrointestinal blood flow and vascular resistance at rest and during exercise in saline control and diltiazem-treated animals. *Significant exercise-induced change; presence of P value indicates significant drug-induced change. (From Flaim et al., 1982, with permission.)*

significantly elevated blood flow in the gut at rest, and reduced vascular resistance both at rest and during exercise when compared to saline. Although exercise significantly lowered gut blood flow in the diltiazem group, no significant change was noted in the saline group. In the hepatic arterial circulation, diltiazem significantly increased exercise blood flow and reduced exercise resistance compared to saline control. In the saline control group, exercise significantly lowered hepatic arterial blood flow, but no such effect was noted in the diltiazem group. In the spleen, exercise significantly reduced blood flow and increased vascular resistance in both the saline and diltiazem treatment groups; however, diltiazem treatment also resulted in a significantly lower resting vascular resistance compared to control saline. Exercise significantly increased blood flow and reduced vascular resistance in all areas of the brain studied (cerebellum, cerebrum, midbrain) whereas diltiazem significantly increased blood flow in the cerebellum at rest compared to saline control but had no significant effect elsewhere (Flaim et al., 1982).

VIII. CONCLUSIONS

In reviewing the literature, it is apparent that the calcium blockers have dramatically different potencies depending upon the type of contractile activity against which their effectiveness is tested. Most agents are more potent for the inhibition of vascular smooth muscle contractile activity, secondary to opening of the potential-dependent calcium channels during potassium stimulation, and less potent for the inhibition of contractile activity secondary to opening of the receptor-operated calcium channels during stimulation by agents such as norepinephrine and other circulating vasoagonists. There appears to be, also, considerable variation in potencies demonstrated by these agents depending upon the type of vascular smooth muscle preparation in which they are tested. In general, the calcium blockers are more potent in vessels of the coronary and cerebral circulations and less potent in vessels from other circulations of the body. These findings suggest that there are significant differences among various vessel types with regard to the mechanisms by which agonists such as norepinephrine can induce contractile activity. Calcium blockers are apparently more effective as inhibitors of transmembrane calcium uptake stimulated by potential changes, than by the binding of agents such as norepinephrine to its receptor site on the membrane. Overlying this diversity at the cellular level in blood vessels, there appears to exist considerable variation in the effects of these agents on the intact circulation.

The vasodilator effects of these agents in the intact animal are modulated by a variety of factors which include not only standard considerations such as species, and the presence or type of anesthesia, but also such considerations as the presence and level of sympathetic tone. Results from most previous studies investigating the effects of these calcium blockers in the intact animal have supported the conclusion that these agents are generally vasodilators, and this effect is most potent in the coronary vascular bed. Our studies in the conscious rat model basically support this conclusion, but results obtained on other circulations are quite different. Our findings suggest strongly that increased sympathetic tone, which would be expected during the calcium blocker-induced decrease in systemic arterial pressure, is involved to varying degees in regulating the regional vascular effects of each of the three calcium blockers studied. Our results further suggest that the regional vasodilator effects of verapamil are most potently reversed by the increase in sympathetic tone, those of nifedipine are less affected, and the effects of diltiazem are the least influenced. These findings suggest that diltiazem (and possibly nifedipine to a lesser degree) may have some inhibitory actions on the relationship between alpha-adnergic nerve and vascular smooth muscle during increased reflex-induced sympathetic activity.

REFERENCES

Altura, B. M. (1966). Differential actions of polypeptides and other drugs on coronary inflow vessels. Am. Heart J. **72,** 709-711.

Bevan, J. A. (1979). Transient responses of rabbit cerebral blood vessels to norepinephrine. Circ. Res. **45,** 566-572.

Bevan, J. A., Garstka, W., Su, C., and Su, M. O. (1973). The bimodal basis of the contractile response of the rabbit ear artery to norepinephrine and other agonists. Eur. J. Pharmacol. **22,** 47-53.

Bohr, D. F. (1963). Vascular smooth muscle: dual effect of calcium. Science **139,** 597-599.

Brody, M. J. (1978). Histaminergic and cholinergic vasodilator systems. In "Mechanisms of Vasodilation" (P. M. Vanhoutte and I. Leusen, eds.), pp. 266–277. Karger, Basel.

Burrows, M. E., and Vanhoutte, P. M. (1981). Pharmacology of arterioles: some aspects of variability in response to norepinephrine, histamine, and 5-hydroxytryptamine. J. Cardiovasc. Pharmacol. 3, 1370–1380.

Deth, R., and Van Breeman, C. (1974). Relative contributions of Ca influx and cellular Ca during drug induced activation of the rabbit aorta. Pflugers Arch. 348, 13–22.

Deth, R., and Van Breeman, C. (1977). Agonist induced release of intracellular calcium in the rabbit aorta. J. Membrane Biol. 30, 363–380.

Duckles, S. P. (1979). Neurogenic dilator and constrictor response of pial arteries in vitro: differences between dogs and sheep. Circ. Res. 44, 482–490.

Duckles, S. P. (1980). Functional activity of the noradrenergic innervation of large cerebral arteries. Br. J. Pharmacol. 69, 193–199.

Duckles, S. P., and Bevan, J. A. (1979). Responses of small rabbit pial arteries in vivo. Blood Vessels 16, 80–86.

Fara, J. W. (1971). Escape from tension induced by noradrenalin or electrical stimulation in isolated mesenteric arteries. Br. J. Pharmacol. 43, 865–867.

Flaim, S. F. (1982). Comparative pharmacology of calcium blockers based on studies of vascular smooth muscle. In "Calcium Blockers: Mechanisms of Action and Clinical Applications" (S. F. Flaim and R. Zelis, eds.), pp. 155–178. Urban and Schwarzenberg, Baltimore.

Flaim, S. F., Annibali, J. A., Newman, E. D., and Zelis, R. (1982). Effects of diltiazem on the cardiocirculatory response to exercise in conscious rat. J. Pharmacol. Exp. Ther. 223, 624–630.

Flaim, S. F., Flaim, K. E., and Zelis, R. (1980). Diltiazem: lack of myocardial β-adrenergic receptor-binding capacity. Pharmacology 21, 306–312.

Flaim, S. F., and Kanda, K. (1982). Comparative pharmacology of calcium blockers based on studies of cardiac output distribution. In "Calcium Blockers: Mechanisms of Action and Clinical Applications" (S. F. Flaim and R. Zelis, eds.), pp. 179–192. Urban and Schwarzenberg, Baltimore.

Flaim, S. F., Swigart, S. C., Ginsburg, R., and Zelis, R. (1980). Rhythmicity in rabbit femoral artery: a model for human coronary spasm. Physiologist **23**, 102.

Flaim, S. F., and Zelis, R. (1982). Effects of diltiazem on total cardiac output distribution in conscious rats. J. Pharmacol. Exp. Ther. **222**, 359-366.

Ginsburg, R., Bristow, M. R., Harrison, D. C., and Stinson, E. B. (1980). Studies with isolated human coronary arteries. Chest **78**, 180-186.

Godfraind, T. (1976). Calcium exchange in vascular smooth muscle, action of noradrenalin and lanthanum. J. Physiol. **260**, 21-35.

Godfraind, T. and Kaba, A. (1972). The role of calcium in the action of drugs on vascular smooth muscle. Arch. Intern. Pharmacodyn. Ther. **196**, 35-49.

Gross, G. J., Buck, J. D., and Warltier, D. C. (1981). Transmural distribution of blood flow during activation of coronary muscarinic receptors. Am. J. Physiol. **240**, H941-H946.

Hackett, J. G., Abboud, F. M., Mark, A. C., Schmid, P. G., and Heistad, D. D. (1972). Coronary vascular responses to stimulation of chemoreceptors and baroreceptors. Circ. Res. **31**, 8-17.

Haeusler, G. (1978). Relationship between noradrenalin induced depolarization and contraction in vascular smooth muscle. Blood Vessels **15**, 46-54.

Henry, P. D. (1980). Comparative pharmacology of calcium antagonists: nifedipine, verapamil and diltiazem. Am. J. Cardiol. **46**, 1047-1058.

Ito, Y., Kitamura, K., and Kuriyama, H. (1979). Effects of acetylcholine and catecholamines on the smooth muscle cell of the porcine coronary artery. J. Physiol. **294**, 595-611.

Hermsmeyer, K. (1971). Contraction and membrane activation in several mammalian vascular muscles. Life Sci. **10**, 223-234.

Katz, B. and Miledi, R. (1967). The timing of Ca action during neuromuscular transmission. J. Physiol. **189**, 535-544.

Kitamura, K. and Kuriyama, H. (1979). Effects of acetylcholine on the smoth muscle cell of isolated main coronary artery of the guinea pig. J. Physiol. **293**, 119-133.

Lee, T. J., Hume, W. R., Su, C., and Bevan, J. A. (1978). Neurogenic vasodilation of cat cerebral arteries. Circ. Res. **42**, 535–542.

McCalden, T. A., and Bevan, J. A. (1980). Asymmetry of the contractile response of the rabbit ear artery to exogenous amines. Am. J. Physiol. **238**, H618–H624.

McCalden, T. A., and Bevan, J. A. (1981). Sources of activator calcium in rabbit basilar artery. Am. J. Physiol. **241**, H129–H133.

Mellander, S., and Johansson, B. (1968). Control of resistance, exchange and capacitance functions in the peripheral circulation. Pharmacol. Rev. **20**, 117–196.

Mueller-Schweinitzer, E. (1980). The mechanism of ergometrine-induced coronary arterial spasm: In vitro studies on canine arteries. J. Cardiovasc. Pharmacol. **2**, 645–655.

Ohhashi, T., and Azuma, T. (1980). Paradoxical relaxation of arterial strips induced by vasoactive agents. Blood Vessels **17**, 16–26.

Owen, D. A. A. (1977). Histamine receptors in the cardio-vascular system. Gen. Pharmacol. **8**, 141–156.

Ratz, P. H., and Flaim, S. F. (1981a). Serotonin-induced tension response in bovine coronary artery (BCA): importance of intracellular calcium release. Fed. Proc. **40**, 451.

Ratz, P. H., and Flaim, S. F. (1981b). Evidence that diltiazem and verapamil may inhibit intracellular calcium release during serotonin stimulation of bovine coronary artery. Circulation **64**, IV–122.

Ratz, P. H., and Flaim, S. F. (1982). Species and blood vessel specificity in the use of calcium for contraction. In "Calcium Blockers: Mechanisms of Action and Clinical Applications" (S. F. Flaim and R. Zelis, eds.), pp. 77–98. Urban and Schwarzenberg, Baltimore.

Ratz, P. H., Flaim, S. F., and Zelis, R. (1980). Excitation-contraction coupling in bovine coronary artery: predominance of potential-dependent calcium channels. Circulation **62**, III–253.

Ress, R. J., and Flaim, S. F. (1982). Differential effects of calcium blockers on calcium influx in vascular smooth muscle: evidence for three calcium influx channels. Circulation **66**, II–141.

Ross, G. (1975). Norepinephrine vasoconstrictor escape in isolated mesenteric arteries. Am. J. Physiol. **228**, 1652–1655.

Ross, G., Stinson, E., Schroeder, J., and Ginsburg, R. (1980). Spontaneous phasic activity of isolated human coronary arteries. Cardiovasc. Res. **14**, 613–618.

Sakai, K. (1980). Role of histamine H_1- and H_2-receptors in the cardiovascular system of the rabbit. J. Cardiovasc. Pharmacol. **2**, 607–617.

Shepherd, J. T., and Vanhoutte, P. M. (1975), "Veins and Their Control." Saunders, Philadelphia.

Sitrin, M. A., and Bohr, D. F. (1971). Ca and Na interaction in vascular smooth muscle contraction. Am. J. Physiol. **220**, 1124–1128.

Somlyo, A. V., and Somlyo, A. P. (1968). Electromechanical and pharmacomechanical coupling in vascular smooth muscle. J. Pharmacol. Exp. Ther. **159**, 129–145.

Steedman, W. M. (1966). Micro-electrode studies on mammalian vascular muscle. J. Physiol. **186**, 382–400.

Steinsland, O. S., Furchgott, R. F., and Kirpekar, S. M. (1973). Biphasic vasoconstriction of the rabbit ear artery. Circ. Res. **32**, 49–58.

Suzuki, H., and Casteels, R. (1979). Effect of histamine on the small arteries in the gracilis muscle of the rabbit. J. Pharmacol. Exp. Ther. **211**, 430–435.

Takata, Y. (1980). Regional differences in electrical and mechanical properties of guinea-pig mesenteric vessels. Jpn. J. Physiol. **30**, 709–728.

Towart, R. (1981). The selective inhibition of serotonin-induced contractions of rabbit cerebral vascular smooth muscle by calcium-antagonistic dihydropyridines. Circ. Res. **48**, 650–657.

Van Breemen, C., and Siegel, B. (1980). The mechanism of α-adrenergic activation of the dog coronary artery. Circ. Res. **46**, 426–429.

Van Nueten, J. M., Van Beck, J., and Vanhoutte, P. M. (1980). Inhibitory effect of lidoflazine on contractions of isolated canine coronary arteries caused by norepinephrine, 5-hydroxytryptamine, high potassium, anoxia, and ergonovine maleate. J. Pharmacol. Exp. Ther. **213**, 179–187.

Van Nueten, J. M., and Vanhoutte, P. M. (1980). Effect of the Ca^{++} antagonist lidoflazine on normoxic and anoxic contracitons of canine coronary arterial smooth muscle. Eur. J. Pharmacol. **64**, 173-178.

Yamashita, K., Takogi, T., and Hotta, K. (1977). Mobilization of cellular calcium and contraction-relaxation of vascular smooth muscle. Jpn. J. Physiol. **27**, 551-564.

Zelis, R., and Flaim, S. F. (1981). Ann. Intern. Med. **94**, 124-126.

Index